Dermoscopy Criteria Review

Notice

Dermoscopy Criteria Review

Robert H. Johr, MD, FAAD
Voluntary Professor Emeritus of Dermatology and
Voluntary Associate Professor Emeritus of Pediatrics
University of Miami Miller School of Medicine
Miami, Florida

Prof. Wilhelm Stolz, MD
Director, Clinic of Dermatology, Allergology and Environmental Medicine
Hospital München Thalkirchner Street and
Professor of Dermatology, Faculty of Medicine
Ludwig-Maximilians-Universität München
Munich, Germany

Associate Editor

James A. Ida, MD, MSPH
Private Practice
Affiliate Dermatologist
Department of Medicine
Northwestern Lake Forest Hospital
Lake Forest, Illinois

New York   Chicago   San Francisco   Athens   London   Madrid   Mexico City
Milan   New Delhi   Singapore   Sydney   Toronto

1 2 3 4 5 6 7 8 9   DSS   24 23 22 21 20 19

ISBN 978-1-260-13624-1
MHID 1-260-13624-8

The book was set in minion pro by Cenveo® Publisher Services.
The editors were Karen G. Edmonson, Robert Pancotti, and Christie Naglieri.
The production supervisor was Richard Ruzycka.
Project management was provided by Revathi Viswanathan, Cenveo Publisher Services.
The text designer was Mary McKeon; the cover designer was W2 Design.

This book is printed on acid-free paper.

Library of Congress Cataloging-in-Publication Data

Names: Johr, Robert, editor. | Stolz, W. (Wilhelm), editor. | Ida, James A.,
   associate editor.
Title: Dermoscopy criteria review / editor, Robert H. Johr,
   Prof. Wilhelm Stolz ; associate editor, James A. Ida.
Description: New York : McGraw-Hill Education, [2020] | Includes index.
Identifiers: LCCN 2018059555 | ISBN 9781260136241 (adhesive-soft : alk.
   paper)
Subjects: | MESH: Dermoscopy | Skin Diseases—diagnosis
Classification: LCC RL105 | NLM WR 141 | DDC 616.5/075—dc23 LC record available at
   https://lccn.loc.gov/2018059555

Contents

Contributors

Aimilios Lallas, MD, MSc, PhD
Department of Dermatology
Aristotle University of Thessaloniki
Thessaloniki, Greece
Chapter 5

Antonella Tosti, MD
Professor
Department of Dermatology and Cutaneous Surgery
University of Miami Miller School of Medicine
Miami, Florida
Chapter 6

Foreword

It has been a pleasure and an honor to be asked to review and write a foreword for this new publication. Drs. Johr and Stolz have once again advanced the field of dermoscopy by providing a step-by-step guide which can take the neophyte dermoscopist to the next level of expertise. They have added an associate editor Dr. James Ida and have chapters which relate to the use of dermoscopy in general/non-neoplastic skin disorders as well as hair disorders.

I have had the gift of learning from Dr. Johr, first in 1996 and frequently since then. Although primarily a pediatric dermatologist, I have always seen selected adults as well. With time I would feel disarmed if I somehow started a clinic without a dermatoscope available to me. Obviously, you do not expect to see a child with a melanoma frequently in a pediatric dermatology practice, yet I have seen more than twenty melanomas in children, many before I became proficient in dermoscopy. In children we frequently make use of dermoscopy in inflammatory and infections disorders as well as hair disorders. Having a long interest in scabies, for the past 15 years I have abandoned skin scrapings for diagnosis, and have relied on dermoscopy alone. I will occasionally do a scraping to prove to parents the diagnosis, as they have often been misdiagnosed by other doctors for weeks and months. Likewise, dermoscopy is essential in rheumatologic conditions (e.g., capillary nail fold visualization) and in hair shaft disorders.

This text is an extraordinary teaching instrument. It lays out with descriptions and dermoscopic figures, the basics of features which lead to the diagnosis or differential diagnosis. This is done in the chapter "Dermoscopy A to Z." What follows is the heart of the learning experience: 105 cases which are sequences of brief history, followed by clinical, then unlabeled dermoscopic photos, and then like peeling back the onion, labeled important dermoscopic features, then the diagnosis, as well as discussion of the important features of the case. An honest description of the limits of dermoscopy is given for many cases. These cases are brief, beautifully photographed, and packed with insight.

I truly wish I had this text available when I first learned dermoscopic analysis. A beginner could learn all of the essentials from this work alone, followed by years of practice. I find it inconceivable today that a trained dermatologist would diagnose and treat melanoma, and fail to use a dermoscopy. Drs. Johr, Stolz, and Ida are to be commended for producing a text which will jump-start those on their venture into dermoscopy!

Ronald C. Hansen MD
Professor (Emeritus) Dermatology and Pediatrics,
University College of Medicine, Tucson, Arizona
Affiliate and Founding Chief of Dermatology,
Phoenix Children's Hospital, Arizona

Preface

The term *dermoscopy* derives from two basic Greek words: *dermà*, meaning "skin," and *skopéō*, meaning "to look or see." As you are likely already aware, however, the *science and practice of dermoscopy* involve so much more than simply "looking at skin." Indeed dermoscopy, which is also called dermatoscopy, has evolved a sort of language all its own. As you will soon learn in the coming chapters, there is a wealth of terms, each important to the practice of dermoscopy, with their own specific meanings and even subtle connotations depending on a given lesion. As with any language, a fluent understanding of the meaning of these terms is essential to becoming a proper speaker. To this end, Chapter 1, "Dermoscopy from A to Z," will be your starting point for a comprehensive overview of the basic terminology and concepts of dermoscopy. For example, it is here where you will be introduced to the essential principles of pattern analysis and the "two-step algorithm." This will serve as your basic approach when analyzing a lesion, such as differentiating melanocytic from nonmelanocytic. Next, and arguably the most critical part of the book, is Chapter 2, "Comprehensive Dermoscopy Criteria Review." In this chapter, representative images and detailed explanations will guide you as you learn the language of dermoscopy. Although the task may be initially daunting, through study, practice, and dedication you will overcome a steep learning curve to master the techniques and language of dermoscopy.

Our goal in writing this book has been to teach you the language and key principles of dermoscopy. Through the use of extensive clinical and dermoscopic images along with detailed explanations and diagnostic clues, you will have the opportunity to self-assess your knowledge and skills as you study. In our era of information overload, we have endeavored to design this book to be short, sweet, and to the point. We hope that you will find it to be an easy, enjoyable, and practical read. Important principles are often repeated in an effort to make them familiar and more easily remembered.

We have included 105 cases that are likely to be seen on a regular basis in a general dermatology practice. For each case, you will find a short history along with a clinical image and an unmarked dermoscopic image. Study the unmarked image and attempt to identify the global and local dermoscopic features. Next, make your diagnosis after identifying

as much detail as you can. Then, turn the page and the dermoscopic image will be presented again, this time marked with circles, boxes, arrows, and/or stars to highlight the important dermoscopic features of each case. On the same page you will find the diagnosis along with a detailed discussion and a few pearls, or key take-away points, for your review. Our goal is to fully demonstrate the global features and local criteria of each lesion. The concept of dermoscopic differential diagnosis is critical and is emphasized throughout the book.

Each case has a discussion of all of its salient features. We achieve this not in long, verbose paragraphs, but rather in outline form to make the information easier to digest. We realize that your time is valuable and want to make the learning and recall process as easy and effective as possible.

Case series are organized into groups, depending on particular common dermoscopic features. For example, there are lesions in which the major feature may be pigment network; dots and globules; regression; pink, blue or black color; or vascular structures. There are similar clinical and/or dermoscopic images grouped together in specific body locations, such as brownish spots on the face or black lesions on the trunk. We have done this to better simulate real-life clinical encounters. One case often flows into the next, and concepts learned in a previous case may inform the analysis of a subsequent case. Finally, each case ends with a series of dermoscopic and/or clinical pearls based on our combined years of experience treating patients in outpatient clinical settings.

We present the many faces of melanoma from head to toe, whether easily diagnosed with well-developed criteria or challenging to the most astute dermoscopist. We include more than 100 clinical and dermoscopic images of melanoma to help you improve your diagnostic skills. In addition, we are especially delighted to include subspecialty expertise in the fields of hair and nail dermoscopy. You will find nail cases as well as chapters on trichoscopy and on dermoscopy in general dermatology. At the end of the book, you will also find a succinct glossary of specific terms and general principles to review at a glance.

In conclusion, we strongly believe in the importance of using dermoscopy routinely in the practice of dermatology. As a cutting-edge, noninvasive technique, dermoscopy uniquely allows us insights into the diagnosis of numerous dermatologic conditions and indeed may be a potentially lifesaving tool to care for our patients. Our book is sprinkled with general principles and specific points that may at times be controversial but are strongly embedded in our core beliefs. Each of us has a profound responsibility for the well-being of every patient who walks through the door. We applaud you as you embark on your journey to learn the techniques and language of dermoscopy!

Dr. Robert H. Johr
Chapel Hill, North Carolina

Dr. Wilhelm Stolz
Munich, Germany

Acknowledgments

My journey continues! I would like to take a moment to express my gratitude to those who have meant so much in putting together this book.

To Professor Wilhelm Stolz, a pioneer in the field of dermoscopy and a loyal friend and colleague for more than 25 years. This book would not have been possible without your contribution of such superb and varied cases.

To Dr. James Ida, our copy editor and all-around language aficionado. Your gift for the written word has been indispensable for the writing of a clear, concise, and readable book. I appreciate your many "posthaste" edits of each case, pithy comments, eye to detail, and overall positive attitude.

To Dr. Antonella Tosti and Dr. Aimilios Lallas for their generous time and contribution of truly fantastic cases without which our text would not be complete.

To Robert Pancotti, Senior Development Editor at McGraw-Hill Medical, for his editorial oversight and meticulous attention to detail throughout the publishing process, and Revathi Viswanathan, Senior Project Manager at Cenveo Publisher Services for transforming our written material into the actual book.

Allow me to also thank Karen Edmonson, Senior Content Acquisitions Editor at McGraw-Hill Medical, for her unwavering support and belief in us. It has truly been a delightful experience to work with Karen on the present book as well as on all of our projects over the years.

Finally, to my wife Irma to whom I owe infinite gratitude. You are my life's best friend. I thank you for your continual sage advice, encouragement, and support.

Dr. Robert H. Johr

I am deeply grateful to my friend and highly esteemed colleague Dr. Robert Johr for the wonderful cooperation and his extremely passionate work on the case presentations that are the core of this book.

Without the very valuable contributions of Dr. James Ida, Dr. Antonella Tosti, Dr. Aimilios Lallas, Robert Pancotti, Revathi Viswanathan, and, especially, Karen Edmonson, writing this book would not have been possible.

For her enthusiasm and skill regarding the beautiful color images, a cornerstone of our text, I would like to thank our nurses in the outpatient clinic: Mss. Carolin Mertens, Delia Nagy, Antje Seehuber, and Vesna Davidovic.

To the many physicians in our clinic who assisted me with my dermoscopy clinic and with the case preparations, most of all Dr. Brigitte Coras-Stepanek, Dr. Stefanie Guther and Dr. Ulrike Weigert, I wish to extend my sincerest thanks.

Special thanks also go to my assistant in our office, Mrs. Leonie Rieger, for her continuous, very helpful support in the management of both patients and staff.

However, first and foremost I would like to express my deepest gratitude to my wife, Karola, who has lovingly shared my many dermoscopic and academic pursuits over the past three decades.

Dr. Wilhelm Stolz

CHAPTER 1

Dermoscopy From A to Z

SYNONYMS

- Dermatoscopy.
- Skin surface microscopy.
- Epiluminescence microscopy (ELM).
- Digital dermoscopy/digital ELM.
- *Auflichtmikroscopie* (German).
- *Dermoscopia/dermatoscopia* (Spanish).
- *Dermoscopy* and *dermatoscopy* are used interchangeably by experienced dermoscopists and in the literature.

DEFINITION

- Dermoscopy is an in vivo, noninvasive technique in which oil or fluid (eg, mineral oil, gel, alcohol, water) is placed on the lesion.
  - Fluid eliminates reflection of light from the surface of the skin, allowing visualization of color and structure in the epidermis, dermoepidermal junction, and papillary dermis.
  - The color and structure visualized cannot be seen with the naked eye or with typical magnification that clinicians use.
  - Polarizing light and digital instrumentation do not require fluid.
- When using polarized light dermoscopy:
  - Light from a polarized light source penetrates the stratum corneum with less scatter.
  - A second polarizer screens out scattered surface light, resulting in the physician seeing primarily light from the deeper structures.
  - This removes the need for contact with the skin and the need for immersion fluids, resulting in faster examination times.
- There is noncontact and contact polarized dermoscopy.
  - Gels can be used with contact polarized dermoscopy to enhance the appearance of vessels or eliminate the negative effects of dry skin.
- There is contact nonpolarized dermoscopy.
  - Some criteria can be better visualized with polarized dermoscopy, such as small vessels and blue-white color.
  - Some criteria can be better visualized with nonpolarized contact dermoscopy, such as milia-like cysts seen in seborrheic keratosis and melanocytic lesions.
  - Crystalline structures (aka shiny white structures) can only be seen with polarized dermoscopy.
  - All the criteria needed to make a dermoscopic diagnosis can be made using any form of the technique.

BENEFITS OF DERMOSCOPY

- Helps to differentiate melanocytic from nonmelanocytic skin lesions.
- Helps to differentiate benign from malignant skin lesions.

- With dermoscopy, the sensitivity to diagnose melanoma is 85% and better compared with 65% to 80% when the technique is not used.
- Increases the diagnosis of early melanoma.
- Increases the diagnosis of amelanotic and hypomelanotic melanoma.
- Increases the diagnosis of melanoma incognito (clinically false-negative melanoma).
- Increases the diagnosis of inflammatory lesions (ie, lichen planus, psoriasis, seborrheic dermatitis, rosacea, discoid lupus erythematosus, granulomatous diseases).
- Increases the diagnosis of infestations (eg, scabies, head lice, crab lice).
- Increases the diagnosis of alopecia (eg. androgenic alopecia, alopecia areata) and hair shaft pathology (eg, monilethrix, trichorrhexis invaginata).
- Helps to avoid unnecessary surgery.
- Helps to plan surgery.
- Helps to work better with a pathologist (asymmetrical high-risk criteria, collision tumors, dermoscopic-pathologic correlation).
- Patient reassurance.
- Allows for follow-up of patients with a single nevus or multiple nevi digitally to find changes over time.

DERMOSCOPIC DIGITAL MONITORING

- There are pigmented skin lesions that are not high-risk enough to warrant immediate histopathologic diagnosis, yet not so banal that there is no concern at all.
- There are melanomas that do not appear to be high-risk clinically or with dermoscopy.
- They are only diagnosed after monitoring for dermoscopic changes over time when comparing baseline with subsequent digital images.
- Short-term monitoring is performed every 3 or 4 months.
  - Any change over time could be a melanoma.
- Long-term monitoring is done at 6-month to yearly intervals.
  - Important changes include asymmetrical enlargement, the appearance of high-risk criteria, new colors, or regression.
- Single or multiple suspicious pigmented skin lesions can be chosen for digital monitoring.

THE 2-STEP ALGORITHM

- The analysis of a suspicious skin lesion is a 2-step process:
  - Step 1: Determine if it is melanocytic or nonmelanocytic.
  - Step 2: If it has the criteria for a melanocytic lesion, the second step is to determine if it is low, intermediate, or high risk using the melanocytic algorithm of your choice.

TABLE 1-1 • ABCD Rule of Dermatoscopy: Identify Criteria and Assign Points to Determine Total Dermatoscopy Score (TDS)
Dermoscopic Criterion Definition Score Weight Factor
Asymmetry: In 0, 1, or 2 perpendicular axes; assess contour, colors, and structures 0-2
Border: Abrupt ending of pigment pattern at periphery in segments 0-8
Color: Presence of up to 6 colors (white, red, light brown, dark brown, blue-gray, and black) 1-6
Dermoscopic structures: Presence of network, structureless (homogeneous) areas, branched streaks, dots, and globules 1-5
Formula for calculating TDS: (A score × 1.3) + (B score × 0.1) + (C score × 0.5) + (D score × 0.5) = TDS. Interpretation of total score: <4.75. Benign melanocytic lesion 4.75-5.45; suspect lesion (close follow-up or excision recommended); >5.45, lesion highly suspect for melanoma

- Pattern analysis was the first melanocytic algorithm developed for this purpose and is most often used by experienced dermoscopists. Variations of pattern analysis have also been developed, including
  - The ABCD rule of dermatoscopy (Table 1-1).
  - The 11-point checklist (Table 1-2).
  - The 7-point checklist (Table 1-3).
  - The 3-point checklist (Table 1-4).

Step 1: Identification of Criteria

Look for the criteria associated with a melanocytic lesion. If one does not find them, the search is on for the criteria associated with seborrheic keratosis, basal cell carcinoma, dermatofibromas, vascular lesions, and others (Table 1-5).

- Not all of the possible criteria are needed to make a diagnosis.
- When there is absence of criteria for a melanocytic lesion, seborrheic keratosis, basal cell carcinoma, dermatofibroma, or vascular lesion, you are now dealing with a melanocytic lesion by default.
- The "default category" is the last criterion used to diagnose a melanocytic lesion (Fig. 1-1).

TABLE 1-2 • 11-Point Checklist
Dermoscopic Criteria
1. Symmetry of pattern (negative feature)
2. Presence of single color (negative feature)
Positive Features
3. Blue-white veil (color)
4. Multiple brown dots
5. Pseudopods (streaks)
6. Radial streaming (streaks)
7. Scar-like depigmentation (bony-white color)
8. Peripheral black dots/globules
9. Multiple (5 or 6) colors
10. Multiple blue/gray dots
11. Broadened network (irregular pigment network)

For melanoma to be diagnosed, both negative features must be absent and 1 or more of the 9 positive features must be present.

TABLE 1-3 • 7-Point Checklist

Dermoscopic Criteria	Scores
1. Irregular pigment network (**major criteria**)	2
2. Bluish-white veil (any blue and/or white color)	2
3. Polymorphous vascular pattern	2
4. Irregular streaks (**minor criteria**)	1
5. Irregular dots/globules	1
6. Irregular blotches	1
7. Regression	1

By simple addition of the individual scores, a minimum total score of 3 is required for the diagnosis of melanoma, whereas a total score of less than 3 is indicative of nonmelanoma.

TABLE 1-4 • 3-Point Checklist to Diagnose High-Risk Lesions (Melanoma, Basal Cells)

Asymmetry of color and/or structure
Irregular pigment network
Blue and/or white color
2 out 3, 3 out 3 → Excise

The 3-point checklist is based on simplified pattern analysis and is intended to be used by nonexpert dermoscopists as a screening technique. Its aim is to diagnose melanocytic and nonmelanocytic potentially-malignant pathology.

TABLE 1-5 • Criteria for Various Lesions

Criteria for a Melanocytic Lesion
Pigment network (trunk and extremities)
Aggregated brown globules.
Homogeneous blue color (blue nevus).
Parallel patterns on acral sites.
By default (when there is an absence of criteria for a melanocytic lesion, seborrheic keratosis, basal cell carcinoma, hemangioma, or dermatofibroma, the lesion should be considered melanocytic by default).
Criteria for a Seborrheic Keratosis
Milia-like cysts
Pseudofollicular/comedo-like openings
Fissures/furrows and ridges/fat fingers
Hairpin vessels
Sharp border demarcation
Criteria for a Basal Cell Carcinoma
Absence of pigment network
Arborizing blood vessels/serpentine vessels
Pigmentation
Ulceration
Spoke-wheel structures
Criteria for a Dermatofibroma
Central white patch
Peripheral pigment network
Criterion for a Vascular Lesion
Vascular spaces called lacunae
Fibrous septae

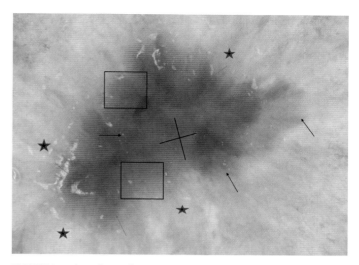

FIGURE 1-1. **Invasive melanoma.** A melanocytic lesion by default, because there is an absence of criteria for a melanocytic lesion, seborrheic keratosis, basal cell carcinoma, dermatofibroma, or hemangioma. There is asymmetry of color and structure (+), bluish-white color (black arrows), milky-red color (red arrows) with polymorphous vessels (boxes). The vessels are dotted, linear and comma shaped. The bony-white color of regression (stars) surround the lesion.

Criteria Defined

Melanocytic lesion

PIGMENT NETWORK/NETWORK

- On the trunk and extremities.
- Shades of black or brown.
- Honeycomb-like, reticular, web-like line segments (elongated and hyperpigmented rete ridges) with hypopigmented holes (dermal papilla).

WHITE/NEGATIVE NETWORK

- Bony-white network-like structures.
- Not a primary criterion used to diagnose melanocytic lesions.
- Can be seen in pink/pigmented nevi, Spitz nevi, melanoma, and dermatofibromas.

PSEUDONETWORK/PSEUDOPIGMENT NETWORK

- Because the skin of the head and neck is thin and does not have well-developed rete ridges, one sees:
  - Appendageal openings/adnexal structures (sebaceous glands, hair follicles).
  - Uniform, round white or yellowish structures.
- When they penetrate areas of diffuse pigmentation, reticular-like structures are formed that are referred to as the *pseudonetwork*.
- Monomorphous appendageal openings can often be seen on the skin of the face without any pigmentation.
- They should not be confused with the milia-like cysts seen in seborrheic keratosis.
- It is not always possible to make the differentiation.
- Consequences could be misdiagnosing lentigo maligna for a seborrheic keratosis.

- This criterion can be seen with nonmelanocytic lesions (ie, actinic keratosis, solar lentigo, lichen planus–like keratosis).
- It is not diagnostic of a melanocytic lesion.

DOTS AND GLOBULES

- Roundish structures distinguished only by their relative sizes.
- Dots (0.1 mm) are smaller than globules (>0.1 mm).
- Black, brown, gray, or red.
  - When black, they can represent atypical melanocytes in the epidermis or transepidermal elimination of pigment.
  - Regular brown dots and globules (brown is the main color to diagnose a melanocytic lesion) represent nests of melanocytes at the dermoepidermal junction.
  - Irregular brown dots and globules represent nests of atypical melanocytes at the dermoepidermal junction.
  - Grayish dots ("peppering") represent free melanin and/or melanophages in the papillary dermis, which can be seen in regression, alone, or in benign pathology such as lichen planus–like keratosis or posttraumatically.
  - Reddish globules (milky-red globules) can be seen in melanoma (neovascularization).
  - It is written and taught that aggregated brown globules identify a melanocytic lesion with no mention of the smaller dots. The reality is that both dots and globules define a melanocytic lesion (Fig. 1-2).

HOMOGENEOUS BLUE PIGMENTATION

- Structureless blue color in the absence of local criteria such as pigment network, dots, or globules (Fig. 1-3).

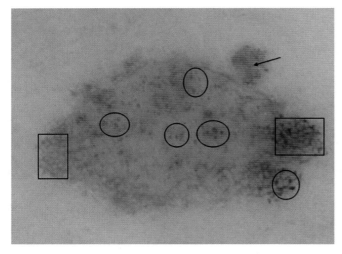

FIGURE 1-2. Acquired nevus. A melanocytic lesion, because it has pigment network (black boxes) and aggregated brown globules (circles). There is a small hemangioma adjacent to the nevus (arrow). (Reproduced with permission from Johr RH and Stolz W. *Dermoscopy: An Illustrated Self-Assessment Guide.* 2nd ed. New York, NY: McGraw-Hill Education; 2015.)

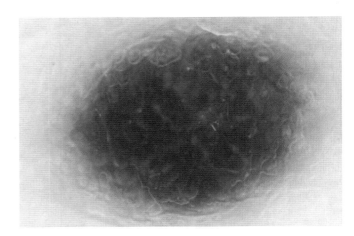

FIGURE 1-3. Blue nevus. The classic homogenous blue color of a blue nevus. (Reproduced with permission from Johr RH and Stolz W. *Dermoscopy: An Illustrated Self-Assessment Guide.* 2nd ed. New York, NY: McGraw-Hill Education; 2015.)

- Different shades of homogeneous blue color usually represents a blue nevus.
- The history is important, because there is a differential diagnosis which could include a lesion as banal as a radiation tattoo to one more ominous such as nodular or cutaneous metastatic melanoma.

PARALLEL PATTERNS/ACRAL PATTERNS/PALMS AND SOLES

- Fissures/furrows and ridges on the skin of the palms and soles (dermoglyphics).
- Can create parallel patterns.
  - Parallel lines can also be seen on all nonglabrous skin/mucosal surfaces (ie, lips, genitalia).

PARALLEL-FURROW PATTERN (BENIGN PATTERN)

- Thin brown parallel lines in the furrows of the skin (crista superficialis limitans).
- Variations include 2 thin lines with or without dots and globules (Fig. 1-4).

LATTICE-LIKE PATTERN (BENIGN PATTERN)

- Thin brown parallel lines in the furrows.
- Thin brown parallel lines running perpendicular to the furrows forming a ladder-like picture (Fig. 1-5).

FIBRILLAR PATTERN (BENIGN PATTERN)

- Fine brown lines.
- Run in an oblique (/////) direction.
- Pressure can change the lattice-like pattern into a fibrillar pattern.

GLOBULAR PATTERN (BENIGN)

- Brown globules without a parallel component.

RETICULAR PATTERN (BENIGN)

- A lesion with only pigment network.

HOMOGENEOUS PATTERN (BENIGN)

- Brown homogeneous color.

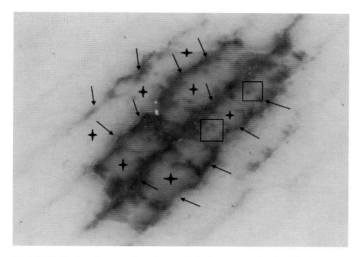

FIGURE 1-4. **Acral nevus.** A melanocytic lesion on acral skin with the benign parallel furrow pattern. Pigmentation is in the thin furrows (arrows) with globules (boxes) in the ridges (stars). (Reproduced with permission from Johr RH and Stolz W. *Dermoscopy: An Illustrated Self-Assessment Guide.* 2nd ed. New York, NY: McGraw-Hill Education; 2015.)

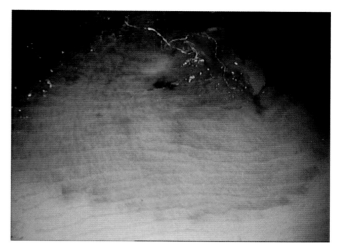

FIGURE 1-6. **Acral melanoma.** The parallel-ridge pattern diagnoses this acral melanoma with pigmentation in the thicker light brown ridges. The thin white lines are the furrows. (Reproduced with permission from Johr RH and Stolz W. *Dermoscopy: An Illustrated Self-Assessment Guide.* 2nd ed. New York, NY: McGraw-Hill Education; 2015.)

PARALLEL-RIDGE PATTERN (THIN/EARLY MELANOMA)

- Pigmentation is in the thicker ridges of the skin (crista profunda intermedia) (Fig. 1-6).
- Sometimes there are monomorphous round white structures in the ridges that represent the acrosyringia of the sweat ducts ("string of pearls").
- The acrosyringia are always in the ridges.
- An important landmark when one has to determine if pigmentation is in the furrows or ridges. Benign (furrows) vs malignant (ridges) pathology.
- Foci of the parallel-ridge pattern can be seen in more advanced acral melanomas with a multicomponent global pattern and melanoma-specific criteria (ie, regression, irregular blotches, blue color, polymorphous vessels).
- Parallel-ridge pattern created by blood (talon noir, black heel) (Fig. 1-7).
- Parallel-ridge pattern in darker-skinned persons (Fig. 1-8).

- Macules seen in the Peutz-Jeghers syndrome.
- This pattern is not 100% diagnostic of melanoma.

DIFFUSE VARIEGATE PATTERN (MELANOMA)

- Irregular pigmented dark blotches.
- Black, brown, or gray.

MULTICOMPONENT PATTERN (MELANOMA)

- Filled with regular and irregular criteria.
- Multiple colors plus areas with acral benign patterns (fibrillar, parallel furrow).

NONSPECIFIC PATTERN (MELANOMA)

- If one cannot determine any of the above benign or malignant patterns, this represents a red flag of concern.

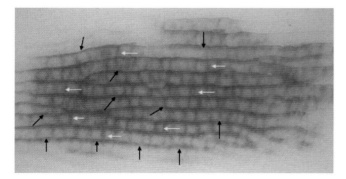

FIGURE 1-5. **Acral nevus.** Brown lines in the furrows (black arrows) and perpendicular to the furrows (yellow arrows) characterize the lattice-like pattern. Pressure on the foot can change this into the fibrillar pattern with fine oblique (/////) lines. (Reproduced with permission from Johr RH and Stolz W. *Dermoscopy: An Illustrated Self-Assessment Guide.* 2nd ed. New York, NY: McGraw-Hill Education; 2015.)

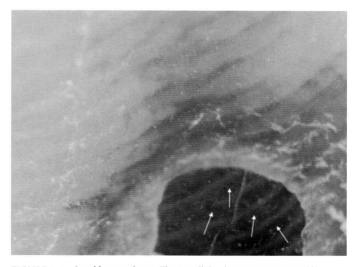

FIGURE 1-7. **Acral hemorrhage.** The parallel-ridge pattern created by blood (white arrows). (Reproduced with permission from Johr RH and Stolz W. *Dermoscopy: An Illustrated Self-Assessment Guide.* 2nd ed. New York, NY: McGraw-Hill Education; 2015.)

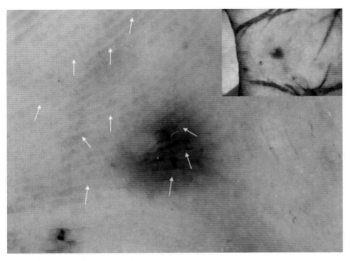

FIGURE 1-8. Acquired nevus. There is an increased incidence of acral melanoma in darker-skinned persons. This nevus on the palm of an African American patient was without change and demonstrates the benign parallel-ridge pattern. Pigmentation is seen in the ridges of the nevus (yellow arrows) and in the ridges of the entire palm (white arrows). (Reproduced with permission from Johr RH and Stolz W. *Dermoscopy: An Illustrated Self-Assessment Guide.* 2nd ed. New York, NY: McGraw-Hill Education; 2015.)

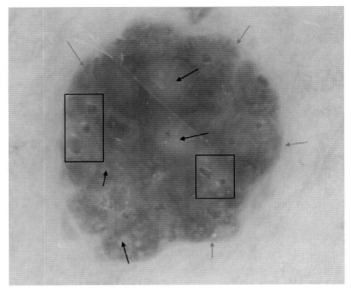

FIGURE 1-9. Seborrheic keratosis. Sharp borders (red arrows), milia-like cysts (black arrows), and pigmented pseudofollicular openings (boxes) characterize this seborrheic keratosis. (Reproduced with permission from Johr RH and Stolz W. *Dermoscopy: An Illustrated Self-Assessment Guide.* 2nd ed. New York, NY: McGraw-Hill Education; 2015.)

PEARLS

- There can be exceptions to every dermoscopic rule.
- The history and clinical appearance of a lesion are important and should not be ignored.
- Negative "gut" feelings should not be ignored.
- If an acral lesion is rapidly changing yet has a benign appearance, it still could be melanoma.
- A supposedly benign acral pattern with irregularity of some components could be high-risk.
- The presence of blood at acral sites (palms, soles, nails) can be associated with melanoma.
- Look carefully for other high-risk criteria when blood is seen.
- If in doubt, cut it out!

Seborrheic keratosis

MILIA-LIKE CYSTS

- Variously sized white or yellow structures.
- Small or large, single or multiple.
- They can appear opaque or bright—like "stars in the sky" (epidermal horn cysts).

PSEUDOFOLLICULAR OPENINGS/COMEDO-LIKE OPENINGS

- Sharply demarcated roundish structures.
- Pigmented or nonpigmented.
- Shapes can vary, not only within a single lesion but from lesion to lesion in an individual patient.

- When pigmented, they can be brownish-yellow or even dark brown and black (oxidized keratin-filled invaginations of the epidermis).
- Pigmented pseudofollicular openings can be hard to differentiate from the pigmented dots and globules of a melanocytic lesion (Fig. 1-9).

FISSURES/FURROWS AND RIDGES

- Fissures/furrows (sulci) and ridges (gyri) seen in seborrheic keratosis can create several patterns.
- Large irregularly shaped keratin-filled fissures are called *crypts.*
  - Fissures/furrows and ridges can also be seen in papillomatous melanocytic lesions.
  - Cerebriform or brain-like in which they resemble a sagittal section through the cerebral cortex.
  - Mountain-like with variously sized or uniformly roundish structures representing mountains (ridges) and fine pigmented lines representing valleys (fissures).
    - Possible to confuse the mountain-and-valley pattern with the globular or cobblestone pattern of a melanocytic lesion.
  - Pigmented lines should not be confused with an irregular pigment network.
  - Hypo- and hyperpigmented ridges can be digit-like (straight, kinked, circular, or branched) and are referred to as "fat fingers."
  - "Fat fingers" might be the only clue that a lesion could be a seborrheic keratosis.
- All these patterns are commonly seen in this ubiquitous most commonly encountered benign skin lesion (Fig. 1-10).

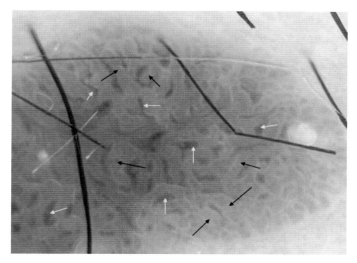

FIGURE 1-10. Seborrheic keratosis. A striking brain-like pattern created by pigmented fissures (yellow arrows) and light ridges (black arrows). Many of the ridges look like "fat fingers." (Reproduced with permission from Johr RH and Stolz W. *Dermoscopy: An Illustrated Self-Assessment Guide.* 2nd ed. New York, NY: McGraw-Hill Education; 2015.)

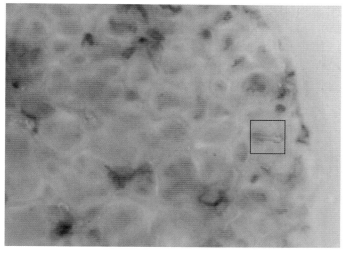

FIGURE 1-11. Seborrheic keratosis. An especially well-formed hairpin vessel in a seborrheic keratosis (black box). (Reproduced with permission from Johr RH and Stolz W. *Dermoscopy: An Illustrated Self-Assessment Guide.* 2nd ed. New York, NY: McGraw-Hill Education; 2015.)

FINGERPRINT PATTERN

- Brown fine/thin parallel line segments that resemble fingerprints.
  - The lines can be arched, swirled, or look like branched fungal hyphae.
  - The lines can fill the lesion or be broken up.
- Differ from the pigment network where the line segments are honeycomb-like or reticular.
  - Network-like structures/pseudonetwork can be seen in seborrheic keratosis created by fissures/furrows and ridges not elongated and hyperpigmented rete ridges of the true pigment network.
- Fingerprint pattern can be seen in flat seborrheic keratosis or in solar lentigines.
- Some authors believe that solar lentigines are flat seborrheic keratosis (see below and Fig. 1-23).

HAIRPIN VESSELS

- Elongated vessels (capillary loops) resembling hairpins (Fig. 1-11).
- May or may not be surrounded by hypopigmented halos.
- Light halo indicates a keratinizing tumor and may be found in keratoacanthomas.
- Irregular and thick hairpin vessels can be seen in melanoma.

MOTH-EATEN BORDERS

- Flat or slightly raised brown seborrheic keratoses and solar lentigines.
- Well-demarcated, concave borders that are felt to resemble a moth-eaten garment.

SHARP DEMARCATION

- The majority of seborrheic keratoses have sharp, well-demarcated borders.
- Not always indicative of melanoma in a pigmented lesion (see Fig. 1-9).

Basal cell carcinoma
ABSENCE OF A PIGMENT NETWORK
Arborizing Vessels
- One of the most sensitive and specific vascular structures seen with dermoscopy.
- Not all basal cell carcinomas contain arborizing vessels.
  - Red tree-like branching telangiectatic blood vessels.
  - Can be thick or thin lines that are in focus because of their superficial location.
- Out-of-focus arborizing vessels are a clue that the lesion might be a melanoma.
  - Most often there are different-caliber vessels in a single lesion.
- Can also be found with:
  - Benign nevi
  - Sebaceous gland hyperplasia
  - Scars
  - Sun-damaged skin
  - Melanoma
  - Desmoplastic melanoma
  - Merkel cell carcinoma
- Serpentine Vessels
  - May be very fine/thin or thick
  - Irregular linear red lines
  - A variation of linear vessels
  - Typically found in flat lesions without arborizing vessels
  - Might be the only clue to suggest the diagnosis

PIGMENTATION

- Basal cell carcinoma may or may not contain pigment (pigmented nests or island of basal cell carcinoma in the dermis) that can range from:
  - Fine dots to large leaf-like structures (bulbous extensions forming a leaf-like pattern).
  - Blue-gray ovoid nets.
  - Multiple blue-gray dots and globules.
  - Colors that can be seen
    - Black
    - Brown
    - Gray
    - Blue
    - Red
    - White
- Not necessary to try to determine if leaf-like structures (maple-leaf–like areas) are present, because in reality this is a difficult task (Fig. 1-12).

ULCERATION

- Single or multiple areas where there is loss of epidermis with oozing blood or congealed blood and crusts (Fig. 1-13).
- Multifocal ulceration is associated with superficial basal cell carcinomas.
- There should be no recent history of trauma.

SPOKE-WHEEL STRUCTURES

- Can be found in up to 10% of basal cell carcinomas.
- Diagnostic of basal cell carcinoma.
  - May or may not be associated with the other criteria used to make the diagnosis.
- Well-defined pigmented radial projections meeting at a darker central globule/central axle/hub.

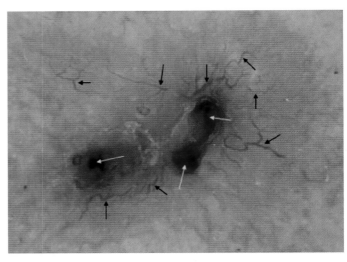

FIGURE 1-13. Basal cell carcinoma. Arborizing vessels (black arrows) and ulcerations (yellow arrows) characterize this nonpigmented basal cell carcinoma. (Reproduced with permission from Johr RH and Stolz W. *Dermoscopy: An Illustrated Self-Assessment Guide.* 2nd ed. New York, NY: McGraw-Hill Education; 2015.)

- Complete or incomplete variations of this structure can be seen, and one often has to use one's imagination to make the identification.
- Streak-like structures referred to as *pseudostreaks* represent incomplete spoke-wheel structures and could be confused with true steaks of a melanocytic lesion.
- Finding spoke-wheel structures might be the only clue to the correct diagnosis.

PEARL

- At times, one cannot differentiate melanoma from basal cell carcinoma. If there is pigment network in any form, then it cannot be a basal cell carcinoma.

Dermatofibroma

CENTRAL WHITE PATCH

- Most typical presentation of this criterion is:
  - Centrally located
  - Scar-like
  - Bony or milky-white
  - Homogeneous area (scarring in this fibrohistiocytic tumor)
- Several variations such as white network-like structures (white/negative network), which can also be seen in Spitz nevi and melanoma.
- Telangiectatic vessels (ie, pinpoint vessels) with different shapes can also be found anywhere in the lesion.
- Not all dermatofibromas have a central white patch.
- The clinically firm feel should be used to help make the diagnosis.

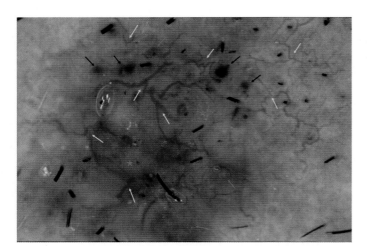

FIGURE 1-12. Basal cell carcinoma. This is a classic pigmented basal cell carcinoma with thick and thin walled branching/arborizing vessels (yellow arrows), bluish-white (red stars), blackish-white, black (black arrows) and brown pigmentation (red arrows).

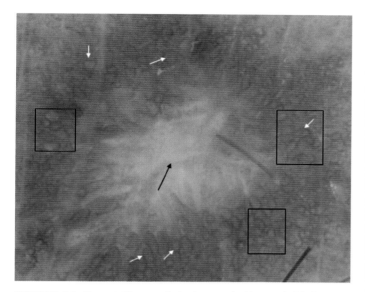

FIGURE 1-14. Dermatofibroma. A classic central white patch (black arrow) and pigment network (black boxes) characterize this dermatofibroma. In this instance, ring-like structures (white arrows) make up the pigment network. Ring-like structures can also be seen in flat seborrheic keratosis. (Reproduced with permission from Johr RH and Stolz W. *Dermoscopy: An Illustrated Self-Assessment Guide.* 2nd ed. New York, NY: McGraw-Hill Education; 2015.)

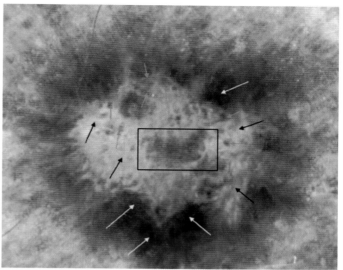

FIGURE 1-15. Atypical dermatofibroma. Regressive melanoma is in the dermoscopic differential diagnoses of this atypical dermatofibroma. There is asymmetry of color and structure, the multicomponent global pattern, irregular pigment network (box), irregular globules (red arrows), and irregular blotches (yellow arrows), multiple colors. This presentation warrants a histopathologic diagnosis. (Reproduced with permission from Johr RH and Stolz W. *Dermoscopy: An Illustrated Self-Assessment Guide.* 2nd ed. New York, NY: McGraw-Hill Education; 2015.)

PIGMENT NETWORK

- Dermatofibromas are one of the types of nonmelanocytic lesions that can have a pigment network; solar lentigines are another.
  - In most cases, a fine peripheral pigment network with thin brown lines is seen.
  - Ring-like structures, which are a variation of a pigment network (Fig. 1-14).
  - Not all dermatofibromas have a pigment network.
- Atypical dermatofibromas with the following features are melanoma simulators that warrant a histopathologic diagnosis:
  - Irregular pigment network
  - Irregular dots/globules/dark blotches
  - Pink color
  - Irregular regression-like white color
  - High-risk vascular structures/polymorphous vessels with different shapes (Fig. 1-15)

Vascular lesions

LACUNAE

- Sharply demarcated bright red to bluish round or oval structures (dilated vascular spaces in the dermis) (Fig. 1-16).
  - Different colors can be seen in a single hemangioma.
  - The deeper the vessels, the darker the color (dark blue).
  - Lacunae should not be mistaken for the milky-red globules seen in pigmented and amelanotic melanoma, which can have out-of-focus reddish globular-like structures.

- Black homogeneous structureless areas represent thrombosis.
- Significant scale or dryness (hyperkeratosis) can be seen in angiokeratomas.
- Patchy white color or blue-white veil (blue and/or white color) can be seen in hemangiomas.
- Linear white lines can fill the lesion and represent fibrous septae.

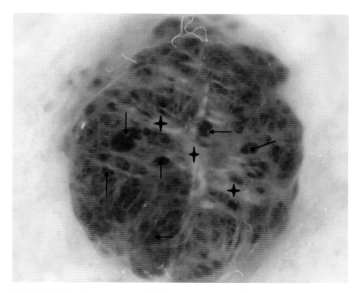

FIGURE 1-16. Hemangioma. Well-demarcated dark red lacunae (arrows) and blue-white color (stars) characterize this classic hemangioma. The linear blue-white color represents fibrous septae. (Reproduced with permission from Johr RH and Stolz W. *Dermoscopy: An Illustrated Self-Assessment Guide.* 2nd ed. New York, NY: McGraw-Hill Education; 2015.)

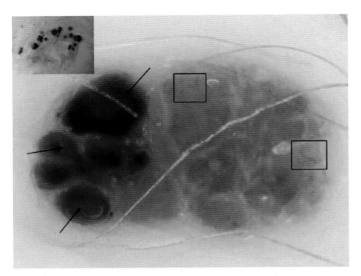

FIGURE 1-17. Cutaneous metastatic melanoma. One of many generalized cutaneous metastatic lesions in a 27-year-old white man with a history of a 7-mm melanoma on his back. There are well-demarcated lacunae-like areas (arrows) and irregular vessels (boxes). Milky-red color fills most of the lesion. A collision tumor, hemangioma, and amelanotic melanoma are in the dermoscopic differential diagnosis. (Reproduced with permission from Johr RH and Stolz W. *Dermoscopy: An Illustrated Self-Assessment Guide.* 2nd ed. New York, NY: McGraw-Hill Education; 2015.)

- Blue and/or white color or fibrous septae should not be mistaken for regression found in melanomas.
- Cutaneous metastatic melanoma can be indistinguishable from a hemangioma
  - A history of a previous melanoma will help make the diagnosis (Fig. 1-17).

PEARL

- There is a significant learning curve with dermoscopy. It is essential to learn the definitions of the criteria and patterns and be able to recognize the classic examples, because there are innumerable variations that one will see in daily practice. This is the weak link in the chain for those who attempt to master this tissue-sparing life-saving technique. One cannot learn dermoscopy by osmosis, and one cannot see what one does not know.

Step 2: Analysis of a Melanocytic Lesion

Pattern Analysis Defined

Identify as many criteria in the lesion as possible, and see if they fit into the known patterns associated with the variants of the following:
- Melanocytic nevi:
  - Congenital
  - Acquired

- Recurrent
- Halo
- Combined
- Blue
- Dysplastic
- Spitz
- Melanoma:
  - In situ
  - Superficial spreading
  - Nodular
  - Hypo- and amelanotic
  - Nail apparatus
  - Acral
- Even though pattern analysis is considered a melanocytic algorithm, the same principles are used to diagnose all the lesions that can be identified with the technique.
  - Melanocytic
  - Nonmelanocytic
  - Benign
  - Malignant
  - Inflammatory

PEARLS

- Do not focus on 1 or 2 criteria and make a diagnosis before checking for all the criteria. You could be lead astray.
- Try to identify all of the criteria in a lesion.
  - High-risk criteria that are present are not always easy to find. Beware!

Pattern Analysis Method

Step 1
- Determine symmetry or asymmetry of color and/or structure using the mirror image technique.
  - Contour of the lesion is not important with this algorithm.
  - The lesion is bisected by 2 lines that are placed 90° to each other.
  - The lines should attempt to create the most symmetry as possible and should be visualized with that point in mind.
  - Is the color and/or the structure on the left half of the lesion a mirror image of the right half?
- Repeat the analysis for the upper and lower half of the lesion.
- Perfect symmetry of color and structure is not often found in nature, and interobserver agreement is not good with this assessment even among experienced dermoscopists.
- Symmetry or asymmetry can also be determined along any axis through the center of the lesion.

- Significant asymmetry of color and/or structure is a very important clue that you might be dealing with high-risk pathology.
- Raise a red flag of concern, and proceed with focused attention to what else you might find.

Step 2
- Determine the global/overall pattern of the lesion. The predominant criteria seen throughout the lesion could be the following:
  - Reticular.
  - Globular.
  - Cobblestone.
  - Homogeneous.
  - Parallel.
  - Starburst.
  - Multicomponent.
  - Nonspecific.
  - There can be combinations of criteria in a single lesion, such as reticular and homogeneous or reticular and globular.
  - The "reticular homogeneous pattern" or "reticular globular pattern."

Step 3
- Identify the local criteria in the lesion:
  - Pigment network
  - Dots and globules
  - Streaks (also called pseudopods and radial streaming)
  - Blotches
  - Blue-white veil
  - Regression
  - Colors
  - Vascular structures

Step 4
- Determine if the criteria are:
  - Regular or irregular
  - Good or bad
  - Low-, intermediate-, or high-risk
- Melanoma-specific criteria are defined as criteria that can be seen in benign and malignant lesions but are more specific for high-risk pathology such as the following:
  - Dysplastic nevi
  - Spitzoid lesions
  - Melanoma
- All of the high-risk criteria can be seen in benign pathology, and one should never tell a patient that they have melanoma 100%.
- Due to the different characteristics of the skin in the following locations, the criteria are different:
  - Head and neck
  - Trunk and extremities
  - Palms, soles, and genital mucosa

- Thinner skin on the head and neck versus the trunk and extremities and thicker skin on the palms and soles with fissures/furrows and ridges.
- The criteria for the head, neck, palms, soles, and genital mucosa are referred to as *site-specific criteria*.

Global Patterns

Reticular
- Pigment network filling most of the lesion.

Globular
- Dots and globules filling most of the lesion.

Cobblestone
- Larger angulated globules resembling street cobblestones filling most of the lesion (Fig. 1-18).

Homogeneous
- Diffuse pigmentation in the absence of local criteria such as pigment network, dots, and globules.

Starburst (spitzoid)
- Streaks and/or dots and globules at the periphery of the lesion (the most common of the 6 patterns found in Spitz nevi).

Multicomponent
- Three or more different areas within a lesion.
- Each zone can be composed of a single criterion or multiple criteria.

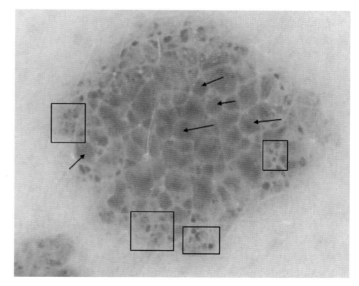

FIGURE 1-18. Acquired nevus. Small brown dots and globules (boxes) and larger angulated brown globules (arrows) characterize this benign nevus. The cobblestone global pattern is seen. The mountain-and-valley pattern seen in seborrheic keratosis is in the dermoscopic differential diagnosis. A positive wobble sign, in which the soft nevus moves from side to side with movement of instrumentation versus a stiff immoveable seborrheic keratosis, helps to make the differentiation. (Reproduced with permission from Johr RH and Stolz W. *Dermoscopy: An Illustrated Self-Assessment Guide.* 2nd ed. New York, NY: McGraw-Hill Education; 2015.)

Nonspecific
- None of the above global patterns can be identified.

Local Criteria

Regular pigment network
- Various shades of brown.
- Honeycomb-like (web-like, reticular) line segments.
- Uniform color, thickness, and holes.
- The lighter holes seen between the line segments represent the dermal papilla.

Irregular pigment network
- Black or brown.
- Line segments that are thickened, branched, and broken up (enlarged, irregular fused rete ridges).
- There may be a diffuse distribution or foci of irregular pigment network.

Regular dots and globules
- Brown roundish structures:
  - Usually clustered.
  - Dots (0.1 mm) are smaller than globules (>0.1 mm).
  - Size, shape, and color are similar with an even distribution in the lesion (nest of melanocytes at the dermoepidermal junction).
- Dots and/or globules only found at the periphery can be seen in Spitz or actively changing nevi.
- Actively changing means if followed digitally, the nevus will invariably enlarge within a short period of time.
- Peripheral dots and globules are usually seen in younger patients with benign pathology.
- Beware of this pattern in a newly acquired nevus in an adult.

Irregular dots and globules
- Black, brown, gray, or red roundish structures.
  - Different sizes, shapes, and shades of color.
  - Usually but not always asymmetrically located in the lesion.

Regular streaks
- Black or brown linear projections of pigment can stand alone.
- Can be associated with a pigment network or dark regular blotch.
- At all points along the periphery of the lesion.
- Pseudopods and radial streaming are similar structures clinically and histopathologically (aggregates of tumor cells running parallel to the epidermis) that can be seen in Spitz nevi or represent the radial growth phase of melanoma that are difficult to differentiate from each another.
- To simplify the identification, the term *streaks* is now used by many but not all experienced dermoscopists to encompass all variations of this criterion.

- The shape of the linear projections does not determine if they are regular or irregular, rather their distribution at the periphery of the lesion.

Irregular streaks
- Black or brown linear projections.
- Can stand alone or be associated with a pigment network or a dark blotch.
- Irregularly distributed at the periphery of a lesion.
- Some but not all points at the periphery, foci of streaks.

Regular blotches
- Black or brown.
- Structureless (ie, absence of network, dots, or globules) areas of color.
- Bigger than dots and globules.
- Uniform shape and color symmetrically located in the lesion (aggregates of melanin in the epidermis and/or dermis).

Irregular blotches
- Black, brown, or gray.
- Irregular in size and shape, asymmetrically located in the lesion.

Blue-white veil
- Irregular, structureless area of confluent blue color.
- Does not fill the entire lesion.
- Overlying whitish ground-glass appearance:
  - Orthokeratosis
  - Acanthosis
  - Hypergranulosis
- Can represent heavily pigmented tumor cells in the dermis.
- In lectures, publications, and books, the use of the term *blue-white veil* is loosely used and quite often does not meet the definition of the criterion. Any blue and/or white color is often called the "veil."

Regression
- Bony or milky-white scar-like depigmentation (fibrosis).
- With or without gray or blue pepper-like granules; "peppering."
- Gray color is much more commonly seen than blue in areas of regression.
- Gray irregular blotches can be associated with peppering.
- Peppering represents free melanin and/or melanophages in the dermis.
- The white color should be lighter than the surrounding skin.
- Regression by itself is an independently potentially high-risk criterion.
- The more regression seen, the greater the chance the lesion is a melanoma.

Blue-white color

- It is not always possible to identify classic regression or classic blue-white veil.
- Blue and/or white color of any intensity, shape, or distribution.
- A red flag of concern should be raised.

Crystalline structures

- Also called shiny white streaks.
- White, shiny, linear structures.
- Only visible with polarized dermoscopy.
- Represents dermal fibrosis/fibroplasia.
- Seen in melanocytic, nonmelanocytic, benign, malignant, and inflammatory pathology.
- Basal cell carcinoma, melanoma, Spitz nevi, dermatofibromas, lichen planus.
- If seen in a melanocytic lesion, it favors the diagnosis of melanoma.

Hypopigmentation

- Commonly seen featureless areas of light brown color in all types of melanocytic lesions, both benign and malignant.
- Multifocal hypopigmentation is a common feature of dysplastic nevi.
- Asymmetrical irregular hypopigmentation seen at the periphery can be seen in melanoma.
- Inexperienced dermoscopists can have trouble differentiating hypopigmentation from the white color seen with true regression.
- An important clue to make the differentiation is that hypopigmentation does not have any gray color or peppering.

Colors seen with dermoscopy

- Eumelanin has a brown color.
- Its location in the skin will determine the colors one sees with dermoscopy (the Tyndall effect).
- Black indicates melanin is superficially located in the epidermis (ie, in the stratum corneum).
- Black color in a nodular lesion usually represents invasive melanoma.
- Black is not always an ominous color but can be seen in benign pathology as well as in melanoma.
- Light and dark brown indicates pigment is at the dermo-epidermal junction.
- Gray in the papillary dermis represents free melanin and melanophages (peppering).
- As the pigment gets into the deeper dermis, it looks blue.
- Red and/or pink color can be created by inflammation or neovascularization.
- Sebaceous material and hyperkeratosis can look yellow.
- The more colors seen, the greater chance one is dealing with high-risk pathology (Figs. 1-19, 1-20, and 1-21).

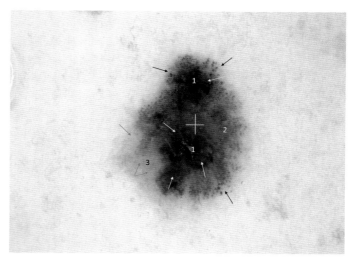

FIGURE 1-19. **Invasive melanoma.** Brown dots and globules diagnose a melanocytic lesion. There is asymmetry of color and structure (+) plus the multicomponent global pattern (1,2,3). Local criteria include irregular brown dots and globules (black arrows), irregular black blotches (yellow arrows), milky-red homogeneous color with a few linear vessels (red arrows) plus 4 colors. All of the criteria are irregular and are therefore considered to be melanoma-specific or high risk.

Polymorphous vascular pattern/polymorphous vessels

- Three or more different shapes of telangiectatic vessels.
- Telangiectatic vessels that can be seen in melanoma are nonspecific; they can also commonly be found in other lesions, including the following:
  - Benign
  - Malignant
  - Inflammatory

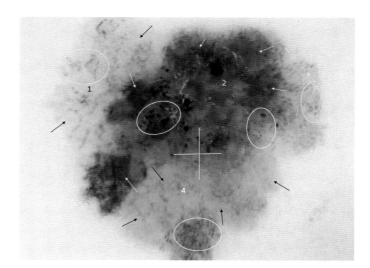

FIGURE 1-20. **Invasive melanoma.** Brown dots and globules diagnose a melanocytic lesion. There is asymmetry of color and structure (+) plus the multicomponent global pattern (1,2,3,4). Local criteria include irregular brown dots and globules (circles), irregular dark brown blotches (yellow arrows), and bluish-white color (star). The classic veil is not seen. Large areas of hypopigmentation (black arrows) plus 5 colors round off the melanoma-specific high risk criteria.

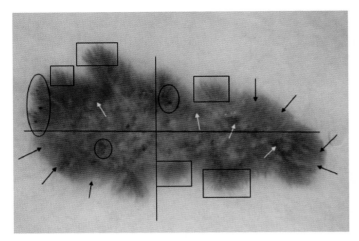

FIGURE 1-21. Melanoma. This is a melanocytic lesion, because there are aggregated brown globules (circles). There is an irregular starburst (spitzoid) global pattern with foci of streaks at the periphery (boxes). Local criteria include: irregular dots and globules (circles), irregular streaks (boxes), and regression. The white and gray blotches (yellow arrows) make up the regression. The black arrows point out where there are no streaks. Five colors, including red, round off the melanoma-specific criteria. (Reproduced with permission from Johr RH and Stolz W. *Dermoscopy: An Illustrated Self-Assessment Guide.* 2nd ed. New York, NY: McGraw-Hill Education; 2015.)

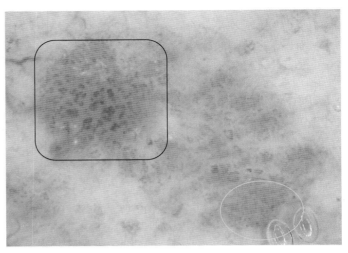

FIGURE 1-22. Bowen disease. A focus of coiled glomerular vessels (black box) and smaller dotted vessels (circle) diagnose a classic Bowen disease. A psoriatic plaque could have the same clinical appearance with pinpoint and/or glomerular vessels. Typically, the vessels fill a psoriatic lesion.

- When identified, they should raise a red flag of concern, including the following:
  - Dotted/pinpoint (dots resembling the head of a pin).
  - Linear (regular and irregular).
  - Arborizing.
  - Serpentine.
  - Glomerular.
  - Irregular torturous/corkscrew (irregular, thick, coiled).
  - Irregular hairpin (irregular and thick hairpin-shaped).
  - Many shapes can be seen that have not been described.
  - One must focus his/her attention to make out the shapes of these small vessels.

Milky-red areas
- Localized or diffuse (seen in pigmented, hypo-, or amelanotic melanoma) pinkish-white color.
- Milky-red/pink color can also be seen in benign pathology, both melanocytic and nonmelanocytic (ie, nevi, acute lichen planus–like keratosis).
- With or without reddish and or bluish out-of-focus/fuzzy globular structures (neovascularization).
- Not to be confused with the in-focus lacunae seen in hemangiomas.

Glomerular vessels
- Diffuse or clustered fine coiled vessels that can be seen in the following:
  - Bowen disease (see Fig. 1-22)
  - Melanoma

- Acute pink lichen planus–like keratosis
- Stasis dermatitis
- Psoriasis
- Pinpoint and larger glomerular vessels represent a variation of the same criterion.

Asymmetrical pigmentation around follicular openings
- Seen only on the face, nose, and ears.
- Irregular brown color outlining parts of the round follicular openings.
- The color does not completely encircle the openings (early proliferation of atypical melanocytes).

Annular-granular pattern/structures
- Seen only on the face, nose, and ears.
- Brown or gray fine dots that surround follicular openings (melanophages and/or atypical melanocytes).
  - This criterion can be seen in the following:
    - Lentigo maligna, lentigo maligna melanoma
    - Pigmented actinic keratosis
    - Posttraumatic
    - Late-stage lichen planus–like keratosis (Fig. 1-23)

Rhomboid structures
- Seen only on the face, nose, and ears.
- Rhomboid shape is a parallelogram with 2 pairs of parallel lines in which the opposite sides have equal length and there are obtuse angles.
- Black, brown, or gray thickening completely surrounding the follicular openings.
- In reality, true rhomboids are not regularly formed.
- Any pigmented thickening around follicular openings is worrisome.

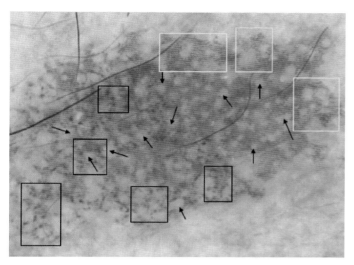

FIGURE 1-23. Lichen planus–like keratosis. Remnants of a fingerprint pattern (yellow boxes) with faint brown parallel lines of a solar lentigo are clues that this is not lentigo maligna. Gray annular-granular pattern (black boxes) around follicular openings (arrows) are also seen. The gray dots represent melanophages and free melanin in the papillary dermis, not atypical melanocytes. A subset of lichen planus–like keratosis is thought to represent an immunologic event against flat seborrheic keratosis of solar lentigines. (Reproduced with permission from Johr RH and Stolz W. *Dermoscopy: An Illustrated Self-Assessment Guide.* 2nd ed. New York, NY: McGraw-Hill Education; 2015.)

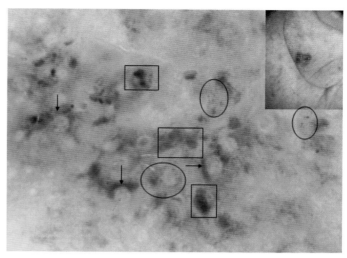

FIGURE 1-24. Lentigo maligna (earlobe). This patient demonstrates variations of the classic criteria. The lesion is suspicious clinically but has a differential diagnosis that includes a seborrheic keratosis. The dermoscopic criteria for a seborrheic keratosis are not present. There are asymmetry of color and structure, asymmetrical pigmentation (black arrows) around follicular openings (red arrows), annular-granular structures (circles), and irregular dark blotches (boxes). One should have a mental checklist of the melanoma-specific criteria for this site-specific area because they are not always easy to find and identify. "One cannot see what one does not know." (Reproduced with permission from Johr RH and Stolz W. *Dermoscopy: An Illustrated Self-Assessment Guide.* 2nd ed. New York, NY: McGraw-Hill Education; 2015.)

Circle within a circle
- Not-well-studied criterion associated with melanoma on the face, nose, and ears.
- Central hair shaft (inner circle).
- Outer ring of gray color (outer circle).
- Gray color can represent atypical melanocytes and/or melanophages.

PEARLS

- A large patch of brown color typically seen on the face of older people cannot be excised to make a histopathologic diagnosis. Commonly, it can have dermoscopic features associated with solar lentigo, actinic keratosis, and melanoma. Use the area and/or areas with atypical features to make an incisional biopsy. For example, biopsy the foci with asymmetrical follicular pigmentation or circle within a circle.

- If you think a lesion is lentigo maligna yet the pathology report does not make the diagnosis, seek another histopathologic opinion or biopsy of another area of the lesion.

- There should always be a good clinico-dermoscopic-pathologic correlation (Fig. 1-24).

Benign pigmented nail bands (melanonychia striata)
- Single or multiple nail involvement with brown longitudinal parallel lines.

- Uniform color, spacing, and thickness.
- Variable presence of a diffuse brown background.
- A single band in a lighter-skinned person with these findings is still worrisome and could represent dysplastic histology or in situ melanoma.

Malignant pigmented nail bands (atypical melanonychia striata)
- Loss of parallelism (broken-up line segments) with brown, black, or gray parallel lines that demonstrate different shades of color, irregular spacing, and thickness (Fig. 1-25).
- High-risk dermoscopic criteria at this location in adults are usually not associated with high-risk pathology when seen in children.
- Disfiguring nail matrix biopsies can usually be avoided.
- Any rapidly changing scenario warrants a histopathologic diagnosis, no matter how old or young the patient.

PEARL

- Digital monitoring is helpful to monitor pigmentation in the nail apparatus.

Fungal melanonychia (Fig. 1-26)
- Relatively rare.
- Twenty-one-plus species of dematiaceous fungi that produce melanin in their cell wall or secrete it extracellularly.
- Eight species of nondematiaceous fungi.

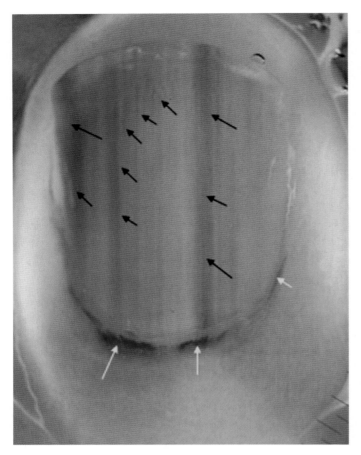

FIGURE 1-25. Acrolentiginous melanoma/nail apparatus melanoma. The pigmented bands are not uniform in color and thickness (black arrows) with loss of parallelism (broken up line segments). Loss of parallelism is created by the atypical melanocytes that produce pigment irregularly. There is also Hutchinson sign (yellow arrows). (Reproduced with permission from Johr RH and Stolz W. *Dermoscopy: An Illustrated Self-Assessment Guide.* 2nd ed. New York, NY: McGraw-Hill Education; 2015.)

- Dematiaceous fungus *Scytalidium dimidiatum* and dermatophyte *Trichophyton rubrum* most frequently isolated agents of fungal melanonychia.
- There can be diffuse melanonychia filling the entire nail or pigmented bands.
- The pigmented bands are wider distally and taper proximally, consistent with distal-to-proximal spread of infection.
- Components of the bands can be rounded proximally.

Micro-Hutchinson sign (Hutchinson sign)
- Pigmentation of the cuticle that can only be seen clearly with dermoscopy.
- A nonspecific dermoscopic finding that is often but not always associated with a nail apparatus melanoma.
- Pigmentation of the cuticle easily seen without dermoscopy.

Nonmelanocytic nail apparatus bands
- The history is important.
- Pregnancy.
- PUVA.

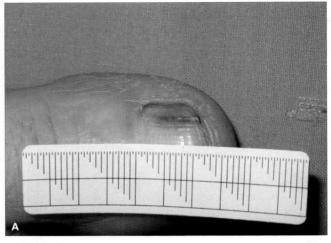
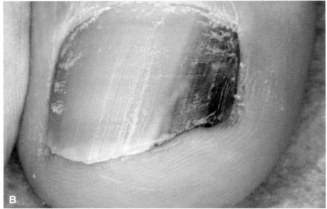

FIGURE 1-26. Fungal melanonychia created by dematiaceous fungi that produce melanin. (Reproduced with permission from Johr RH and Stolz W. *Dermoscopy: An Illustrated Self-Assessment Guide.* 2nd ed. New York, NY: McGraw-Hill Education; 2015.)

- Occupational exposure.
- Medications (chemotherapeutic agents, multiple nails).
- Racial longitudinal melanonychia (multiple nails).
- Nail trauma or inflammation (nail biting, friction, paronychia).
- Exposure to exogenous pigments (chromonychia), tobacco, dirt, potassium permanganate, tar, iodine, silver nitrate (usually can be easily scratched off).

Uniform grayish lines/bands
- Can be seen in the following:
  - Lentigo
  - Ethnic pigmentation
  - Drug-induced pigmentation
  - Postinflammatory
  - Laugier-Hunziker syndrome
- Represents epithelial hyperpigmentation without melanocytic hyperplasia.

Nail apparatus blood/subungual hematoma
- The color of blood seen in the nail apparatus depends on how long the blood has been there.
- Fresh blood looks red or purple/violaceous.

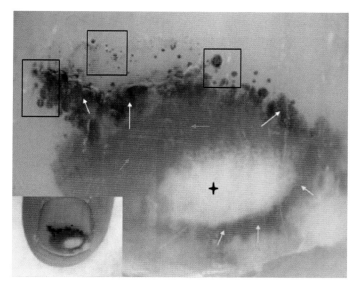

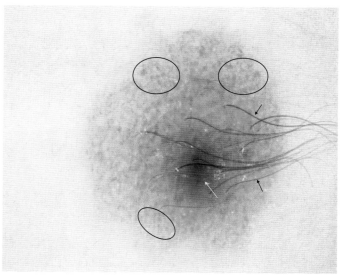

FIGURE 1-27. Subungual hematoma. Different colors plus purple blood pebbles (boxes) characterize this posttraumatic lesion. The white color (star) is secondary to trauma, not regression. The brown blotches (red arrows) and purple blotches (white arrows) result from the breakdown of blood. No melanoma-specific criteria are seen. (Reproduced with permission from Johr RH and Stolz W. *Dermoscopy: An Illustrated Self-Assessment Guide.* 2nd ed. New York, NY: McGraw-Hill Education; 2015.)

FIGURE 1-28. Congenital melanocytic nevus. Poorly defined regular brown dots and globules forming the globular global pattern (circles) fill the lesion plus a focus of terminal hairs (black arrows) characterize this banal small congenital melanocytic nevus. The regular blue blotch (yellow arrow) represents pigmentation deeper in the dermis.

- Older blood can look yellowish brown or black.
- A well-demarcated homogeneous area with parallel lines at the distal edge and globule-like blood spots/pebbles (Fig. 1-27).
- Digital dermoscopy is helpful to follow nail apparatus blood that should slowly move distally over several months.

PEARLS

- Presence of blood does not rule out melanoma.
- Search carefully for high-risk criteria that might also be present.
- Finding the Hutchinson sign and the malignant parallel-ridge pattern on the surrounding skin adjacent to the nail can help make the diagnosis of nail apparatus melanoma.
- An experienced surgeon and dermatopathologist plus a well-placed generous biopsy specimen are essential to make the correct diagnosis of nail apparatus pigmentation.

Common Dermoscopic Patterns

Congenital nevi
- Diffuse homogeneous brown color.
- Patchy or diffuse pigment network (target network may or may not be seen as network holes, each with a small centrally located brown dot or pinpoint vessel).
- Globular and/or cobblestone pattern (target globules may or may not be seen as globules with a smaller centrally located dot or vessel).

- Islands of normal skin and islands of criteria, such as network, dots, and globules.
- Multicomponent pattern with 3 or more distinct areas of criteria.
- Dark coarse terminal hairs with or without surrounding hypopigmentation (perifollicular hypopigmentation) (Fig. 1-28).
- Milia-like cysts and pseudofollicular openings most often found in seborrheic keratosis can be seen.

Acquired nevi
- Light/dark brown or pink color.
- Regular pigment network filling the lesion.
- Sharp border demarcation.
- Globular or cobblestone global patterns (the most common patterns seen in children).
- Symmetry of color and structure.
- Comma-shaped blood vessels.
- Hypopigmentation.
- Milia-like cysts, pseudofollicular openings, fissures, and ridges can be seen.
- Pink nevi can be featureless or feature-poor and have a white/negative network.
- A solitary flat pink lesion is more worrisome than multiple soft and compressible pink lesions.

PEARL

- Dermoscopy might not be helpful to diagnose pink macules and papules, which can be melanocytic, nonmelanocytic, benign, malignant, or inflammatory (Fig. 1-29).

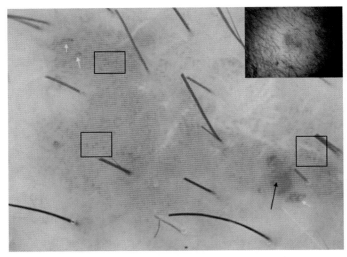

FIGURE 1-29. Acute pink lichen planus–like keratosis. Small papule found only after a complete skin examination. There are different shades of pink color, pinpoint vessels (boxes), and comma-shaped vessels (yellow arrows) plus a milky-red area (black arrow). Amelanotic melanoma and Merkel cell carcinoma are in the clinical and dermoscopic differential diagnosis. (Reproduced with permission from Johr RH and Stolz W. *Dermoscopy: An Illustrated Self-Assessment Guide.* 2nd ed. New York, NY: McGraw-Hill Education; 2015.)

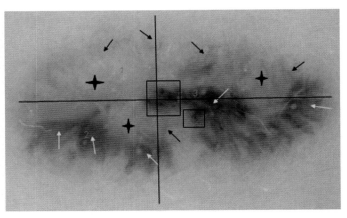

FIGURE 1-30. Recurrent nevus. Asymmetry of color and structure (+), the multicomponent global pattern (1, 2, 3) irregular brown globules (boxes), irregular dark blotches (yellow arrows), and scar tissue (stars) with arborizing vessels (black arrows) characterize this recurrent nevus. Regressive melanoma is in the dermoscopic differential diagnosis. Review the original pathology report to confirm the benign nature of this lesion. (Reproduced with permission from Johr RH and Stolz W. *Dermoscopy: An Illustrated Self-Assessment Guide.* 2nd ed. New York, NY: McGraw-Hill Education; 2015.)

Blue nevi
- Blue, blue-gray, or blue-black homogeneous color (see Fig. 1-3).
- Variable number of subtle blue globular-like structures.
- Regression with white or gray areas commonly seen.
- Radiation tattoo, nodular, and cutaneous metastatic melanoma are in the clinical and dermoscopic differential diagnosis.
- The history is essential to help make the correct diagnosis.

Combined nevi
- Light/dark brown homogeneous color +/− other local criteria (regular nevus) and central blue blotch (blue nevus) with a "fried egg" clinical appearance.
- Diffuse brown homogeneous color with a blue border.
- Diffuse blue homogeneous color with a brown border.
- Variable combinations of blue and brown color.

Recurrent nevi/pseudomelanoma
- Sharp border.
- Irregular pigment network; irregular streaks.
- Irregular dots and globules.
- White scar-like areas with arborizing vessels.
- Any combination of criteria can be seen.
- Pigmentation centrally located in the scar; if the pigmentation goes out of the scar, rule out melanoma.
- The history of previous surgery and histopathology is important (Fig. 1-30).

Dysplastic nevi
- ABCD/ABCDE clinical lesions can look banal or high-risk with dermoscopy.
- Being indistinguishable from melanoma.

- Evolving/changing (E) might be the only clue that a lesion is high-risk.
- Asymmetry of color and structure.
- Irregular pigment network.
- Irregular blotches.
- Irregular dots and globules.
- Multifocal hypopigmentation (Fig. 1-31).
- Regression, blue-white color/blue-white veil, polymorphous vessels, and streaks are not usually seen.
- May look more malignant than benign, but not definitely malignant.

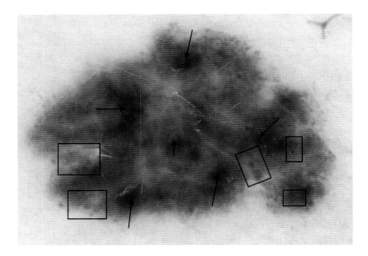

FIGURE 1-31. Dysplastic nevus. Foci of irregular brown dots and globules (boxes), irregular dark blotches (black arrows), and multifocal hypopigmentation (red arrows). It might be hard to differentiate the hypopigmentation from regression. (Reproduced with permission from Johr RH and Stolz W. *Dermoscopy: An Illustrated Self-Assessment Guide.* 2nd ed. New York, NY: McGraw-Hill Education; 2015.)

- Patients with multiple dysplastic nevi usually do not have many that look very atypical with dermoscopy.
- Look for the clinical and/or dermoscopic "ugly duckling" to consider for biopsy or digital follow-up.
- Pink dysplastic nevi can be feature-poor or featureless with low- or high-grade histopathology.

Spitz nevi
- There are 6 patterns seen in Spitz nevi:
  - Starburst
  - Globular
  - Homogeneous
  - Pink
  - Black pigment network
  - Atypical
- *Spitzoid* is the term used when any of the different 6 patterns is seen.
- Starburst is the most common pattern (Fig. 1-32).
  - Streaks and/or dots and globules at the periphery.
  - Light/dark brown, black, or blue color centrally.
  - A white/negative network can be seen within the lesion.
  - Regular or irregular pattern depends on the location of the streaks.
- Regular starburst pattern has symmetrical streaks around the lesion.
- Irregular starburst pattern has foci of streaks at the periphery.
- Symmetrical and asymmetrical starburst patterns can be seen in melanoma.
- Globular is the second most common spitzoid pattern.
  - Filled with regular or irregular brown dots and/or globules.
  - Blue color is the clue that the lesion might be a Spitz nevus.

- Homogeneous pattern.
  - Featureless brown color.
- Pink pattern.
  - Featureless pink papule.
    - Can have polymorphous vessels.
    - Not to be mistaken for amelanotic melanoma.
    - Not to be mistaken for a pyogenic granuloma.
- Black network pattern.
  - The lesion is composed totally of a prominent black pigment network.
  - Ink-spot lentigo and melanoma are in the differential diagnosis.
- Atypical pattern.
  - This can have any combination of melanoma-specific criteria similar to superficial spreading melanoma.
  - The histopathologic diagnosis is usually a surprise.
- White network/negative network can sometimes be identified.
  - This is an important clue that the lesion is spitzoid.

PEARL
- Any spitzoid pattern requires a histopathologic diagnosis, especially in adults. Monitoring these lesions with digital dermoscopy has been reported, but it is foolhardy and puts the patient's life at risk (ie, missing spitzoid melanoma)!

In situ melanoma (trunk and extremities)
- May or may not demonstrate the clinical ABCD criteria.
- Flat or slightly raised lesion.
- Asymmetry of color and structure.
- Black and/or dark brown irregular pigment network.
- Irregular dots and globules.
- Irregular dark blotches.
- Hypopigmentation.
- Lacks the criteria for deeper melanoma (pink, red, gray, or blue color; polymorphous vessels or regression).
- May look more malignant than benign, but not definitely malignant (Fig. 1-33).

Superficial spreading melanoma
- Starts in an existing nevus or de novo.
- Demonstrates the clinical ABCD criteria.
- Contains a variable number of the melanoma-specific criteria found on the trunk and extremities (see Figs. 1-19, 1-20, and 1-21).

Nodular melanoma
- Starts in an existing nevus or de novo.
- May or may not be fastgrowing.
- Pigmented, hypomelanotic, or amelanotic.

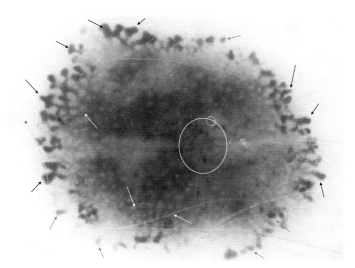

FIGURE 1-32. Spitz nevus. This is the classic symmetrical starburst/spitzoid pattern. Streaks (black arrows) in the form of pseudopods and brown globules (red arrows) are found at all points of the periphery. Foci of regular pigment network (white arrows) plus a focus or irregular brown dots and globules (yellow circle) are also identified.

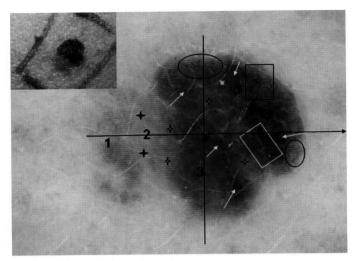

FIGURE 1-33. In situ melanoma. This is a melanocytic lesion, because it shows a pigment network (black box) and aggregated brown lobules (circles). There is asymmetry of color and structures (+), the multicomponent global pattern (1, 2, 3), irregular pigment network (black box), irregular brown dots and globules (circles), irregular dark blotches (yellow arrows), and white network (white box). The hypopigmentation (black stars) should not be confused with regression. There is diffuse erythema (red stars) and only 3 other colors. (Reproduced with permission from Johr RH and Stolz W. *Dermoscopy: An Illustrated Self-Assessment Guide.* 2nd ed. New York, NY: McGraw-Hill Education; 2015.)

- Can have symmetrical pigmentation and shape.
- Can be mistaken clinically for a banal nevus (especially in the pediatric population) or squamous cell carcinoma.
- Usually lacks the clinical ABCD criteria.
- Due to the absence of the radial growth phase, there is a scarcity of local criteria (network, globules, streaks).
- Remnants of local criteria may or may not be present at the periphery of the lesion.
- Large intense irregular dark black blotches.
- Multiple deeper-skin colors seen such as blue, white (regression), pink (inflammation), milky-red (neovascularization).
- Polymorphous vessels.

PEARLS

- The clinical appearance of a lesion (flat, palpable, or nodular, presence or absence of the ABCD criteria) plus the colors and structures seen with dermoscopy can help estimate if you are dealing with a thin, intermediate, or thick melanoma.
- Flat melanomas are usually in situ or early invasive with black and/or brown color plus well-developed local criteria.
- Thick melanomas tend to be elevated or nodular and can have a paucity or absence of local criteria such as pigment network, dots and globules plus blue-white color, regression, multiple other colors, and polymorphous vessels.

Amelanotic melanoma

- Flat, palpable, or nodular.
- Partially pigmented, hypopigmented, pink or red.
- May or may not have the melanoma-specific criteria typically seen in pigmented melanomas.
- Different shades of pink color and polymorphous vessels.
- Milky-red areas are important clues to the correct diagnosis.
- Pediatric patients have a high proportion of amelanotic melanomas (Fig. 1-34).
- Amelanotic melanoma should always be in the differential diagnosis of a Merkel cell carcinoma, pyogenic granuloma, or pink Spitz nevus.

Desmoplastic melanoma

- Rare variant of cutaneous melanoma.
- Diagnosis often delayed.
- Most common clinical presentation palpable and/or indurated lesion on sun-exposed skin.
- Histopathology can be pure desmoplastic melanoma (DM) or mixed DM (associated with another subtype of melanoma, eg, lentigo maligna).
- Dermoscopically, one can find one or more melanoma-specific criteria.
- Regression/white scar-like areas/peppering/gray color.
- Multiple colors.
- Polymorphous vessels.
- Milky-red areas with or without milky-red globules.
- Pink color/vascular flush.
- Crystalline structures.

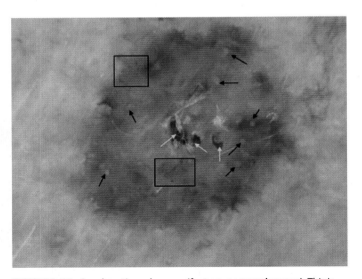

FIGURE 1-34. Amelanotic melanoma (feature-poor melanoma). This is a melanocytic lesion, because it has aggregated brown globules (boxes). There is an absence of melanoma-specific criteria found on the face with different shades of pink and brown color plus ulceration (yellow arrows). Follicular openings (black arrows) should not be confused with the milia-like cysts of a seborrheic keratosis. (Reproduced with permission from Johr RH and Stolz W. *Dermoscopy: An Illustrated Self-Assessment Guide.* 2nd ed. New York, NY: McGraw-Hill Education; 2015.)

- A high index of suspicion and dermoscopic clues can increase the clinical diagnosis of dermoplastic melanoma.

Pediatric melanoma
- Pediatric melanoma is rare, yet the incidence is steadily increasing each year.
- Dermoscopic features of superficial spreading, pigmented nodular, or amelanotic melanoma.
- A significant number do not present with the ABCD clinical features.
- In many cases, the conventional ABCD criteria are inadequate in children.
- Amelanosis, symmetry, regular borders, diameter less than 6 mm, bleeding, uniform color, variable diameter, and de novo development are common.

PEARLS

- Additional ABCD detection criteria include amelanotic, bleeding bump, color uniformity, de novo, and diameter.
- At any age, E for evolution or any change is significant, no matter what a lesion looks like.

Cutaneous metastatic melanoma
- Dermoscopy might not be as helpful to make the diagnosis as the history of a melanoma being previously excised.
- Single or multiple.
- Pigmented and/or nonpigmented macules, papules, and ulcerated or nonulcerated nodules can be seen in the same patient.
- Any combination of criteria can be seen.
- Benign patterns such as a hemangioma-like cutaneous metastatic melanoma (see Fig. 1-17).

Feature-poor melanoma
- Melanoma without well-developed melanoma-specific criteria (Fig. 1-34).
- Melanoma incognito/false-negative melanoma.
- Clinically, the lesion does not look like melanoma.
- With dermoscopy, there may be clues to help make the diagnosis.
- Clues to help make the diagnosis:
  - History of dermoscopic change over time.
  - A spitzoid pattern in a lesion that does not look spitzoid clinically.
  - Areas of regression as the major high-risk criterion.
  - Polymorphous vessels in a pink lesion.
- The "Little Red Riding Hood Sign" is when the lesion looks clinically benign from a distance but not close up with dermoscopy.

PEARL

- Dermoscopy should not only be used on clinically suspicious lesions if one wants to diagnose melanoma incognito.

Featureless melanoma
- Melanoma with no dermoscopic criteria at all.
- Usually a pink or hypopigmented lesion.

Nevi/melanomas associated with decorative tattoos
- It is best not to cover melanocytic lesions with decorative tattoos.
- Malignant change could be camouflaged.
- The infiltration of tattoo pigment into melanocytic lesions can obscure dermoscopic features and makes an accurate dermoscopic diagnosis difficult.
- Laser removal of tattoos covering melanocytic lesions has been reported with invasive melanoma.
- It is not known if lasers have the potential to change benign nevi into melanoma.
- After laser therapy, black pigment in tattoos can be found in regional lymph nodes and makes the diagnosis of metastatic melanoma problematic.

PEARLS

- Avoid covering melanocytic lesions with decorative tattoos until there is more scientific evidence that it is a safe procedure.
- One should excise a melanocytic lesion before covering the area with a tattoo.

Merkel cell carcinoma
- Relatively rare tumor.
- Nonspecific clinical findings.
- Very few studied dermoscopically.
- High mortality rate.
- Often delay in diagnosis due to low index of suspicion.
- Amelanotic tumors are in the clinical and dermoscopic differential diagnosis (eg, basal cell carcinoma, amelanotic melanoma, Bowen disease, acute lichen planus–like keratosis, and other benign lesions).
- Variety of vascular patterns.
- Milky-red areas with/or without milky-red globules.
- Polymorphous vessels (several different shapes).
- Arborizing vessels (similar to basal cell carcinoma).
- Pinpoint and glomerular vessels (similar to Bowen disease).

Nail apparatus melanoma

- Amelanotic reddish diffuse color/amelanotic tumor.
- Diffuse melanonychia with different shades of black, brown, or gray color.
- Irregular pigmented bands (eg, different colors, irregular spacing, thickness, loss of parallelism) (see Fig. 1-25).
- A single uniform band does not rule out melanoma.
- Irregular dots and globules.
- Blood can be found associated with other criteria.
- Nail plate destruction with advanced disease.
- With or without Hutchinson sign.
- The malignant parallel-ridge pattern can be seen on the adjacent skin.

Ink spot lentigo

- Black macule or macules on sun-exposed areas.
- Prominent thickened black pigment network.
- Usually a very easy clinical and dermoscopic diagnosis.
- Melanoma could be in the clinical and dermoscopic differential diagnosis.
- Look for melanoma-specific criteria that should not be present in an ink spot lentigo.

Solar lentigo

- Macules and/or patches.
- Different shades of homogeneous brown color.
- Moth-eaten concave borders.
- Fingerprint pattern with wavy parallel linear line segments can form arches, swirls, be hyphae-like.

Actinic keratosis

- Nonpigmented actinic keratosis:
  - Scaly surface.
  - Pinkish pseudonetwork and round white globules (follicular openings).
  - The pink pseudonetwork with roundish white structures has to be described as having a "strawberry-like" appearance.
- Pigmented actinic keratosis:
  - Mimics lentigo maligna.
  - Asymmetrical follicular pigmentation.
  - Annular-granular structures.
  - Rhomboid structures.

Bowen disease (in situ squamous cell carcinoma)

- Usually solitary pink or reddish scaly macule, papule, nodule, patch, plaque.
- On sun-exposed areas in elderly patients.
- Pinpoint and/or glomerular vessels.
- Clusters and/or diffuse distribution of vessels throughout the lesion.
- With or without homogeneous brown color and/or dark dots and globules (pigmented Bowen disease).

Clear cell acanthoma

- Rare tumor, very few have been studied.
- Pink macule or papule.
- One to 2 cm reddish-moist nodule with scale.
- Trunk and lower extremities.
- Diagnostic dermoscopic findings:
  - Linear and/or curvilinear glomerular and/or pinpoint vessels.
  - String of pearls necklace-like circular arrangement of glomerular and/or pinpoint vessels.

Keratoacanthoma/invasive squamous cell carcinoma

- Centrally located yellowish keratinous material/central keratin.
- White structureless zones.
- White circles.

- Irregular hairpin/coiled and/or linear vessels at the periphery.

Sebaceous gland hyperplasia

- Delled yellow papules seen clinically.
- Multiple grouped white or yellow globules.
- Basal cell carcinoma–like arborizing vessels.
- The vessels have been termed *crown vessels* or *wreath-like vessels.*
- Supposedly never to reach the center of the lesion.
- This is a misnomer, because in reality the vessels rarely meet this criterion and can be found anywhere in the lesion.

PEARLS

- The globules are the main dermoscopic feature used to differentiate sebaceous gland hyperplasia from basal cell carcinoma.
- Typically the vessels are thick. If there are fine arborizing and serpentine vessels, even with the typical colored globules, basal cell carcinoma should be considered.
- If in doubt, cut it out!

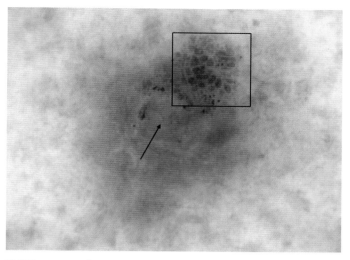

FIGURE 1-35. Collison tumor—squamous cell carcinoma and seborrheic keratosis. A rapidly growing nodule (arrow) representing a squamous cell carcinoma and the mountain-and-valley pattern of a seborrheic keratosis (box) characterize this lesion. The cobblestone pattern of a nevus is in the dermoscopic differential diagnosis. (Reproduced with permission from Johr RH and Stolz W. *Dermoscopy: An Illustrated Self-Assessment Guide.* 2nd ed. New York, NY: McGraw-Hill Education; 2015.)

Collision tumor

- Lesion with the dermoscopic criteria for 2 different pathologies.
- Rarely, one can find a triple collision lesion with 3 different pathologies.
- Collision tumors are commonly seen.
- Diagnostic criteria can be side by side, or one can be seen within the other.
- Examples include the following:
  - Seborrheic keratosis, basal cell carcinoma
  - Seborrheic keratosis, in situ or invasive squamous cell carcinoma
  - Seborrheic keratosis, amelanotic or pigmented melanoma
  - Seborrheic keratosis, eccrine porocarcinoma
  - Basal cell carcinoma, seborrheic keratosis, clear cell acanthoma
- Any combination is possible (Fig. 1-35).

Other Diagnoses Made With Dermoscopy

Scabies

- Burrows appear as discrete linear/S- or zigzag-shaped whitish scaly areas.
- Mites can be seen as a small triangle/gray delta structure/ jet with contrail pattern that corresponds to the front section of the body with its mouth/biting apparatus and legs.
- Higher magnification and oil/gel increase the visibility of the mite, stool, and eggs.

Lichen Planus

- Peppering.
- Brown blotches.
- White reticular areas (Wickham striae).
- Crystalline structures can be seen with polarized dermoscopy (Wickham striae).
- White network is in the dermoscopic differential diagnosis of Wickham striae.

Warts

- Red and/or black dots (thrombosed capillaries).
- With or without a white halo.

Psoriasis

- Red scaly plaque/plaques.
- Diffuse distribution of glomerular and/or pinpoint vessels as opposed to a patchy distribution of similar vessels in Bowen disease.
- Distribution of lesions will help differentiate psoriasis from Bowen disease.
- Both can have single or multiple lesions.

Nail Folds

- Normal capillary loops are hairpin-shaped and run perpendicular to the cuticle.

Scleroderma Pattern

- The triad of:
  - Rarefied capillaries (<6 loops per mm)
  - Thin loops, megacapillaries
  - Pearly shining sclerosis "cotton balls"

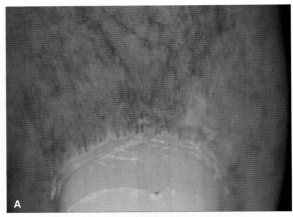

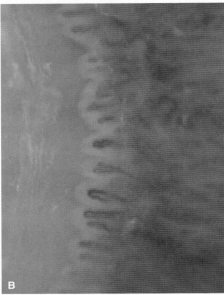

FIGURE 1-36. Nail fold capillaries in cutaneous lupus. Uniform hairpin-shaped capillary loops are replaced with large (mega) irregularly shaped capillary loops that still have a hairpin shape. The surrounding skin is atrophic with diffuse telangiectatic vessels. (Reproduced with permission from Johr RH and Stolz W. *Dermoscopy: An Illustrated Self-Assessment Guide.* 2nd ed. New York, NY: McGraw-Hill Education; 2015.)

Dermatomyositis

- Mega/enlarged, twisted, branched loops, microhemorrhage

Lupus Erythematosus

- Considerable variation of loops, branching, twisted microhemorrhage (Fig. 1-36).

INFESTATIONS

Pediculosis Capitis

- Direct visualization of the parasite and nits.
- It is possible to see if the nits are full (vital nits) or empty, which helps determine the success or failure of treatment.

Pediculosis Pubis

- It is possible to easily see the parasite attached to adjacent pubic hairs or hairs at other sites (eg, eyelashes).

Trichoscopy

- The use of dermoscopy to evaluate scalp skin and hair follicles.
- Any form of dermoscopy can be used (polarized, nonpolarized, contact, noncontact with or without fluid).
- Structures that can be visualized include the following:
  - Hair shafts
  - Hair follicle openings
  - Perifollicular epidermis
  - Cutaneous microvasculature

Criteria Seen With Trichoscopy

- Anisotrichosis: hair diameter variability greater than 20%.
- Black dots (cadaverized hairs): black dots inside follicular openings and represent fragmented and destroyed hair shafts.
- Brown halo (peripilar sign): brown macules surround emergence of the hair shafts from the scalp (follicular ostia) secondary to inflammation.
- Circle hairs: thin short vellus hairs that form a circle.
- Coiled hairs: telogen/catagen broken hairs that coil back.
- Comma hairs: short C-shaped broken hair shafts with ectothrix parasitization.
- Corkscrew hair: short spiral shape broken hair shafts.
- Coudability hairs: hairs of normal length with a narrow proximal shaft.
- Empty follicles: skin-colored small depressions without hairs.
- Exclamation mark hairs: tapered telogen hairs with a light, thin tip at the level of the skin.
- Follicular keratotic plugging: keratotic masses plugging follicular ostia.
- Follicular red dots: erythematous concentric structures in and around follicular ostia representing dilated vessels and extravasated blood.
- Hair tufting: multiple hairs (6) emerging from the same ostium.
- Honeycomb network–like structures: created by homogeneous brown rings; not a true pigment network created by elongated and hyperpigmented rete ridges.
- Morse code–like hairs (aka, bar-code hairs); irregular broken and curved or angulated hairs. There are white spots where the hair bend.
- Peripilar casts: concentrically arranged scales encircling emerging hair shafts.
- Peripilar sign: brown halo surrounding follicular opening caused by inflammation.
- Peripilar white halo: gray-white halo surrounding follicular ostia created by fibrosis.
- Twisted red loops: multiple red dots at low magnification (×10, ×20) and polymorphous beaded lines at higher magnification (×40) representing capillaries in the papillary dermis.

- White dots: interfollicular acrosyringia and follicular openings.
- White patches: well-demarcated irregular white patches seen in scarring alopecia devoid of follicular openings.
- Yellow dots: round or polycyclic yellow to yellow-pink dots representing infundibula plugged with sebum and keratin. May be devoid of hairs or contain miniaturized, cadaverized, or dystrophic hairs.

ACQUIRED HAIR/SCALP DISEASES

Seborrheic Dermatitis Versus Psoriasis

- Vascular patterns help make the diagnosis.
- Psoriasis has pinpoint or glomerular vessels similar to skin plaques.
- Seborrheic dermatitis lacks pinpoint or glomerular vessels but has arborizing and polymorphous vessels.

Tinea Capitis

- Patchy alopecia, erythema, scale, cervical/posterior auricular/occipital adenopathy.
- Comma hairs.
- Morse code-like/bar-code hairs.
- Corkscrew hairs: more commonly seen in African American children.
- Black dots.
- Broken and dystrophic hairs.

Trichosporosis (Piedra)

- Superficial mycosis of the hair shafts:
  - White piedra (*Trichosporon beigelii, Trichosporon inkin*)
  - Hair shafts coated with yellow to beige sheaths
  - Distal fusiform nodules
  - Black piedra (*Piedraia hortae*)
  - Dark nodules along the hair shafts

Trichomycosis Capitis

- *Corynebacterium* species
- Scalp, axilla, pubic hairs
- Yellow sheaths attached to the hair shafts

Androgenic Alopecia

- Anisotrichosis
- Brown halo (peripilar sign)
- Yellow dots
- Honeycomb network
- White dots
- Circle vellus hairs
- Empty follicles

Alopecia Areata

- Yellow dots
- Black dots (cadaverized hairs)

- Circle hairs
- Exclamation mark hairs (mostly along the edges of the patches of alopecia)
- Coudability hairs
- Clustered vellus hairs
- Pseudomonilethrix hairs characterized by constrictions in the hair shaft
- Multiple depressed follicular osteo
- Fibrosis with white dots in long-standing cases
- Alopecia areata incognito:
  - Subtype of alopecia areata with rapidly developing diffuse alopecia
  - Mimics telogen effluvium
  - Diffusely distributed yellow dots
  - Large number of short-growing hairs (2-4 mm)

Trichotillomania

- Coiled hairs (not seen in alopecia areata)
- Broken hairs with different lengths
- Black dots
- Yellow dots
- Absence of exclamation mark hairs characteristic of alopecia areata

Traction Alopecia

- Marginal alopecia
- Traction due to hair styles
- Common in African Americans
- Hair casts around hair shafts at the periphery

Trichorrhexis Nodosa

- Mechanical, chemical, thermal damage
- White nodules along the hair shafts
- Fractured and frayed ends have a brush-like appearance

Bubble Hair

- High temperature from hair styling.
- Gas formation creates bubbles that appear as white oval spaces with a Swiss-cheese appearance.

Trichoptilosis (Split Ends)

- Longitudinal splitting at the distal ends of the hair shafts
- Two or multiple frayed ends at different lengths

Scarring Alopecia

- Primary and secondary types (eg, lichen planopilaris, frontal fibrosing alopecia, discoid lupus, folliculitis decalvans)
- Decreased hair density
- Pinpoint white dots (follicular and acrosyringeal openings)
- Loss of follicular openings
- Cicatricial white patches

Congenital Hair Shaft Abnormalities

Monilethrix

- Hair shaft beading.
- Elliptical nodes (normal shaft diameter).
- Narrow internodes (dystrophic hairs).
- Elliptical nodes regularly separated by narrow internodes.
- Regular bended ribbon sign.
- Hair shafts bend regularly at multiple locations in different directions.
- Trichorrhexis invaginata should be in purple color like the one above it Monilethrix ("bamboo hair"):
  - Seen in Netherton syndrome (autosomal recessive, ichthyosiform erythroderma, atopic diathesis, trichorrhexis invaginata).
  - Invagination of the distal portion of the hair shaft into its proximal portion forming a ball in cup appearance.
  - Bamboo/golf tee/matchstick hairs.

Pili annulati

- Alternating light and dark bands are seen clinically.
- Light bands represent air-filled cavities.

Pili torti

- Flattened hair shafts
- Twisting at irregular intervals

Pili trianguli and Canaliculi

- "Uncombable" hair; dry, unruly hair
- Triangular or reniform hair shafts
- Flattened hairs with longitudinal groves

Pili bifurcati and Multigemini

- Hair shafts grow from the same papilla
- Split from a single tip
- Double tip (bifurcati)
- Several tips (multigemini)

QUESTIONS

1. **Which criteria can be used to diagnose a melanocytic lesion?**
   a. Milia-like cysts and pigmented pseudofollicular openings
   b. Arborizing vessels, ulceration, and pigmentation
   c. A central white patch plus fine peripheral pigment network
   d. Lacunae and black homogenous blotches
   e. Pigment network, brown globules, homogeneous blue color, or parallel patterns

2. **Diagnosing a melanocytic lesion by default means that:**
   a. There are high-risk criteria at the periphery of the lesion that are hard to identify.
   b. There are criteria for a seborrheic keratosis or basal cell carcinoma associated with pigment network and brown globules.
   c. There is an absence of criteria to diagnose a melanocytic lesion, seborrheic keratosis, dermatofibroma, pyogenic granuloma, or ink spot lentigo; therefore, the lesion should be considered melanocytic.
   d. There is an absence of criteria to diagnose a melanocytic lesion, seborrheic keratosis, basal cell carcinoma, dermatofibroma, or hemangioma; therefore, the lesion should be considered melanocytic.
   e. None of the above.

3. **Which criteria can be used to diagnose a seborrheic keratosis?**
   a. Milky-red areas, irregular streaks, and pigmented follicular openings
   b. Streaks, irregular blotches, and regression

   c. Furrows, ridges, sharp border demarcation, milia-like cysts, pseudofollicular openings, fat fingers, and hairpin vessels
   d. Rhomboid structures and/or circle within a circle
   e. Diffuse brown color, glomerular vessels, and milia-like cysts

4. **Which criteria can be used to diagnose a basal cell carcinoma?**
   a. Pigment network and arborizing vessels
   b. Arborizing and pinpoint vessels plus multifocal hypopigmentation
   c. The absence of a pigment network, arborizing vessels, pigmentation, ulceration, spoke-wheel structures
   d. Glomerular vessels, ulceration, and blue ovoid nests of pigmentation
   e. Islands of black blotches, arborizing vessels, and moth-eaten borders

5. **Vascular lesions can contain the following criteria:**
   a. Out-of-focus lacunae-like globules
   b. A variable number of red, sharply demarcated vascular spaces called *lacunae* and *fibrous septae*
   c. Ten to 20 major and minor lacunae and thromboses
   d. A minimal of 2 well-developed glomerular vessels
   e. Fibrous septae, peppering, and blue dark lacunae

6. **Dermatofibromas can be associated with the following criteria:**
   a. Pigment network, arborizing vessels, and central white patch
   b. A central white patch that is never located at the periphery

c. A central white patch and peripheral pigment network

d. A complete absence of blood vessels and a few milia-like cysts

e. Multifocal hypopigmentation, arborizing vessels, and a central bluish white veil

7. **Melanoma-specific criteria on the trunk and extremities can contain this combination of criteria:**

a. Asymmetry of color and structure, a cobblestone global pattern, and regular globules or blotches

b. A multicomponent global pattern, symmetry of color and structure, regular network, regular globules, and regression

c. Polymorphous vessels, arborizing vessels, 2 colors, and regular streaks

d. Irregular network, irregular globules, irregular blotches, and regression

e. Rhomboid structures and the parallel-ridge pattern

8. **Dysplastic nevi typically have the following combination of criteria:**

a. Symmetry of color and structure and no melanoma-specific criteria

b. Asymmetry of color and structure, irregular network, regular blotches, and regular streaks

c. Multifocal regression, peppering, regular pigment network, regular dots and globules

d. Pinpoint, arborizing, and glomerular vessels plus several melanoma-specific criteria

e. Asymmetry of color and structure plus several melanoma-specific criteria

9. **Which statement is true about Spitz nevi?**

a. They can have 10 different patterns.

b. A spitzoid lesion only refers to the starburst or pink patterns.

c. Melanoma is not in the differential diagnosis of regular starburst pattern.

d. In an adult, most spitzoid lesions do not need to be excised.

e. Symmetrical and asymmetrical starburst patterns can be seen in melanoma.

10. **Which of the following statements best describes the criteria seen in superficial spreading melanomas?**

a. Criteria associated with a benign nevus are never seen.

b. They contain several well-developed melanoma-specific criteria such as symmetry of color and structure and one prominent color.

c. Usually they have several well-developed melanoma-specific criteria such as asymmetry of color and structure, multicomponent global pattern, regular network, regular globules, and regular streaks.

d. They contain a variable number of melanoma-specific criteria such as asymmetry of color and structure, multicomponent global pattern, irregular local criteria, 5 or 6 colors, and polymorphous vessels.

e. They are usually feature-poor or featureless.

ANSWERS

1. **E.** Criteria to diagnose a melanocytic lesion include any variation of pigment network (regular and/or irregular), multiple brown dots and/or globules, homogeneous blue color of a blue nevus, and parallel patterns seen on acral skin. The default category is the last way to diagnose a melanocytic lesion. Milia-like cysts and follicular openings can be seen in melanocytic lesions but are not primary criteria to make the diagnosis. Answers A, B, and C diagnose a basal cell carcinoma, dermatofibroma, and hemangioma.

2. **D.** Diagnosing a melanocytic lesion by default means that one does not see criteria for a melanocytic lesion, seborrheic keratosis, basal cell carcinoma, dermatofibroma, or hemangioma. Default is an absence of criteria. One has to memorize all the criteria from each specific potential diagnosis to be able to diagnose a melanocytic lesion by default. Dermoscopy cannot be mastered by osmosis. It is essential to study and practice the technique routinely in one's daily practice. Ink spot lentigo and pyogenic granuloma are not in this algorithm.

3. **C.** All the criteria used to diagnose seborrheic keratosis are commonly seen in daily practice. Melanoma-specific criteria can also be seen in atypical seborrheic keratosis. Beware of seborrheic keratosis–like melanomas. Milky-red areas, irregular streaks, regression, rhomboid structures, and circle within a circle are all melanoma-specific criteria that are more sensitive and specific for melanoma but could be found in seborrheic keratosis. Glomerular vessels are a primary criterion to diagnose Bowen disease and are not seen in seborrheic keratosis.

4. **C.** Basal cell carcinomas are usually a clinical diagnosis, and dermoscopy is used to confirm one's clinical impression (on-the-spot dermoscopic second opinion). By definition, if one sees pigment network, the lesion could not be a basal cell carcinoma. A subset of melanomas can be undistinguished from basal cell

carcinoma with pigmentation and arborizing vessels. Pinpoint and glomerular vessels could be seen, but they would be outshadowed by arborizing vessels. If not, one could be dealing with a basal cell–like melanoma. Moth-eaten borders are seen in lentigines and flat seborrheic keratosis; never in basal cell carcinomas.

5. **B.** The hallmarks of vascular lesions are lacunae; vascular spaces with well-demarcated sharp borders. There is no set number of lacunae needed to make the diagnoses. At times one has to use one's imagination to decide if the margins fit the criteria for vascular spaces. Different shades of red, blue, and even black are typically seen. Black homogeneous color usually represents thrombosis. Major and minor lacunae do not exist. Fibrous whitish septae and/or bluish-white color are routinely seen in typical hemangiomas. At times it is not possible to differentiate lacunae and red color of a hemangioma from the milky-red areas that can contain out-of-focus reddish globules seen in melanoma.

6. **C.** Dermatofibromas are ubiquitous benign tumors, and in most cases dermoscopy is not needed to make the diagnosis. A central white patch and pigment network, the primary criteria to make the diagnosis, may or may not be present. It might not be possible to differentiate an atypical dermatofibroma from a melanoma if melanoma-specific criteria are identified. There are innumerable ways that the central white patch can appear, and in many cases it is not centrally located. Telangiectatic vessels with polymorphous shapes are commonly seen, but basal cell–like arborizing vessels would make the diagnosis of a dermatofibroma unlikely.

7. **D.** Irregularity is the name of the game if criteria are to be considered melanoma-specific. Melanoma-specific criteria can be seen in both benign and malignant pathology but are more sensitive and specific for melanoma. There is not a single melanoma-specific criterion that is pathognomonic for melanoma. One should learn one's definitions and study as many classic textbook examples as possible. Rhomboid structures help diagnose melanoma on the face, and the parallel-ridge pattern can be seen in acral melanomas.

8. **E.** Dysplastic nevi are ubiquitous in the light-skinned population and can be indistinguishable clinically and dermoscopically from melanoma. They usually look more benign than malignant with dermoscopy; however, there are melanomas that do not have well-developed melanoma-specific criteria. Vessels of any kind are not typically seen except in pink feature-poor dysplastic nevi. They can have a variable number of melanoma-specific criteria (eg, irregular pigment network, irregular dots and/or globules, irregular blotches) that are not as well-developed as those seen in melanoma. Streaks, regression, and many colors are not usually seen and should raise a red flag of concern that the lesion might be a melanoma.

9. **E.** Spitzoid lesions are always a red flag for concern. Even symmetrical patterns can be seen in melanoma. There are only 6 patterns (starburst, globular, homogeneous, pink, black network, atypical). One often has to use one's imagination to diagnose a spitzoid lesion. Since symmetrical and asymmetrical spitzoid patterns can be found in melanoma, they should all be excised in children as well as in adults. A dermatopathologist who specializes in melanocytic lesions is good, although one who has expertise in spitzoid lesions is ideal. Even experienced dermatopathologists have trouble differentiating atypical spitzoid lesions from melanoma, and atypical spitzoid lesions have the potential to metastasize to regional lymph nodes and kill the patient.

10. **D.** Superficial spreading melanoma can have it all as far as the spectrum of melanoma-specific criteria goes. The criteria can be well-developed or difficult to identify. Criteria associated with benign melanocytic lesions can also be seen. The more high-risk criteria identified in the lesion, the greater the chance that one is dealing with a melanoma. Nodular and amelanotic melanoma are more likely to be feature-poor or featureless.

Comprehensive Dermoscopy Criteria Review

SYMMETRY AND ASYMMETRY

Mirror Image Technique

- The lesion is bisected by 2 lines that are placed 90° to each other.
- One does not physically place lines over the lesion; the lines are visually imagined.
- The lines should be placed to create as much symmetry as possible.
- Are the color and/or the structure on the left half of the lesion a mirror image of the right half?
- Repeat the analysis for the upper and lower half of the lesion.

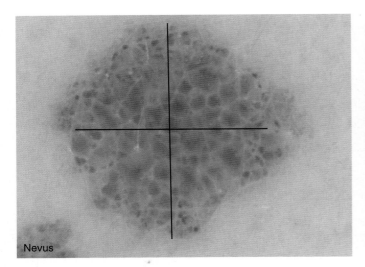
Nevus

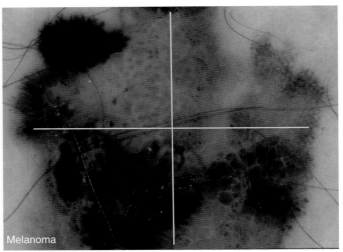
Melanoma

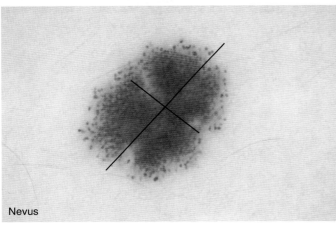
Nevus

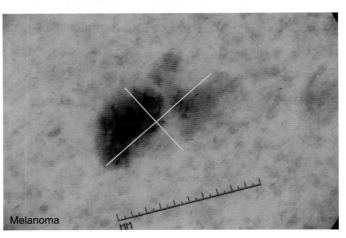
Melanoma

TABLE 2-1 • Global Patterns: Global pattern is the overall dermoscopic picture of a lesion.
Reticular
Pigment network filling most of the lesion.
Globular
Dots and globules filling most of the lesion.
Cobblestone
Larger angulated globules resembling street cobblestones filling most of the lesion.
Homogeneous
Diffuse pigmentation in the absence of local criteria such as pigment network, dots, and globules.
Starburst (spitzoid)
Streaks and/or dots and globules at the periphery of the lesion.
Multicomponent
Three or more different areas within a lesion. Each zone can be composed of a single criterion or multiple criteria.

RETICULAR GLOBAL PATTERN
Pigment Network Filling Most of the Lesion

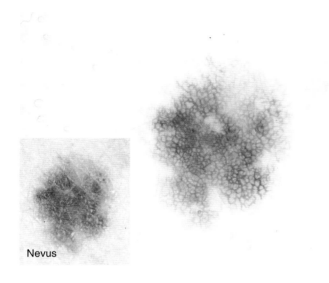

Nevus

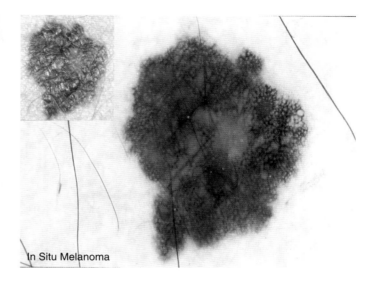

In Situ Melanoma

GLOBULAR GLOBAL PATTERN
Dots and Globules Filling Most of the Lesion

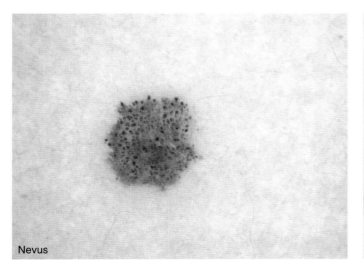

Nevus

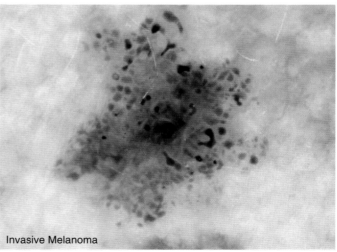

Invasive Melanoma

COBBLESTONE GLOBAL PATTERN
Larger Angulated Globules Resembling Street Cobblestones Filling Most of the Lesion

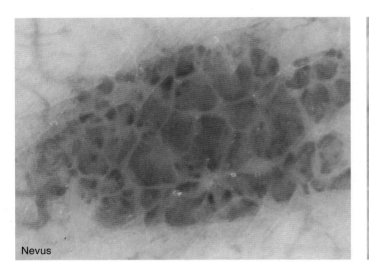

Nevus

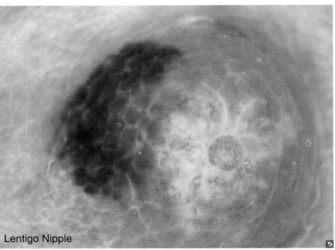

Lentigo Nipple

HOMOGENEOUS GLOBAL PATTERN
Diffuse Pigmentation in the Absence of Local Criteria Such as Pigment Network, Dots, and Globules

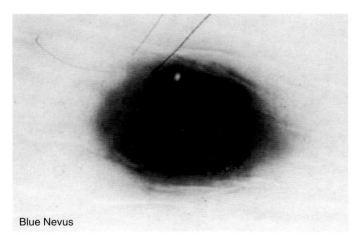

Blue Nevus

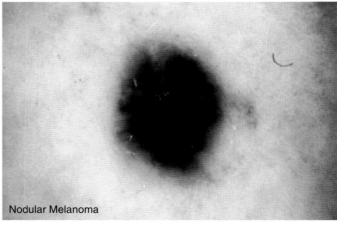

Nodular Melanoma

STARBURST (SPITZOID)

Streaks (black arrows) and/or Dots and Globules (red arrows) at the Periphery of the Lesion

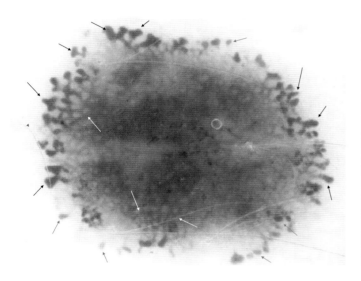

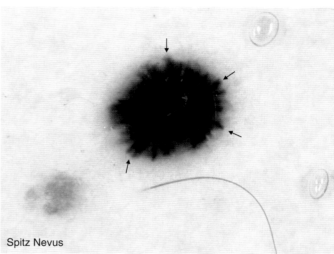

Spitz Nevus

MULTICOMPONENT GLOBAL PATTERN

- Three or more different areas within a lesion.
- Each zone can be composed of a single criterion or multiple criteria.

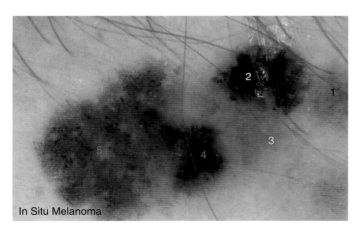

In Situ Melanoma

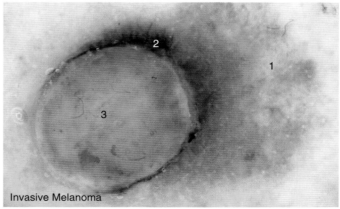

Invasive Melanoma

REGULAR PIGMENT NETWORK

- On the trunk and extremities
- Shades of brown honeycomb-like, reticular, web-like line segments (elongated and hyperpigmented rete ridges) with hypopigmented holes (dermal papilla)
- Uniform color, thickness, and holes

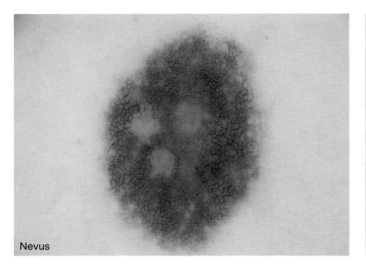

Nevus

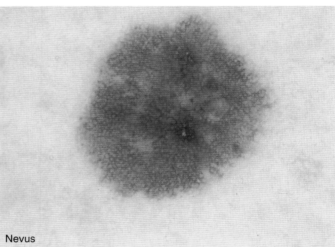

Nevus

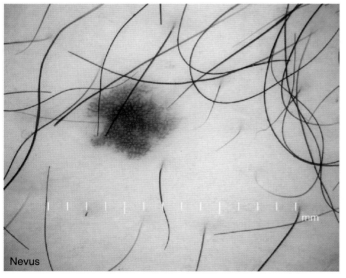

Nevus

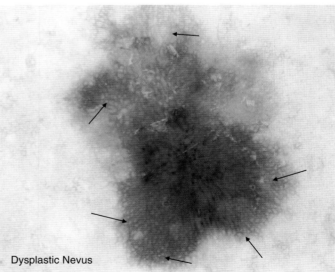

Dysplastic Nevus

IRREGULAR PIGMENT NETWORK

- Shades of brown.
- Line segments that are thickened, branched, and broken up (enlarged, fused rete ridges).
- There may be a diffuse distribution or foci of irregular pigment network.

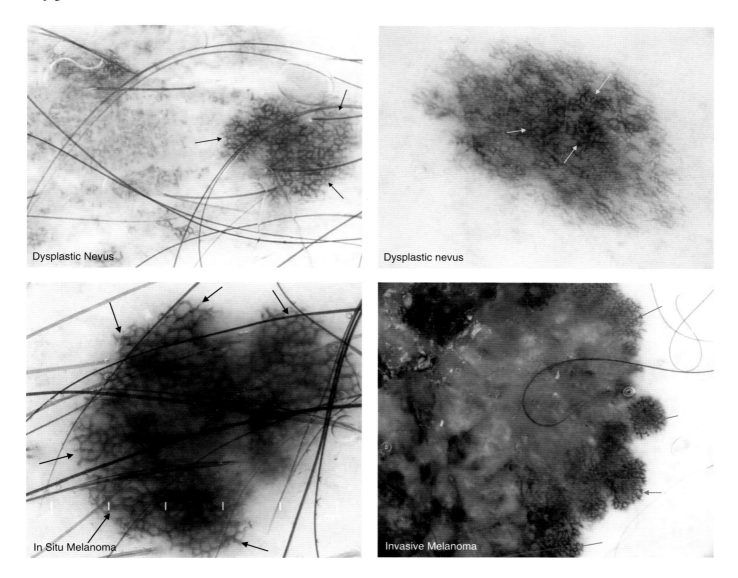

Dysplastic Nevus

Dysplastic nevus

In Situ Melanoma

Invasive Melanoma

TARGET NETWORK

- Brown globules or dotted vessels within the "holes" of the network (melanocytic nests or capillaries in the dermal papilla).
- Typically a single brown globule or single vessel is seen in each papilla.
- Target network can be seen throughout a lesion or be spotty.
- Target network is thought to be a feature of congenital nevi.

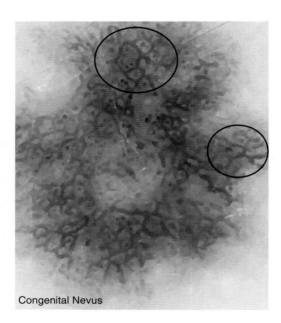

Congenital Nevus

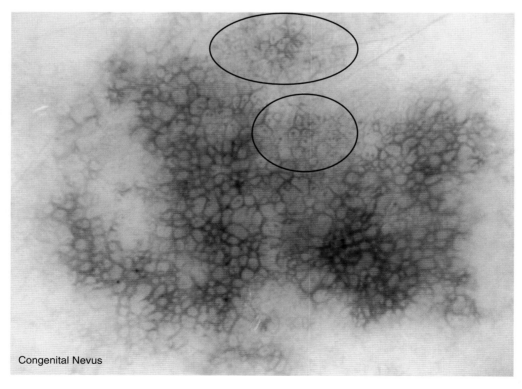

Congenital Nevus

PSEUDONETWORK/PSEUDOPIGMENT NETWORK

- The skin of the face, nose, and ears is thin and does not have well-developed rete ridges.
- Appendageal openings/adnexal structures (sebaceous glands, hair follicles) appear as uniform round white or yellowish structures.

- When they penetrate areas of diffuse pigmentation, reticular-like structures are formed that are referred to as the *pseudonetwork*.
- Not to be confused with the pigment network found on the trunk and extremities.

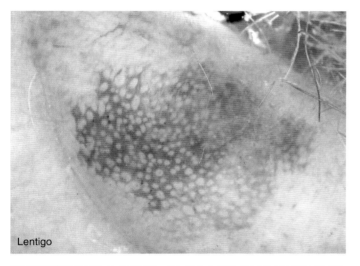

Lentigo

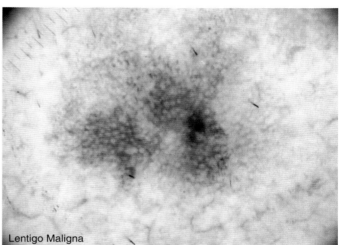

Lentigo Maligna

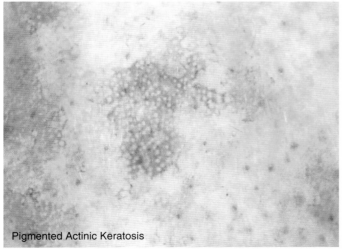

Pigmented Actinic Keratosis

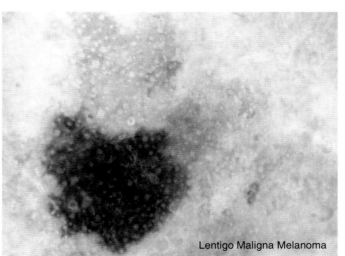

Lentigo Maligna Melanoma

WHITE NETWORK/NEGATIVE NETWORK

- Bony/milky-white reticular network-like structures (increased granular layer, thin lighter elongated rete ridges may be accompanied by large dark melanocytic nests).
- The opposite of brown pigment network.
- May be localized/asymmetrically located or diffuse.

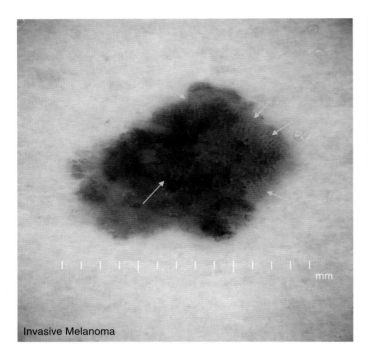

Invasive Melanoma

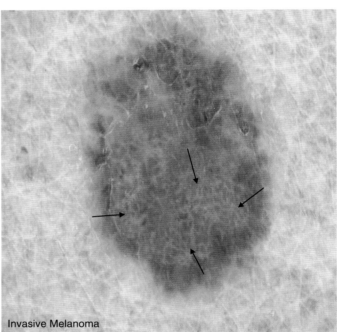

Invasive Melanoma

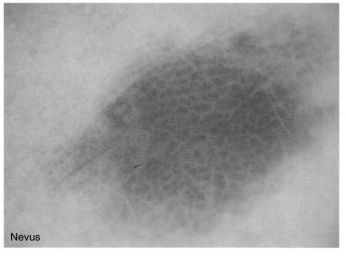

Nevus

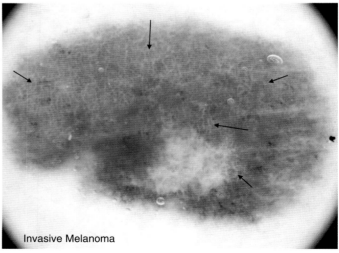

Invasive Melanoma

REGULAR BROWN DOTS AND GLOBULES

- Brown roundish structures (nests of melanocytes at the dermoepidermal junction).
- Size, shape, and color are similar.

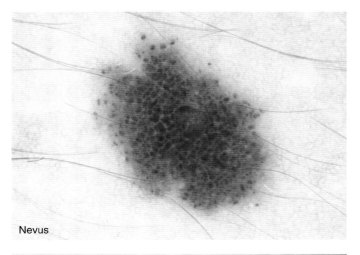

Nevus

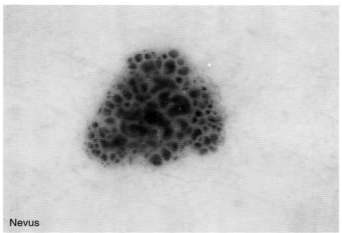

Nevus

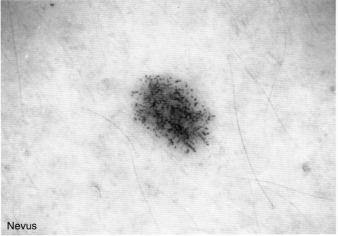

Nevus

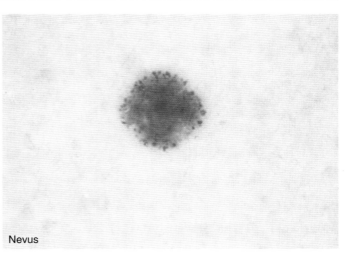

Nevus

IRREGULAR BROWN DOTS AND GLOBULES

- Brown roundish structures.
- Irregular size, shape, and shades of brown color.
- Uneven distribution in the lesion (irregular nests of atypical melanocytes at the dermoepidermal junction).

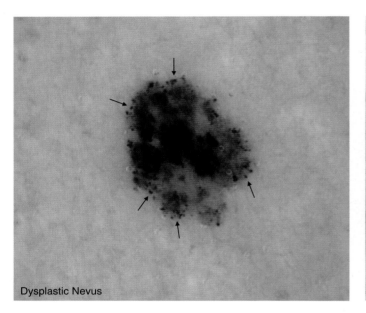

Dysplastic Nevus

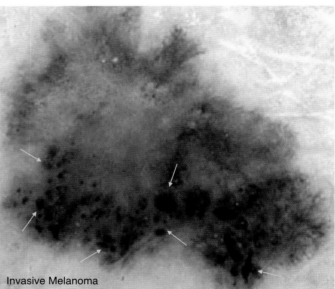

Invasive Melanoma

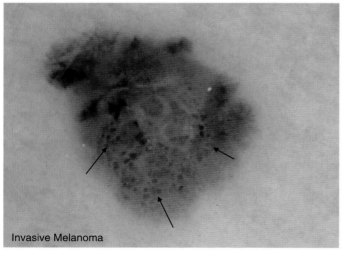

Invasive Melanoma

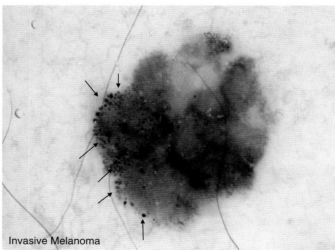

Invasive Melanoma

REGULAR BLOTCH

- Dark black or brown.
- Structureless (absence of network, dots, or globules) areas of color.
- Bigger than dots and globules.

- Uniform shape and color symmetrically located in the lesion (aggregates of melanin can be located in all levels of the skin).
- When black and shiny can represent pigmented parakeratosis ("black lamella").

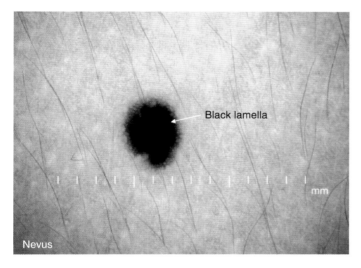

Black lamella

mm

Nevus

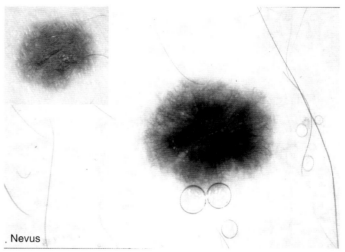

Nevus

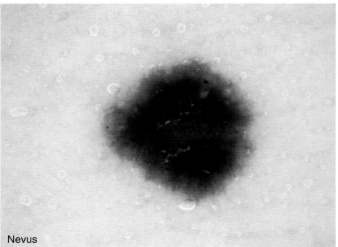

Nevus

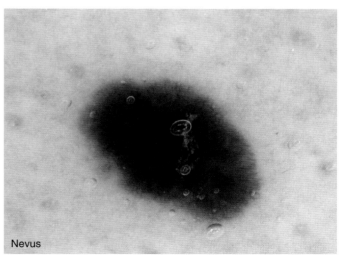

Nevus

IRREGULAR BLOTCH

- Dark shades of black, brown, or gray structureless areas of color.
- Irregular in size and shape (dense aggregates of atypical melanocytes in the epidermis and/or dermis).
- Asymmetrically located in the lesion.

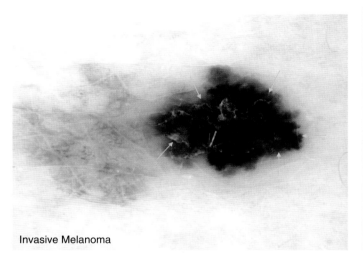

Invasive Melanoma

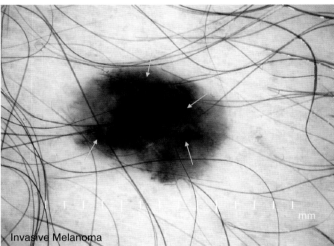

Invasive Melanoma

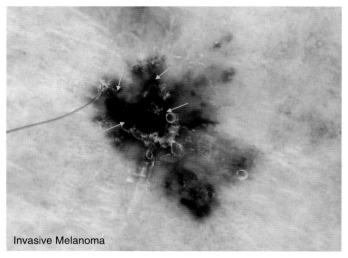

Invasive Melanoma

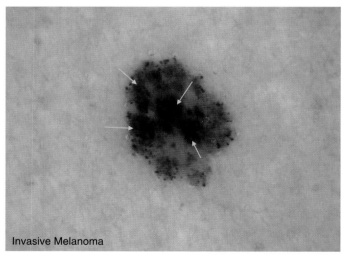

Invasive Melanoma

REGULAR STREAKS

- Black or brown linear projections of pigment.
- At all points along the periphery of the lesion.
- Shape does not determine whether streaks are regular or irregular.
- Can be freestanding or associated with a pigment network or dark blotch (confluent junctional nests of melanocytes running parallel to the epidermis).

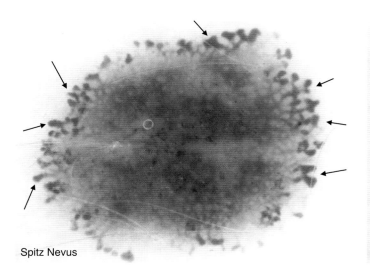

Spitz Nevus

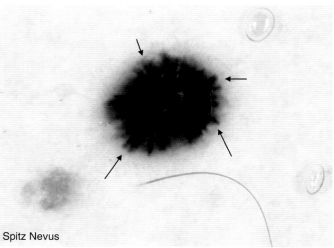

Spitz Nevus

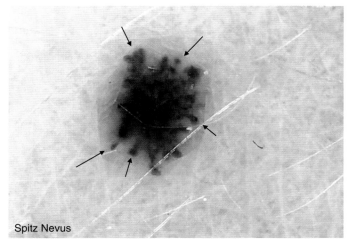

Spitz Nevus

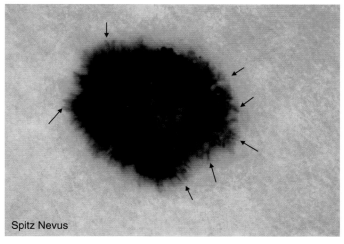

Spitz Nevus

IRREGULAR STREAKS

- Black or brown linear projections of pigment (radial growth phase of melanoma).
- Irregularly distributed at the periphery of a lesion.
- Some but not all points at the periphery "foci of streaks."
- Shape does not determine whether streaks are regular or irregular.

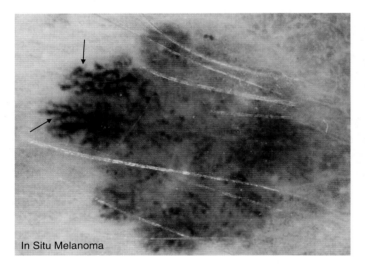

In Situ Melanoma

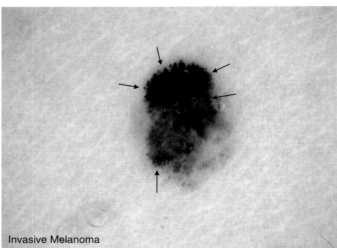

Invasive Melanoma

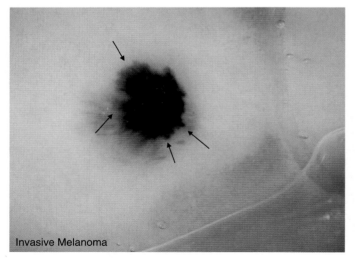

Invasive Melanoma

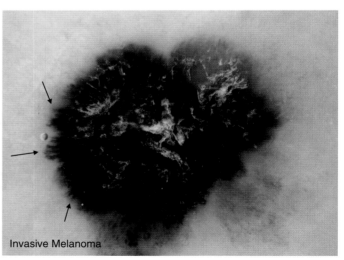

Invasive Melanoma

REGRESSION

- Bony/milky-white irregular scar-like depigmentation (fibrosis).
- With or without blue granules/dots (melanosis) or gray pepper-like granules "peppering" (free melanin and/or melanophages in the dermis).
- The white color should be lighter than the surrounding skin.
- Milky-red/pink color can be seen in areas of regression.

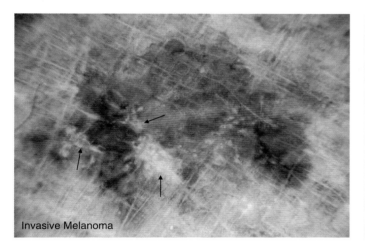

Invasive Melanoma

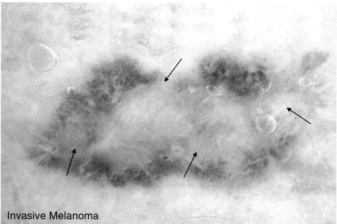

Invasive Melanoma

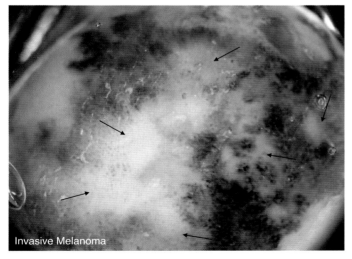

Invasive Melanoma

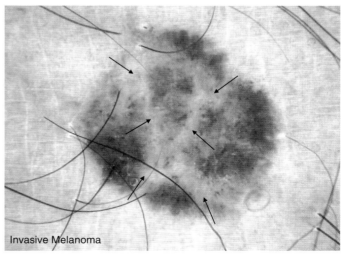

Invasive Melanoma

PEPPERING

- Gray pepper-like granules "peppering" (free melanin and/or melanophages in the dermis).
- Can be associated with regression or inflammation.

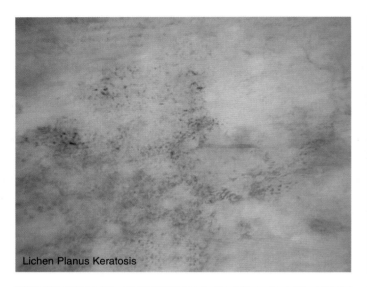

Lichen Planus Keratosis

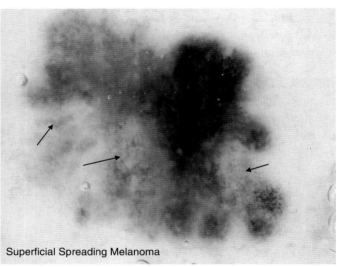

Superficial Spreading Melanoma

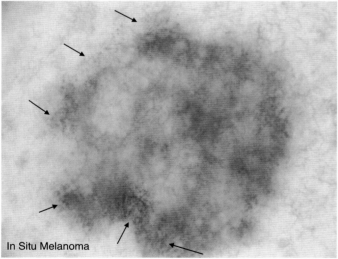

In Situ Melanoma

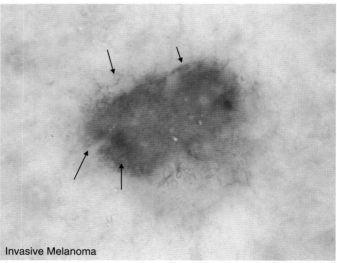

Invasive Melanoma

HYPOPIGMENTATION

- The bony-white color of regression should be differentiated from tan hypopigmentation/light brown color.
- Hypopigmentation may or may not contain local criteria (pigment network, dots, and globules).

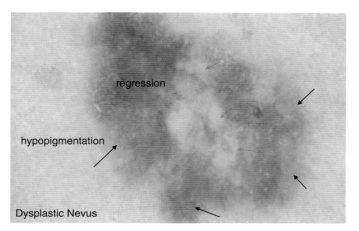

regression

hypopigmentation

Dysplastic Nevus

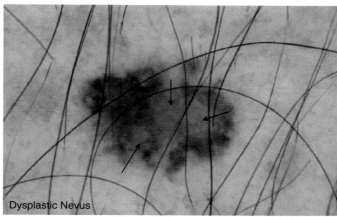

Dysplastic Nevus

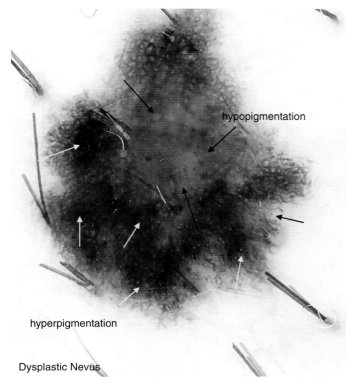

hypopigmentation

hyperpigmentation

Dysplastic Nevus

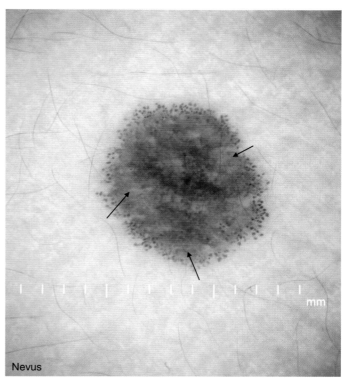

mm

Nevus

CRYSTALLINE STRUCTURES/SHINY WHITE STREAKS

- Collagen bundles have birefringent properties that cause a rapid randomization of polarized light, explaining why collagen is more conspicuous under polarized dermoscopy.

- Skin lesions with an increased amount of collagen (fibroplasia) will often reveal shiny bright white linear streaks and/or white blotches, which are termed *crystalline structures*.
- These structures are not visible with nonpolarized dermoscopy.

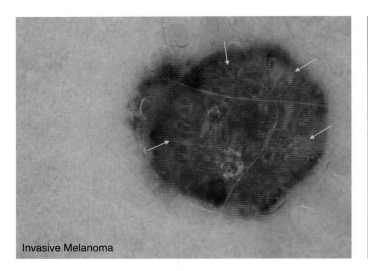

Invasive Melanoma

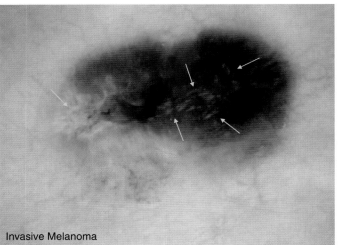

Invasive Melanoma

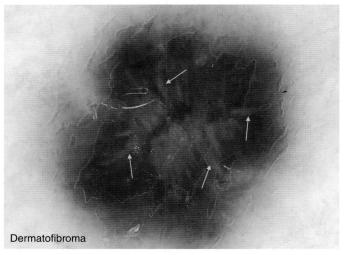

Dermatofibroma

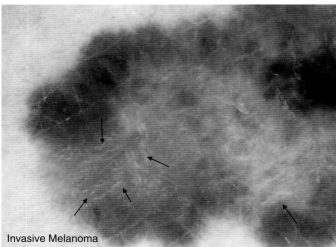

Invasive Melanoma

BLUE-WHITE VEIL

"Veil"

- Irregular, structureless area of confluent blue color that does not fill the entire lesion.

- Overlying whitish ground glass appearance (orthokeratosis acanthosis hypergranulosis).
- Can represent heavily pigmented tumor cells in the dermis.

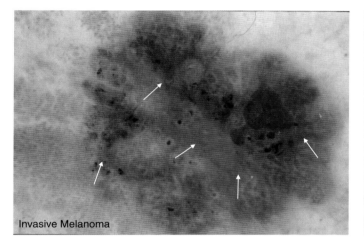

Invasive Melanoma

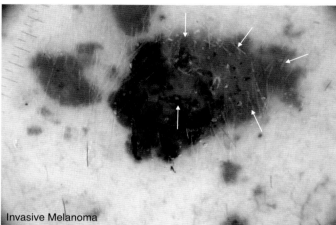

Invasive Melanoma

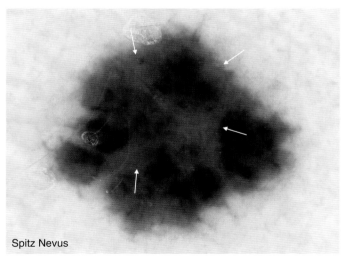

Spitz Nevus

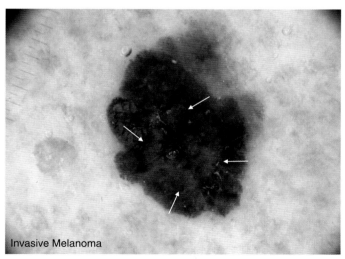

Invasive Melanoma

ASYMMETRICAL FOLLICULAR PIGMENTATION

- Seen only on the face, nose, and ears ("site-specific").
- Irregular brown color outlining parts of the round follicular openings.
- The color does not completely encircle the openings (early proliferation of atypical melanocytes).

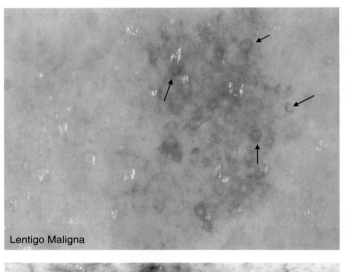

Lentigo Maligna

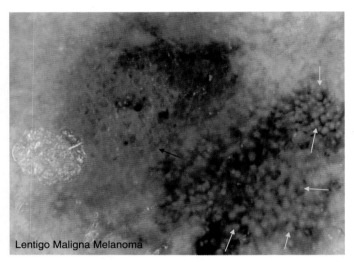

Lentigo Maligna Melanoma

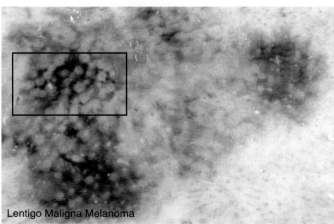

Lentigo Maligna Melanoma

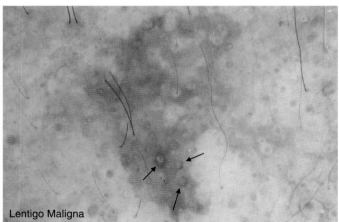

Lentigo Maligna

RHOMBOID STRUCTURES

- Seen only on the face, nose, and ears ("site-specific").
- Rhomboid is a parallelogram with unequal angles and sides.
- Black or brown pigmentation surrounding the entire follicular opening.
- In reality, true rhomboids are not regularly formed.

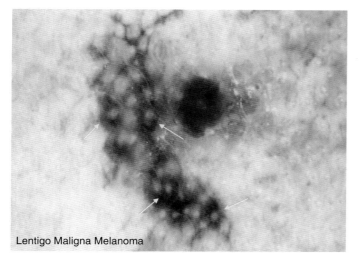

Lentigo Maligna Melanoma

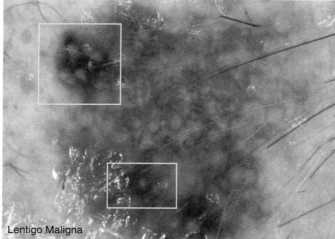

Lentigo Maligna

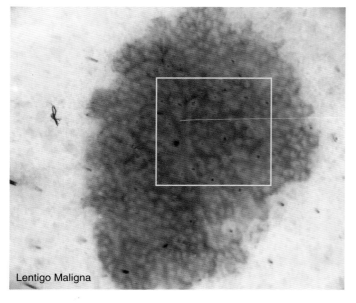

Lentigo Maligna

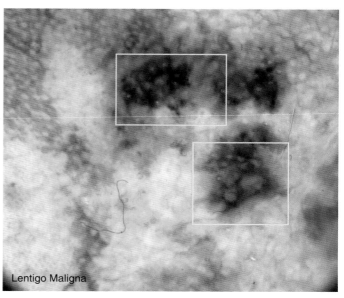

Lentigo Maligna

ANNULAR-GRANULAR STRUCTURES

- Seen only on the face, nose, and ears ("site-specific").
- Brown or gray fine dots that surround follicular openings (melanophages and/or atypical melanocytes).

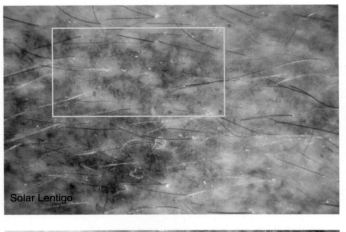

Solar Lentigo

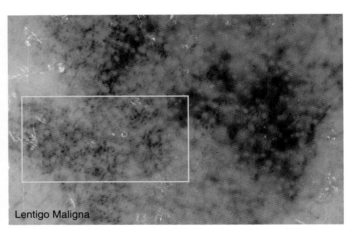

Lentigo Maligna

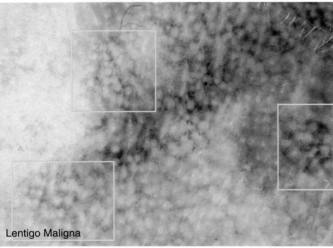

Lentigo Maligna

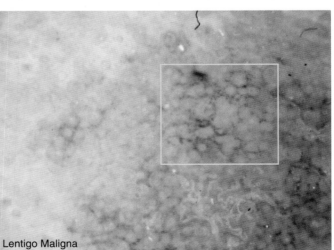

Lentigo Maligna

CIRCLE WITHIN A CIRCLE

- Seen only on the face, nose, and ears ("site-specific").
- A poorly studied structure composed of a central hair shaft (inner circle) and gray pigmentation (atypical melanocytes and/or peppering) that surrounds the hair shaft (outer circle).

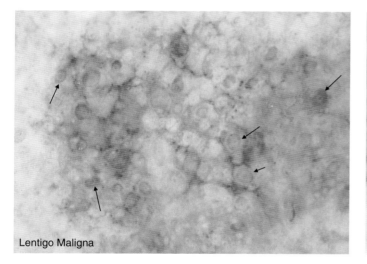

Lentigo Maligna

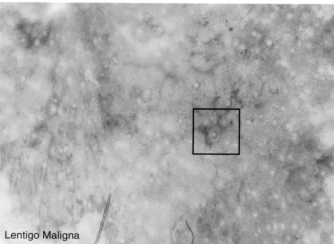

Lentigo Maligna

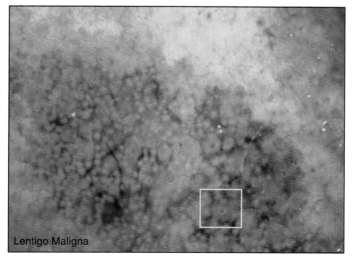

Lentigo Maligna

FINGERPRINT PATTERN

- Brown fine/thin parallel line segments that resemble fingerprints (pigmented acanthotic rete ridges).
- Can be swirled, whirled, or arched.
- Focal/broken up or fill the lesion.
- Differ from the pigment network where the line segments are honeycomb-like or reticular.

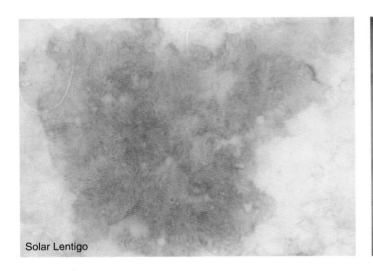

Solar Lentigo

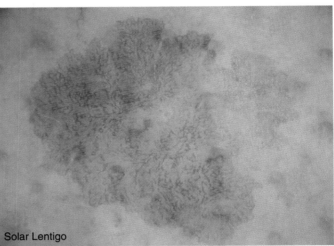

Solar Lentigo

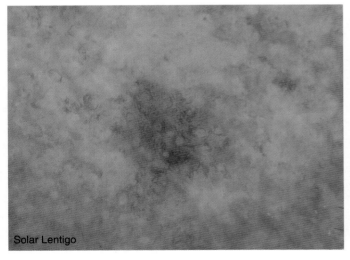

Solar Lentigo

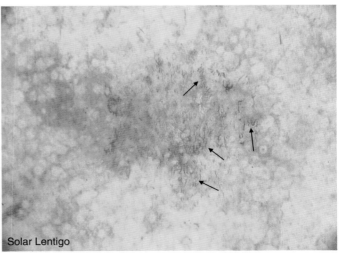

Solar Lentigo

MOTH-EATEN BORDERS

Well-Demarcated, Concave Borders That Are Felt to Resemble a "Moth-Eaten" Garment

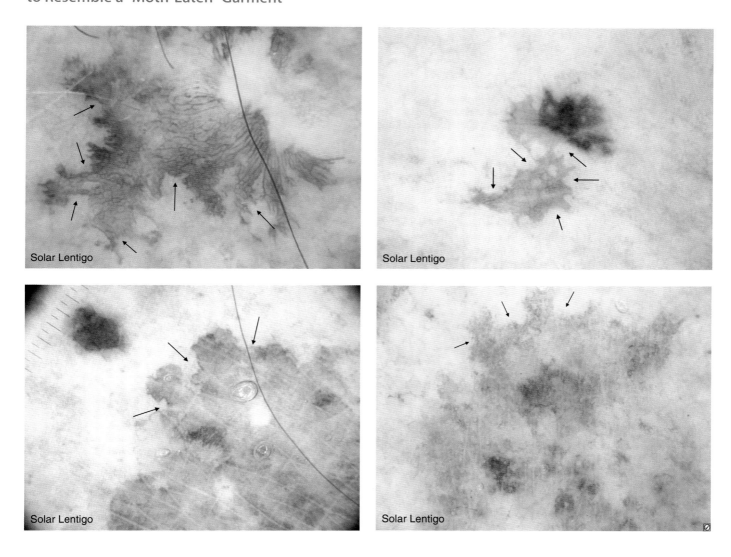

Solar Lentigo

Solar Lentigo

Solar Lentigo

Solar Lentigo

ACROSYRINGIA

"String of Pearls"

- Seen only at acral sites ("site-specific").
- Monomorphous round white structures in the ridges may or may not be seen.

- Represent the intraepidermal section of the sweat ducts.
- Said to look like a "string of pearls."
- Always in the ridges; never in the furrows.

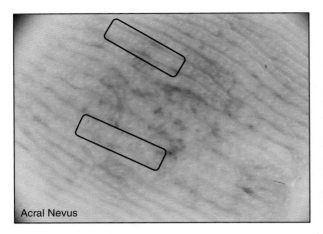

Acral Nevus

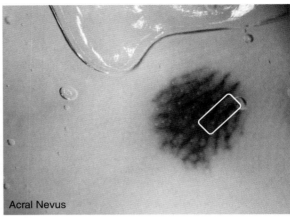

Acral Nevus

PARALLEL-FURROW PATTERN

- Seen only at acral sites ("site-specific").
- Most common benign acral pattern.
- Single thin or thick brown parallel lines in the furrows of the skin (crista superficialis limitans).

- Variations include two brown lines on both sides of the hypopigmented furrows with or without brown dots and globules.

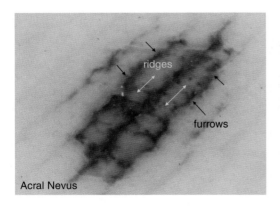

Acral Nevus

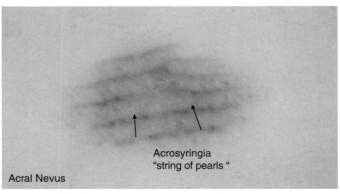

Acral Nevus

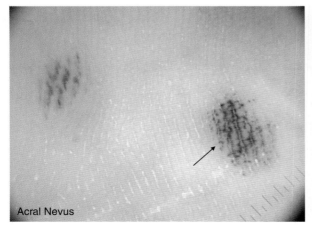

Acral Nevus

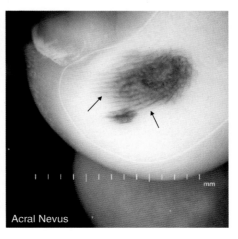

Acral Nevus

LATTICE-LIKE PATTERN

- Seen only at acral sites ("site-specific").
- Benign pattern.
- Brown parallel lines in the furrows.
- Brown lines running perpendicular to the furrows forming a ladder-like picture.

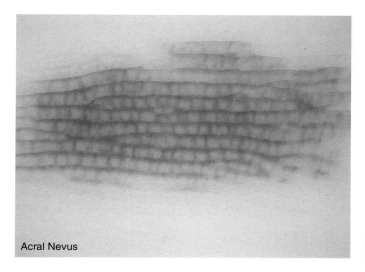

Acral Nevus

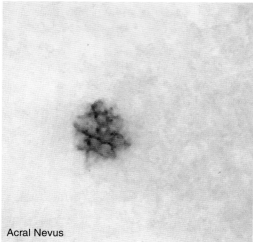

Acral Nevus

FIBRILLAR PATTERN

- Seen only at acral sites ("site-specific").
- Benign pattern.
- Uniform brown lines that run in an oblique (////////) direction.

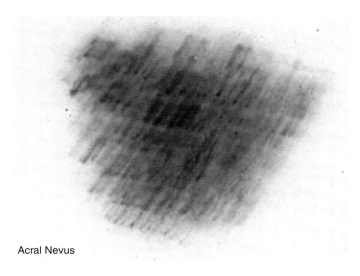

Acral Nevus

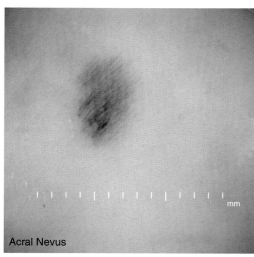

Acral Nevus

PARALLEL-RIDGE PATTERN

- Seen only at acral sites ("site-specific").
- Malignant pattern.
- Not diagnostic of melanoma.

- Pigmentation is in the thicker ridges of the skin (crista profunda intermedia).
- Acrosyringia always are in the ridges and can be a clue where pigmentation is.

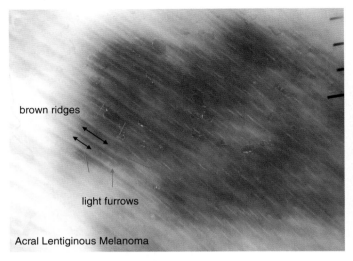

Acral Lentiginous Melanoma

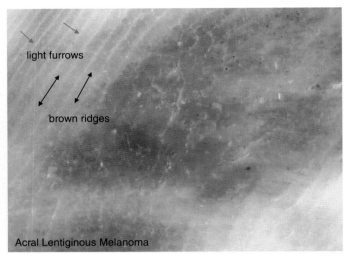

Acral Lentiginous Melanoma

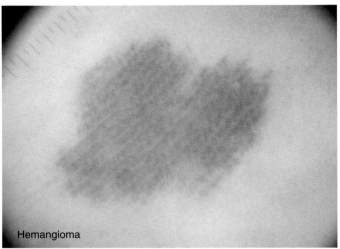

Hemangioma

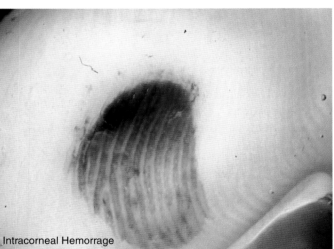

Intracorneal Hemorrage

TABLE 2-2 • Melanonychia Striata

Benign Pattern
- Single or multiple nail involvement with brown or gray longitudinal parallel lines.
- Uniform color, spacing, and thickness.
- May or may not have diffuse brown background color.

Malignant Pattern
- Brown, black, or gray parallel lines.
- Different shades of color, irregular spacing, and thickness.
- Loss of parallelism (broken-up line segments caused by irregular pigmentation produced by malignant melanocytes).
- Hutchinson sign created by pigment spread to the surrounding skin.

MELANONYCHIA STRIATA

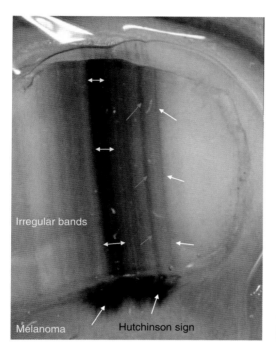

Irregular bands

Melanoma · Hutchinson sign

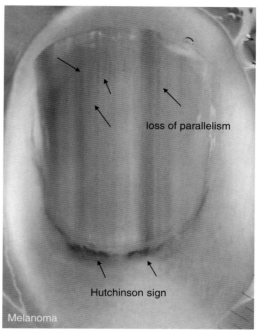

loss of parallelism

Hutchinson sign

Melanoma

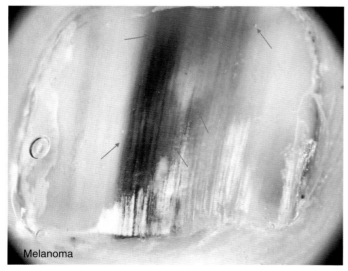

Melanoma

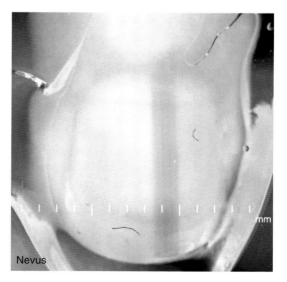

Nevus

mm

SUBUNGUAL HEMORRHAGE

- Typically contains purplish irregular homogeneous color.
- May also have black, bluish-white homogeneous color and other colors of heme oxidation (ie, green, yellow).
- Well-demarcated lateral and proximal borders.
- Purplish filamentous distal border.
- Blood spots/blood pebbles look like irregular purple dots and globules.

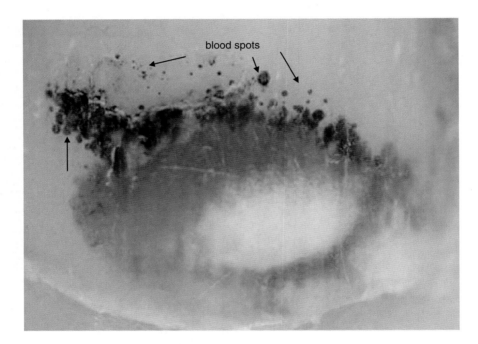

blood spots

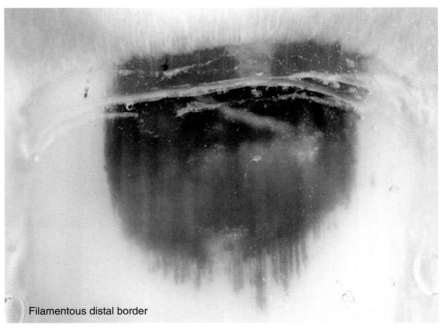

Filamentous distal border

MILIA-LIKE CYSTS

- Variously sized white or yellow structures.
- Small or large, single or multiple.
- They can appear opaque or bright like "stars in the sky" (epidermal horn cysts).
- Milia-like cysts can be seen not only in seborrheic keratosis but also in benign and malignant melanocytic lesions.

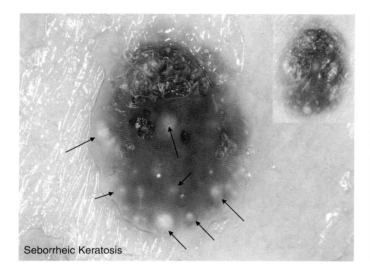

Seborrheic Keratosis

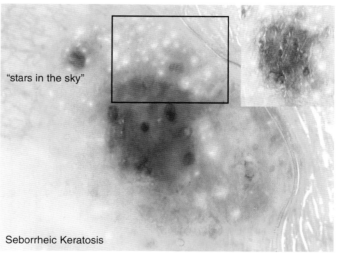

"stars in the sky"

Seborrheic Keratosis

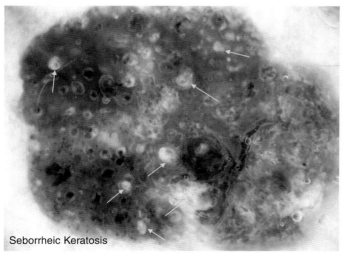

Seborrheic Keratosis

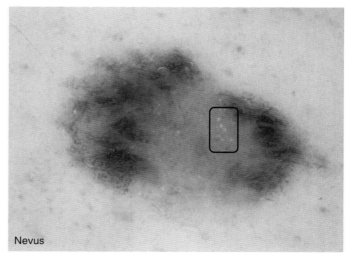

Nevus

PSEUDOFOLLICULAR OPENINGS/ COMEDO-LIKE OPENINGS

- Sharply demarcated roundish structures (keratin-filled invaginations of the epidermis).
- Pigmented or nonpigmented.
- When pigmented, they can be brownish-yellow or even dark brown and black.

- Shape and size can vary.
- Larger keratin-filled irregularly shaped openings are called crypts.
- Pseudofollicular openings can be seen not only in seborrheic keratosis but also in benign and malignant melanocytic lesions.

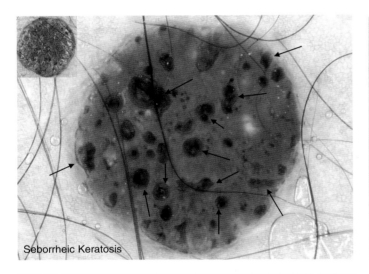

Seborrheic Keratosis

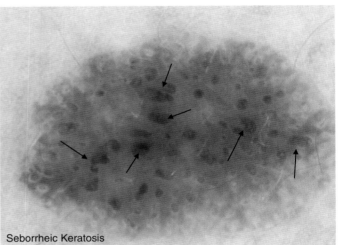

Seborrheic Keratosis

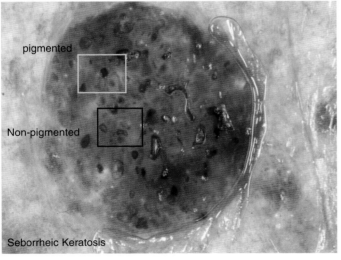

pigmented

Non-pigmented

Seborrheic Keratosis

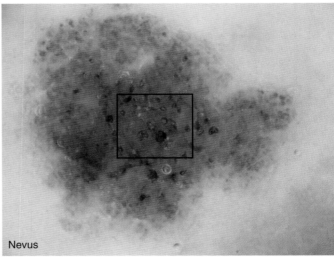

Nevus

FISSURES AND RIDGES

- Fissures/sulci (invaginations of the epidermis) and ridges (gyri) can create several patterns.
- Cerebriform/ brain-like and resembles a sagittal section through the cerebral cortex.

- Hypo- and hyperpigmented ridges can be digit-like (straight, kinked, circular, or branched) and are referred to as "fat fingers."
- Fissures and ridges can be seen not only in seborrheic keratosis but also in benign and malignant melanocytic lesions.

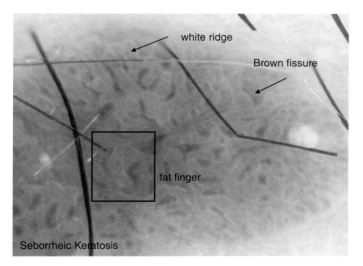

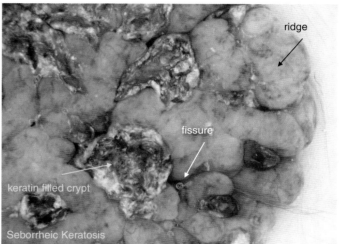

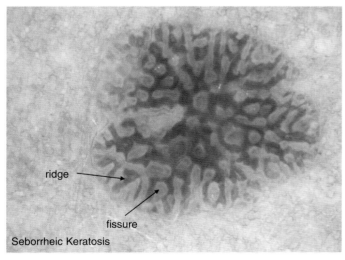

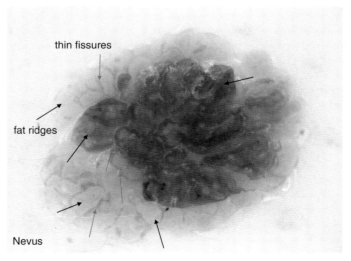

ULCERATION

- Single or multiple irregular areas.
- Clearly bloody or with congealed blood/crusts.

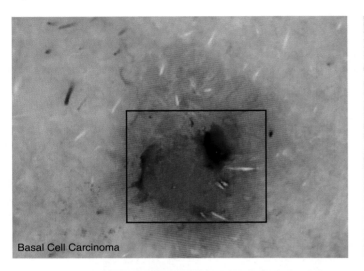

Basal Cell Carcinoma

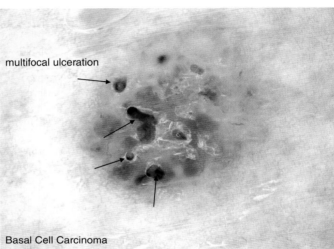

multifocal ulceration

Basal Cell Carcinoma

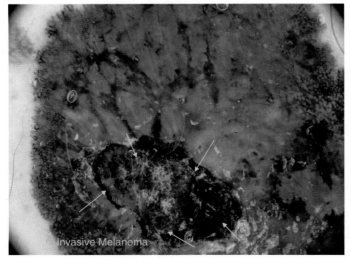

Invasive Melanoma

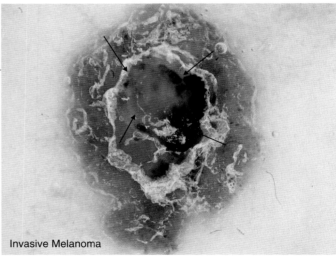

Invasive Melanoma

CENTRAL WHITE PATCH

- Most typical presentation of this criterion is a centrally located homogeneous bony-white scar-like area (fibroplasia).
- Several variations such as white network-like structures (negative network).
- May be very irregular and indistinguishable from the scarring/regression seen in melanoma.

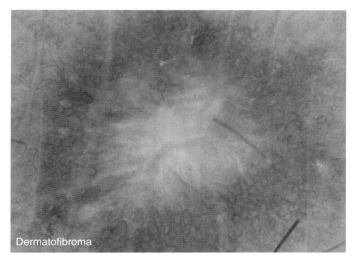

Dermatofibroma

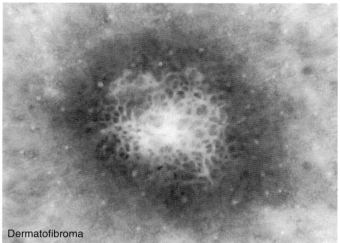

Dermatofibroma

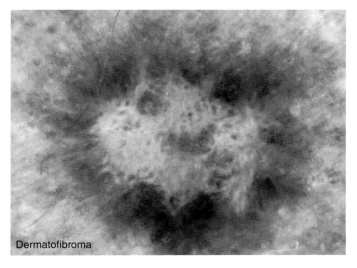

Dermatofibroma

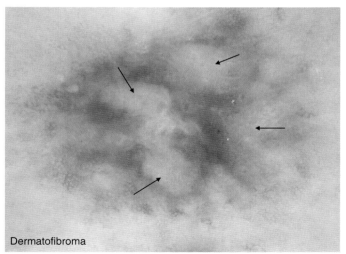

Dermatofibroma

SPOKE-WHEEL STRUCTURES

- Well-defined pigmented radial projections meeting at a darker central globule (nests of basal cell carcinoma emanating from the undersurface of the epidermis).
- Complete or incomplete variations of this structure can be seen.

- One often has to use the imagination to make the identification.
- Diagnostic for basal cell carcinoma.

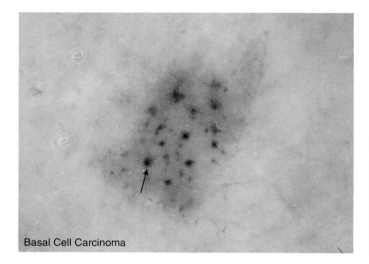

Basal Cell Carcinoma

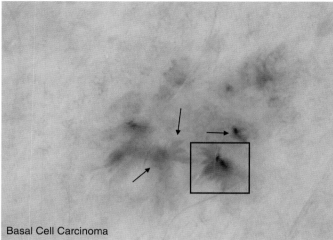

Basal Cell Carcinoma

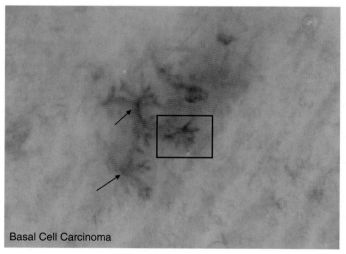

Basal Cell Carcinoma

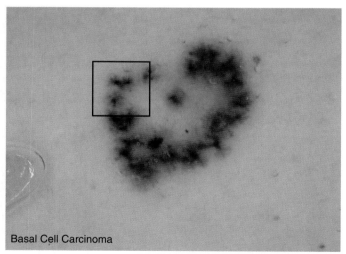

Basal Cell Carcinoma

TABLE 2-3 • Vascular Structures
• Lacunae
• Hairpin
• Comma
• Arborizing
• Serpentine
• Linear
• Dotted (pinpoint)
• Glomerular
• String of pearls
• Corkscrew
• Polymorphous
• Milky-red areas/pink (with or without globules)

LACUNAE

- Sharply demarcated/in-focus bright red to bluish round/oval structures (dilated vascular spaces in the dermis).
- Patchy white color or bluish-white color (fibrous septa) commonly seen.

- Black homogeneous structureless areas represent thrombosis.
- Not to be confused with out-of-focus milky-red globules seen in melanoma.

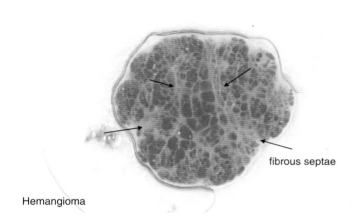

fibrous septae

Hemangioma

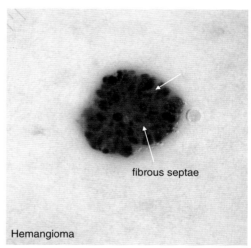

fibrous septae

Hemangioma

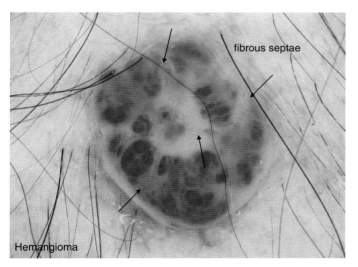

fibrous septae

Hemangioma

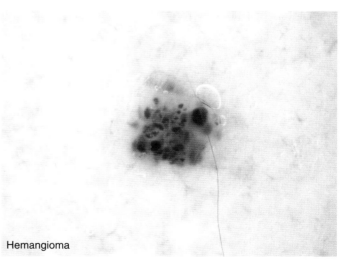

Hemangioma

HAIRPIN VESSELS

- Elongated telangiectatic vessels (capillary loops) resembling hairpins.
- May or may not be surrounded by hypopigmented halos.
- Irregular and thick hairpin vessels can be seen in squamous cell carcinoma and melanoma.

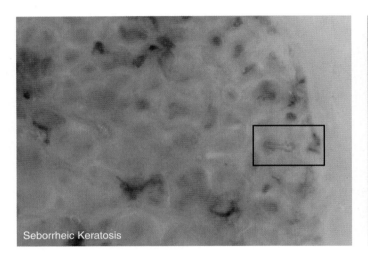
Seborrheic Keratosis

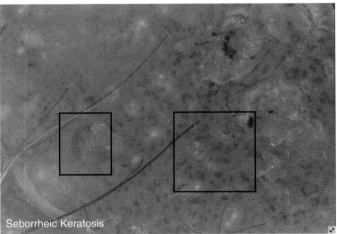
Seborrheic Keratosis

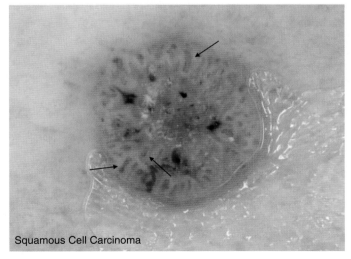
Squamous Cell Carcinoma

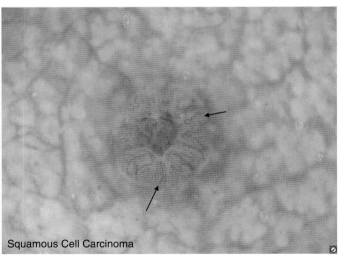
Squamous Cell Carcinoma

COMMA VESSELS
Resembling the Shape of a Comma

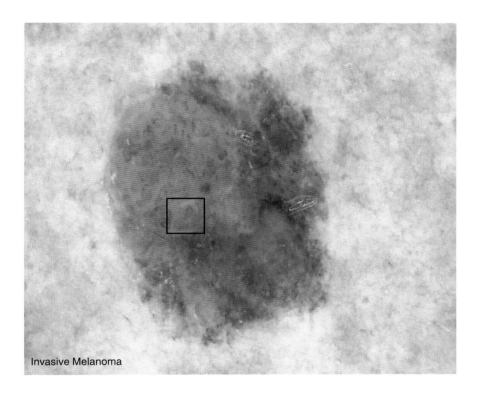

Invasive Melanoma

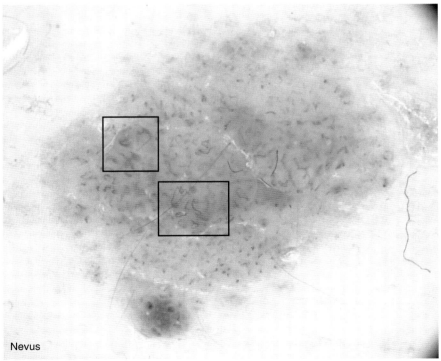

Nevus

ARBORIZING VESSELS

- Red tree-like branching telangiectatic blood vessels.
- In-focus vessels because they are on the surface of the lesion.
- Can be thick or thin.
- Most often there are different caliber vessels in a single lesion.

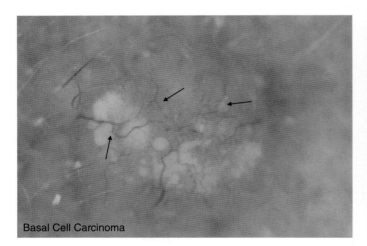

Basal Cell Carcinoma

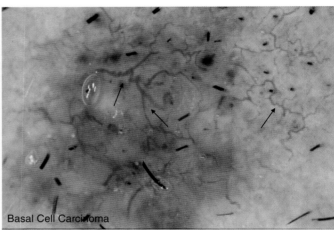

Basal Cell Carcinoma

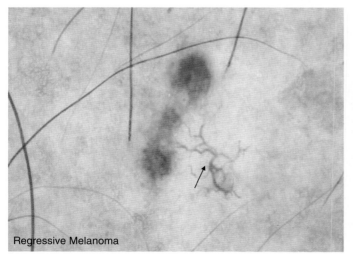

Regressive Melanoma

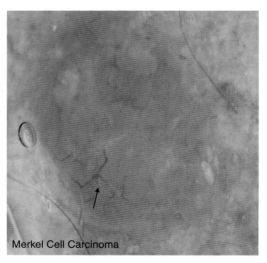

Merkel Cell Carcinoma

SERPENTINE VESSELS

- May be very fine/thin or thick.
- Irregular linear red lines.
- A variation of linear vessels.

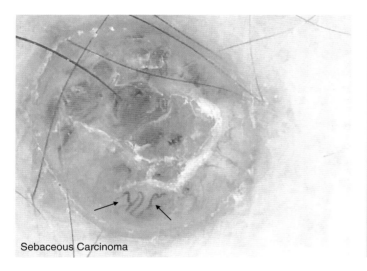

Sebaceous Carcinoma

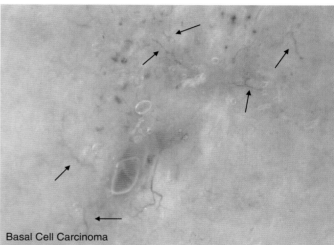

Basal Cell Carcinoma

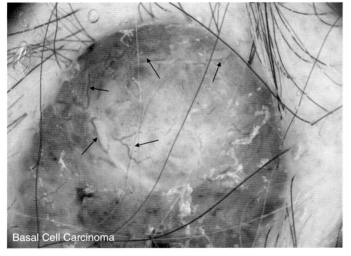

Basal Cell Carcinoma

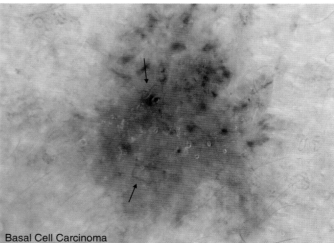

Basal Cell Carcinoma

LINEAR VESSELS

- Straight thin and/or thicker red lines.
- Not curved like serpentine vessels.

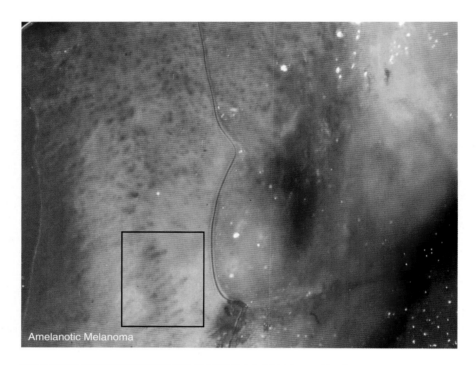

Amelanotic Melanoma

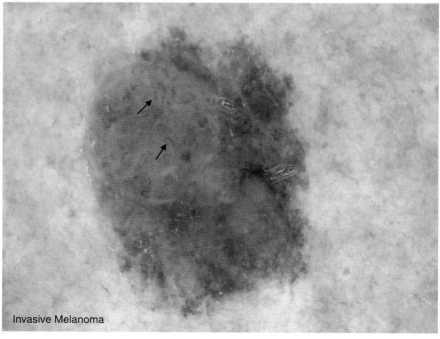

Invasive Melanoma

DOTTED/PINPOINT VESSELS

- Small telangiectatic vessels resembling tiny dots.
- Can be diffuse, grouped, or isolated.

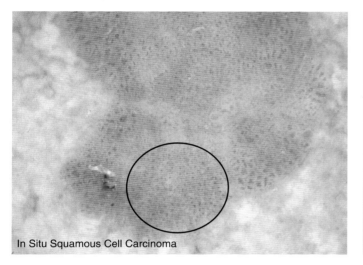

In Situ Squamous Cell Carcinoma

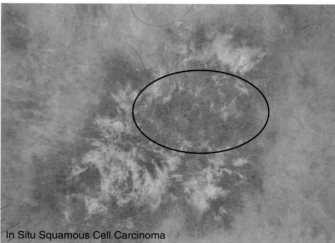

In Situ Squamous Cell Carcinoma

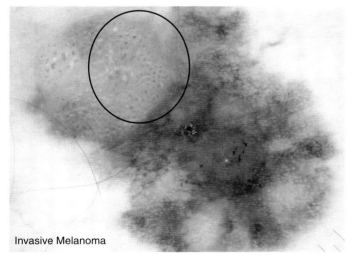

Invasive Melanoma

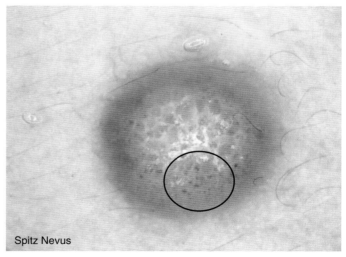

Spitz Nevus

GLOMERULAR VESSELS
Diffuse or Clustered Fine Coiled Telangiectatic Vessels

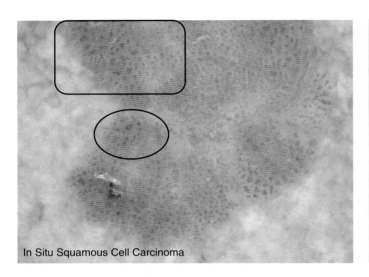

In Situ Squamous Cell Carcinoma

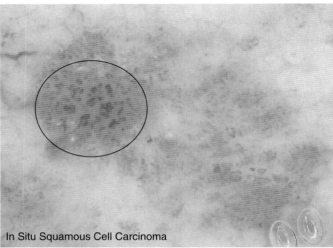

In Situ Squamous Cell Carcinoma

STRING OF PEARLS

- Pinpoint and/or glomerular vessels.
- Following a linear, curvilinear, serpiginous, or necklace-like distribution.
- Diagnostic of clear cell acanthoma (CCA).

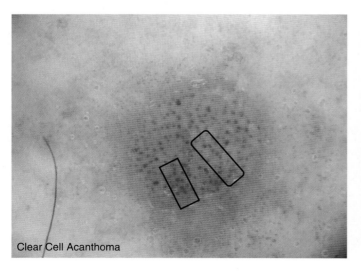

Clear Cell Acanthoma

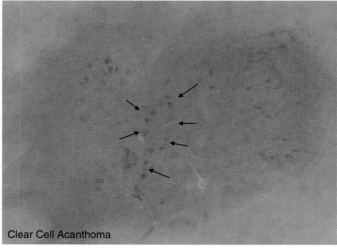

Clear Cell Acanthoma

CORKSCREW VESSELS
Irregular Thick Coiled Vessels

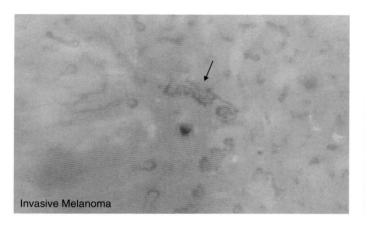

Invasive Melanoma

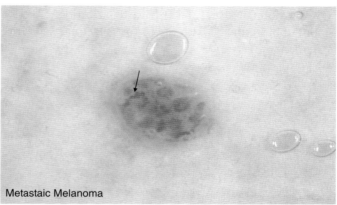

Metastaic Melanoma

POLYMORPHOUS VESSELS

- More than 3 different shapes.
- Any combination of vessels: arborizing, dotted, glomerular, linear, serpentine, hairpin, comma, corkscrew.

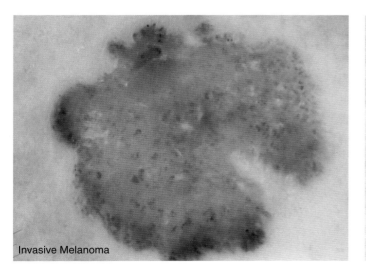

Invasive Melanoma

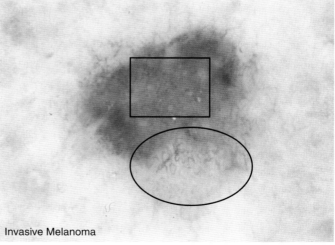

Invasive Melanoma

MILKY-RED AREAS

- Localized or diffuse pinkish-white color.
- With or without reddish and/or bluish out-of-focus/ fuzzy globular structures (neovascularization).
- Not to be confused with the in-focus lacunae seen in hemangiomas.

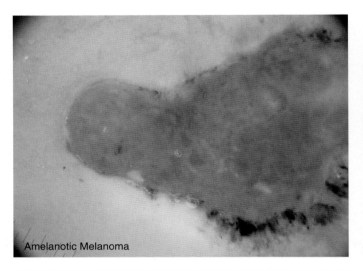

Amelanotic Melanoma

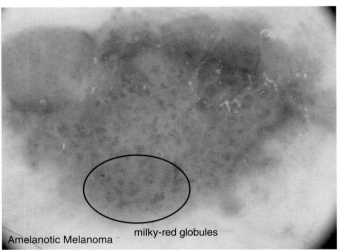

Amelanotic Melanoma   milky-red globules

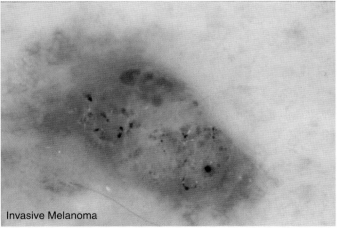

Invasive Melanoma

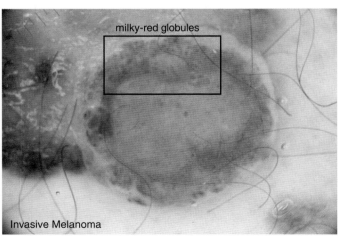

milky-red globules

Invasive Melanoma

PIGMENTATION SEEN IN BASAL CELL CARCINOMA

- Colors that can be seen: black, brown, gray, blue, red, white (nests of pigmented malignant basal cells in the dermis).
- Fine dots to large leaf-like structures (bulbous extensions forming a leaf-like pattern).

- Not necessary to try to determine whether leaf-like structures are present, since in reality this is a difficult task.
- Blue-gray ovoid nests.
- Multiple blue-gray globules.

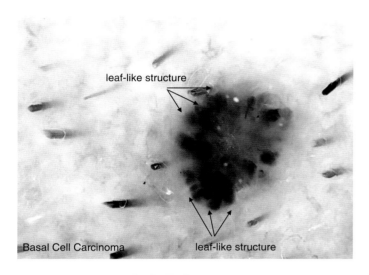

Basal Cell Carcinoma

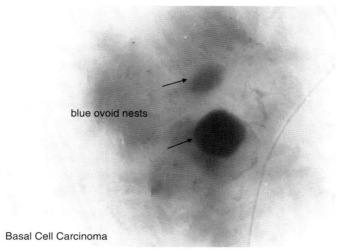

Basal Cell Carcinoma

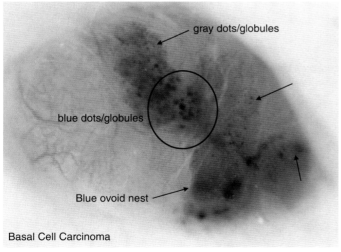

Basal Cell Carcinoma

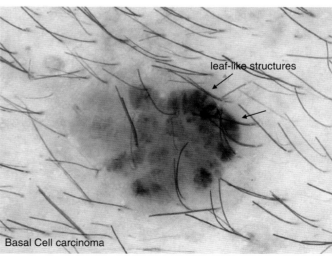

Basal Cell carcinoma

TABLE 2-4 • Melanoma-Specific Criteria, Head and Neck

- Asymmetrical follicular pigmentation
- Rhomboid structures
- Annular-granular structures
- Circle within a circle

TABLE 2-5 • Melanoma-Specific Criteria, Trunk and Extremities

- Asymmetry of color and structure
- Multicomponent global pattern
- Irregular pigment network
- Irregular dots and globules
- Irregular blotches
- Irregular streaks
- Regression
- Shiny white streaks
- Polymorphous vessels
- Milky-red area
- 5-6 colors

TABLE 2-6 • Melanoma-Specific Criteria, Palms and Soles

- Parallel-ridge pattern
- Multicomponent pattern
- Multicolor pattern

CHAPTER 3

Benign and Malignant Melanocytic Lesions

General Instructions

- For each case, there is a short history along with a clinical and an unmarked dermoscopic image.
- Study the unmarked dermoscopic image and try to identify the global and local dermoscopic features.
- Make your diagnosis.
- Next, turn the page and the dermoscopic image will be presented again, this time marked with all the salient dermoscopic findings.
- On the same page you will also find the diagnosis along with a detailed discussion and a few pearls for your review.

CASE 1

HISTORY

This 88-year-old woman has a biopsy-proven basal cell carcinoma under a dark plaque. Clinically, both lesions seem to be connected.

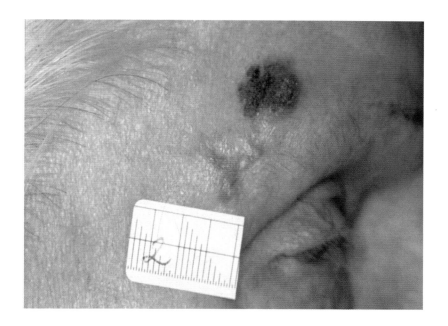

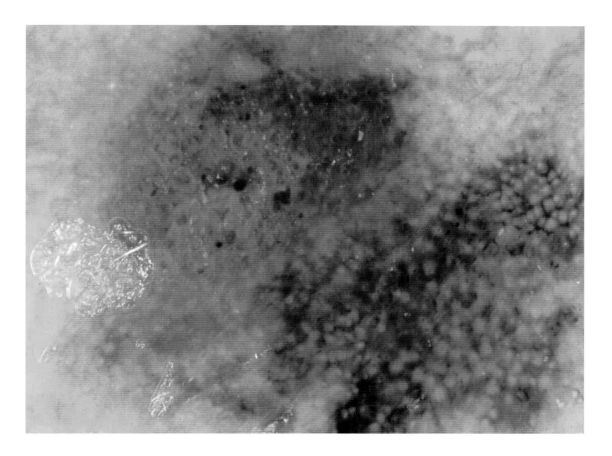

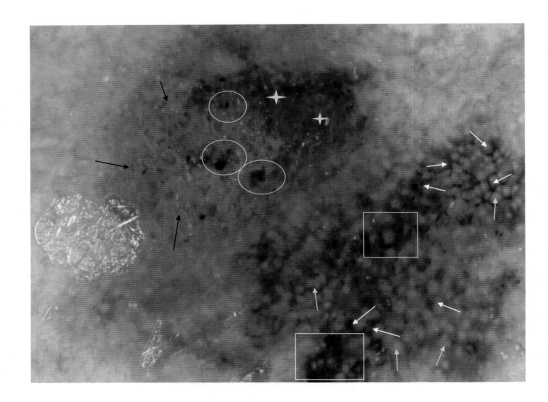

DERMOSCOPIC CRITERIA

- Round follicular openings (yellow arrows)
- Asymmetrical follicular pigmentation (white arrows)
- Rhomboid structures (yellow box)
- Irregular blotch with follicular openings (white box)
- Irregular blotch without follicular openings (stars)
- Irregular dots and globules (yellow circles)
- Milky-red areas (black arrows)

DIAGNOSIS:
Lentigo Maligna Melanoma

DISCUSSION

- Asymmetrical follicular pigmentation, rhomboid structures, annular-granular structures, and circle within a circle are the main criteria associated with melanoma on the face.
- Asymmetrical follicular pigmentation can also be seen in pigmented actinic keratosis and pigmented Bowen disease.
- The first step in the progression of melanoma on the face is represented by asymmetrical follicular pigmentation.
- The follicular openings should not be confused with milia-like cysts seen in seborrheic keratosis.
- The next step in the progression of melanoma on the face is the formation of rhomboid structures.
- True rhomboid forms (parallelogram with unequal angles and sides) are not necessary to identify.
- Any pigmented thickening that completely surrounds follicular openings should be considered rhomboid structures.

- The irregular black blotch with follicular openings is the first sign of dermal invasion (lentigo maligna melanoma).
- The irregular black blotch without follicular openings represents complete obliteration of follicular openings, indicating further dermal invasion.

PEARLS

- This is a collision tumor, representing a basal cell carcinoma and melanoma.
- The diagnosis of melanoma on the face is not always this easy.
- It is essential to learn the definitions of the 4 main criteria associated with melanoma on the face and be able to recognize them.
- Dermoscopy is essential to help make the diagnosis in most cases of early lentigo maligna and offers patients their best chance for survival.

CASE 2

HISTORY

This lesion had been ignored for many years. Itch was the reason the patient finally went to see his family physician, who referred him to a dermatologist for evaluation.

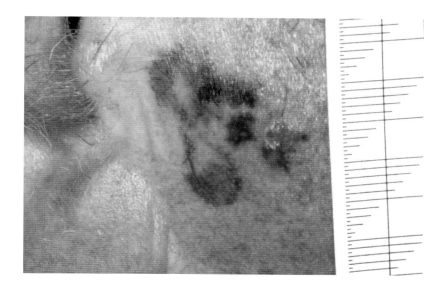

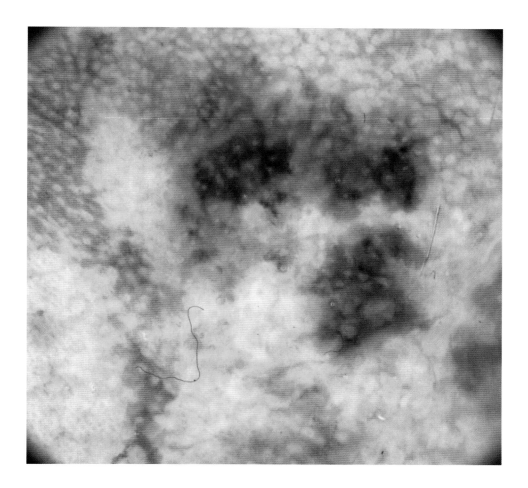

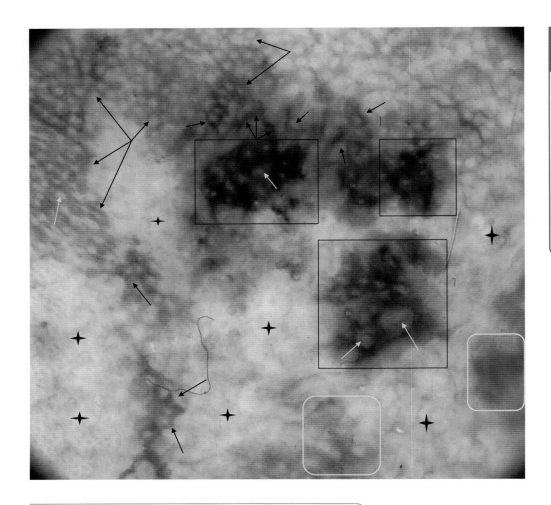

DIAGNOSIS:

Lentigo Maligna Melanoma

DISCUSSION

- Clinically and with dermoscopy, this melanoma should be easy to diagnose.
- The melanoma-specific criteria are well-developed and easy to identify.
- There are areas of confluent, asymmetrical follicular pigmentation.
- Three areas of confluent rhomboid structures (pigmentation completely surrounding the follicular openings) are seen in the center of the lesion.
- The rhomboid structures may also be described as irregular blotches where the follicular openings are preserved.
- The dark blotches represent areas of invasion, supporting a diagnosis of lentigo maligna melanoma.

- The bony-white color identifies areas of regression that correlate with what is seen clinically.
- There are 2 foci of peppering, also associated with regression.

PEARLS

- This is a representative case to use as reference when identifying the high-risk criteria needed to diagnose melanoma of the head and neck.
- Incisional biopsies should be performed in the exact location that melanoma-specific criteria are found in the lesion (ie, asymmetrical follicular openings).

CASE 3

HISTORY

This poorly defined, ominous discoloration on the face of a 79-year-old woman has changed slowly over the past 5 years.

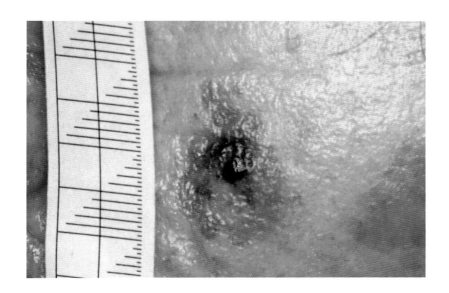

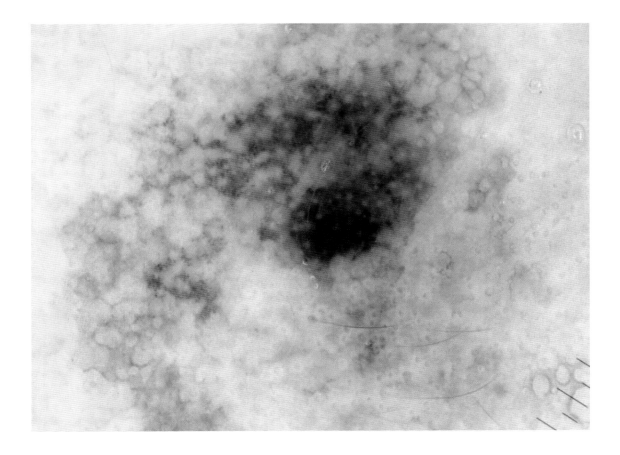

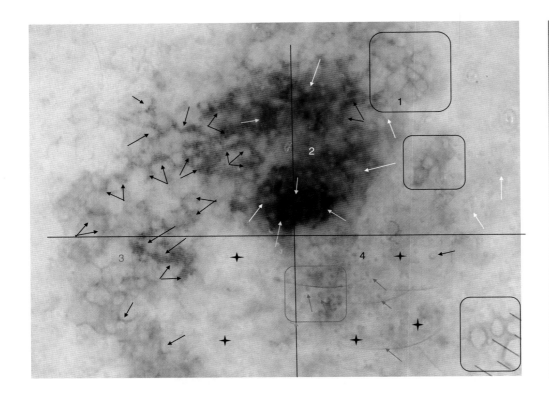

DIAGNOSIS:
Lentigo Maligna Melanoma

DISCUSSION

- Three melanoma-specific criteria found in this lesion are *not* site specific and may be found anywhere on the body.
- Asymmetry of color and structure (the left side of the lesion is not a mirror image of the right side; the top half is not a mirror image of the bottom half).
- Multicomponent global pattern with 3 different zones of criteria.
- Six colors.
- The site-specific melanoma-specific criteria are well-developed.
- Asymmetrical follicular pigmentation is created by grayish dots (annular-granular structures) and homogeneous dark brown color.
- Annular-granular structures and asymmetrical follicular pigmentation are associated with lentigo maligna.
- The irregular dark blotches and regression point to a diagnosis of invasive melanoma (lentigo maligna melanoma).
- The regression area is composed of 3 colors: white (scarring), blue (melanosis), and gray (peppering).
- Of note, blue color points to pigmentation deeper in the skin (called the Tyndall effect).
- The area with blue color is filled with follicular openings and sparse hairs. This is an unusual presentation of these 2 common criteria.

PEARLS

- If your incisional biopsy is within the area of regression, you could miss the correct diagnosis.
- Sampling from within the dark blotch will yield the best likelihood to diagnose this invasive melanoma.

CASE 4

HISTORY

This was one of several tan spots on the face of a 48-year-old woman who presented for a routine skin examination.

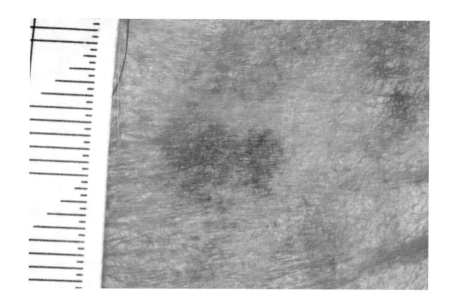

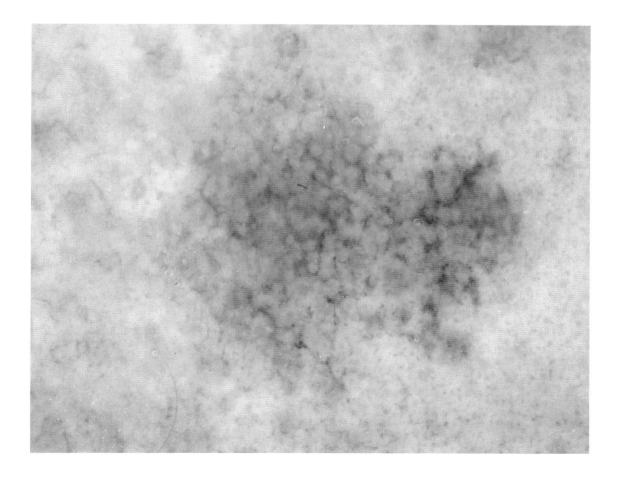

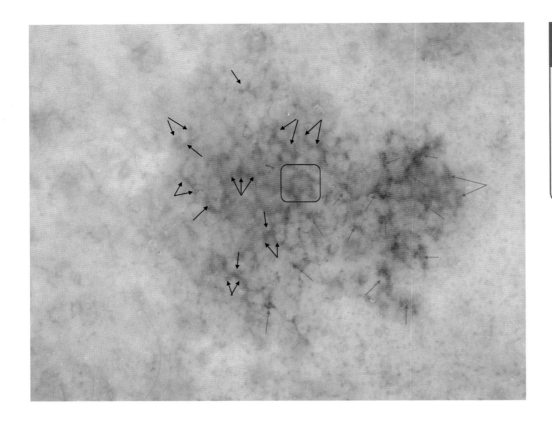

DIAGNOSIS:
Lentigo Maligna

DISCUSSION

- Clinically on first examination, this tan macule appears low-risk. However, dermoscopy clearly demonstrates the features of melanoma.
- The left side of the lesion has areas with asymmetrical follicular pigmentation.
- Asymmetrical follicular pigmentation can be diagnosed without seeing the follicular openings clearly.
- Follicular openings may or may not be well-developed or easy to identify. In this case they are not well-developed.
- The right side of the lesion has foci of annular-granular structures.
- At times it might be difficult to differentiate annular-granular structures from the peppering that can be seen in areas of regression.

- The bony-white color of regression is not present.
- The criteria associated with a soar lentigo (moth-eaten borders, fingerprint pattern) are absent.
- Of note, a pigmented actinic keratosis could have the same dermoscopic features.

PEARLS

- Before you look at a banal-appearing pigmented skin lesion in this location with dermoscopy, you should be thinking to yourself, "Will I see the criteria associated with a solar lentigo or lentigo maligna?"
- Use dermoscopy not only to look at atypically pigmented skin lesions.
- You don't want to miss melanoma "incognito" (melanomas without clinical features of melanoma).

CASE 5

HISTORY
The patient has multiple seborrheic keratoses distributed across sun-exposed areas. Clinically, this lesion did not stand out from the others.

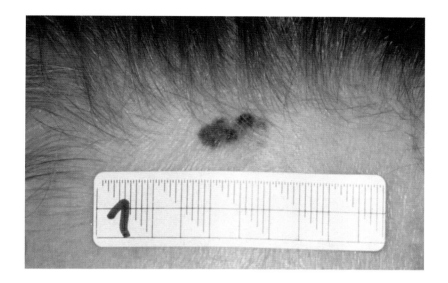

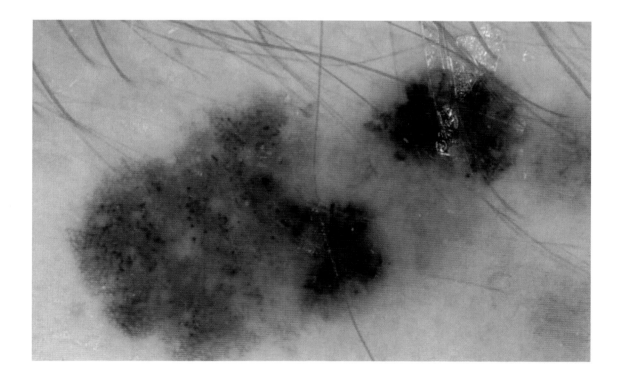

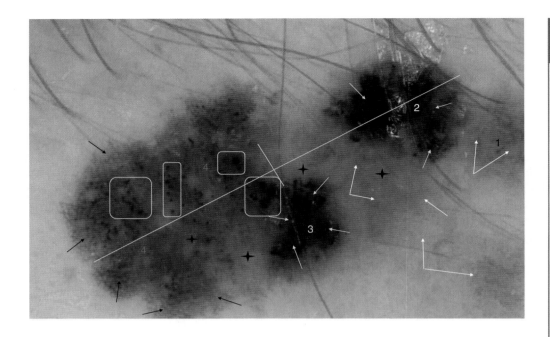

DIAGNOSIS:
In Situ Melanoma

DISCUSSION

- Asymmetrical follicular pigmentation, annular-granular structures, rhomboid structures, and circle within a circle, all typical features of melanoma, are not always present in melanomas of the head and neck.
- All subsets of melanoma can present on the head and neck.
- The dots and globules found here help us diagnose a melanocytic lesion.
- The lack of milia-like cysts, pseudofollicular openings, fissures and ridges, "fat fingers," and hairpin vessels steer our diagnosis away from that of a seborrheic keratosis.
- There is asymmetry of color and structure (the long axis of this lesion should be used to visualize the bisecting lines to make this determination).
- Multicomponent global pattern has 3 or more sections that look different. Sections with a single criterion and/or sections with multiple criteria.
- Regular pigment network (uniform line segments and holes).
- Irregular dots and globules (different sizes and shapes are scattered throughout the lesion).

- Irregular black blotches (different sizes and shapes with asymmetrical location within the lesion).
- The bluish-white color does not fit the definition of the "veil" often seen in invasive melanoma.
- White color of regression should be whiter/lighter than the surrounding skin.
- It is not uncommon to see normal skin within benign and malignant skin lesions.
- Large areas of hypopigmentation at the periphery of a lesion are considered high-risk criterion that can be seen in melanoma.

PEARLS

- Simply identifying criteria within a lesion is not enough.
- Always determine if they are regular or irregular, low- or high-risk, "good" or "bad."
- Blue and/or white color in any form should always be a red flag for concern.
- Be aware that melanoma may include clinical and/or and dermoscopic features of seborrheic keratosis.

CASE 6

HISTORY
This 49-year-old woman was unconcerned about this lesion. Nevertheless, a biopsy was recommended.

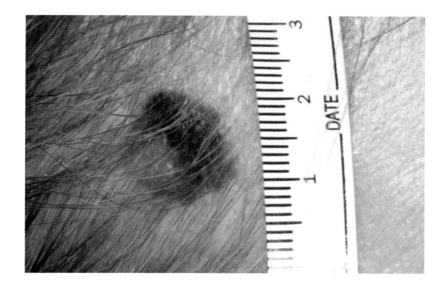

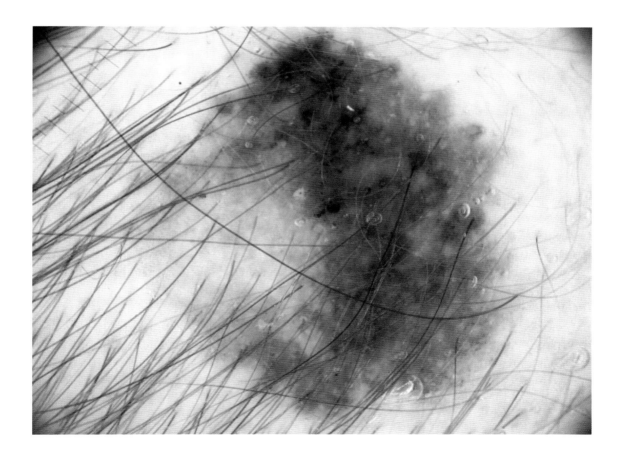

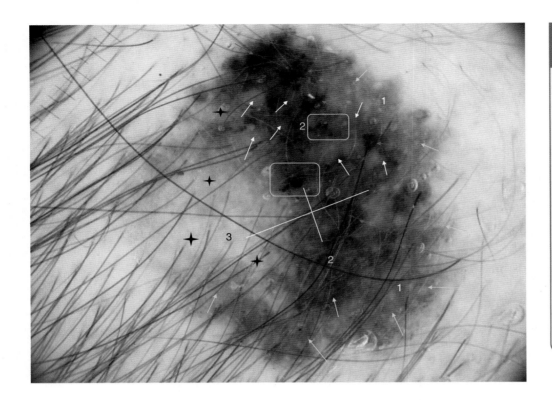

DERMOSCOPIC CRITERIA

- Asymmetry of color and structure (+)
- Multicomponent global pattern (1,2,3)
- Irregular dots and globules (yellow boxes)
- Irregular blotches (red arrows)
- Regression with bony-white color (black stars)
- Regression with peppering (yellow arrows)
- Six colors (black, light/dark brown, gray, blue, white)

DIAGNOSIS:
Superficial Spreading Melanoma

DISCUSSION

- Clinically, but not dermoscopically, this lesion looks similar to Case 5. One should quickly decide if this is a melanocytic or nonmelanocytic lesion.
- The large area with white color is an important clue that this could be a regressive melanoma.
- Foci with a few irregular brown dots and globules identify a melanocytic lesion.
- Significant asymmetry of color and structure plus the multicomponent global pattern are high-risk criteria that suggest this melanocytic lesion could be a melanoma.
- Two distinct forms of regression fill this lesion.
- Bony-white color (scarring) on the left side and diffuse grayish color (peppering) on the right side.
- Centrally, there is a mix of irregular black blotches and bluish-white color.
- However, a classic veil is not identified.

- Topping off the high-risk criteria is the presence of 6 colors: black, light and dark brown, gray, blue, white.
- The white and/or gray color of regression is an independent, high-risk criterion.
- The more regression that fills a lesion, the greater the possibility that it is a melanoma.
- Regression can also be seen in benign melanocytic and nonmelanocytic lesions.

PEARLS

- Don't forget following sayings to help remember 2 important general dermoscopic principles:
  - "If there's blue, they might sue."
  - "If there's white, control your fright."
- Regardless, blue or white color in any form should always be a red flag for concern.

CASE 7

HISTORY
After severe seborrheic dermatitis on the scalp cleared with topical steroids, this lesion was found on a 76-year-old man.

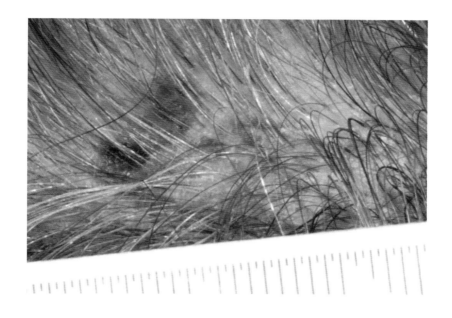

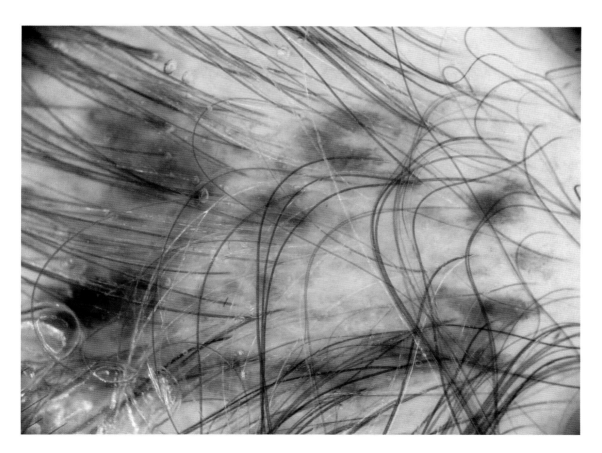

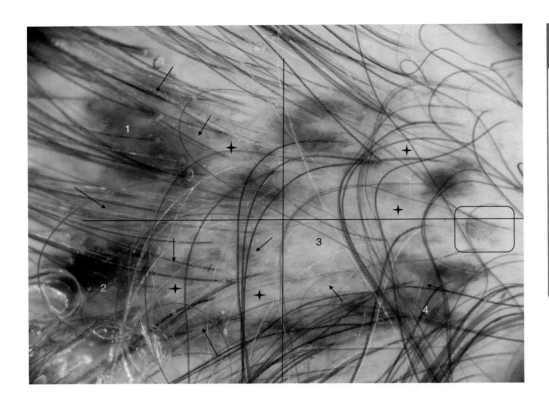

DIAGNOSIS:
Superficial Spreading Melanoma

DISCUSSION

- There is a questionable focus of pigment network that would define this as a melanocytic lesion.
- This could also be considered to be a melanocytic lesion by default.
- Given an absence of criteria to diagnose a melanocytic lesion, seborrheic keratosis, basal cell carcinoma, dermatofibroma, or hemangioma, a lesion should be considered to be melanocytic by default.
- "If there's white control your fright."
- With the majority of the lesion being filled with regression, this is a melanoma until proven otherwise with a histopathologic diagnosis.
- The melanoma-specific criteria include the multicomponent global pattern, asymmetry of color and structure, the large area of regression, and the presence of 5 colors.
- The regression area is composed of bony-white color (scarring) and foci of gray color (peppering made up of free melanin and melanophages in the dermis).

- There is also a suggestion of milky-red/pink color.
- "If there's pink, stop and think!"
- Milky-red/pink color (representing inflammation or neovascularization) in any form should always be a red flag for concern.
- Milky-red/pink color is often seen in invasive melanomas.
- The irregular foci of light and dark brown homogeneous color are often found in dysplastic nevi and melanoma.

PEARLS

- Criteria can be well-developed or poorly developed, or a lesion can be considered to be featureless.
- Before diagnosing a low-risk lesion, make sure that you do not miss a focus of high-risk criteria.
- Amelanotic melanoma is commonly feature-poor or featureless.

CASE 8

HISTORY
This is one of many banal-appearing nevi found on the face, scalp, and neck of a 29-year-old woman.

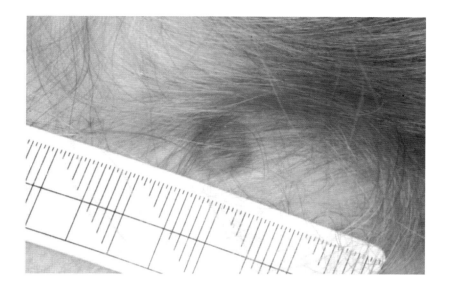

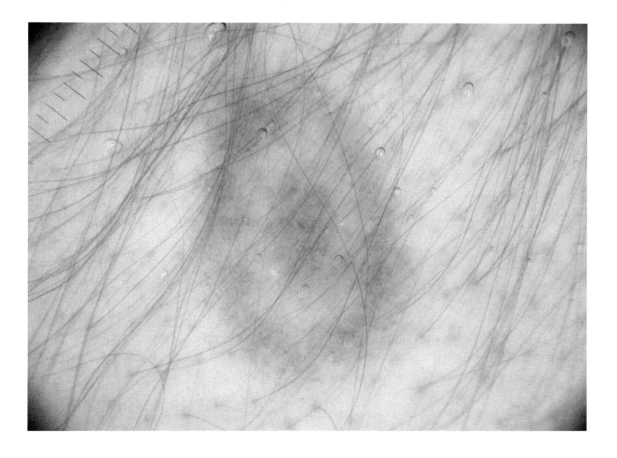

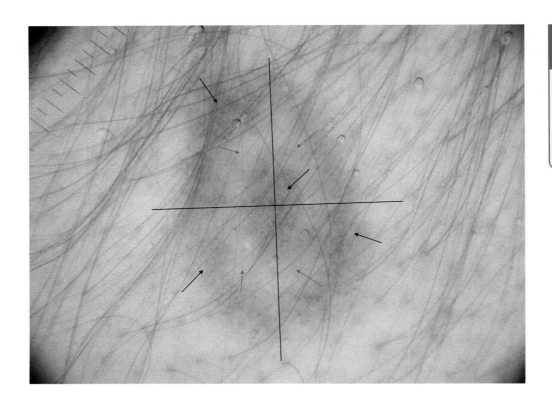

DIAGNOSIS:
Nevus

DISCUSSION

- This is a perfectly symmetrical lesion.
- A very fine, regular pigment network is seen at the lesion periphery, putting a melanocytic lesion at the top of the differential diagnostic list.
- Of note, pigment network may also be found in solar lentigines and dermatofibromas.
- There is a uniform central island composed of very fine regular pigment network, similar to that seen at the periphery.
- The white color filling the inner part of the lesion is not bony-white, and therefore does not reflect the scarring seen in regression.
- At times, it might be difficult to differentiate the light color of normal skin within a lesion from the scarring of regression or hypopigmentation.
- In this case, the light central color is identical to that of the surrounding skin.
- This global pattern is referred to as a *targetoid nevus*.

- In analogous fashion, a ring of regular pigment network at the periphery and light color filling the lesion has been described as a "crown of thorns" nevus and is benign.
- Typically the pigment network is better developed than in this case.
- The crown of thorns pattern is most commonly found on the scalp in children. Less commonly, it may be found on the trunk in adults.

PEARLS

- One expects to see a uniform globular pattern or the crown of thorns pattern in nevi on the scalp in children.
- Any other pattern should be a red flag for concern.
- The scalp is a common place to find dysplastic nevi in children.

HISTORY
A 48-year-old man noticed the color changing in this lesion on his leg.

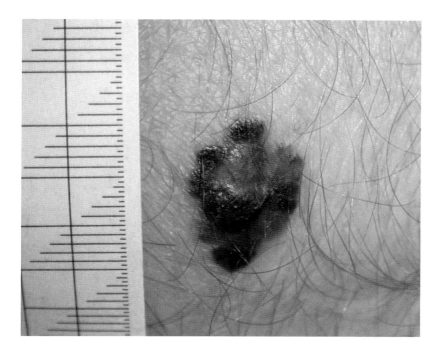

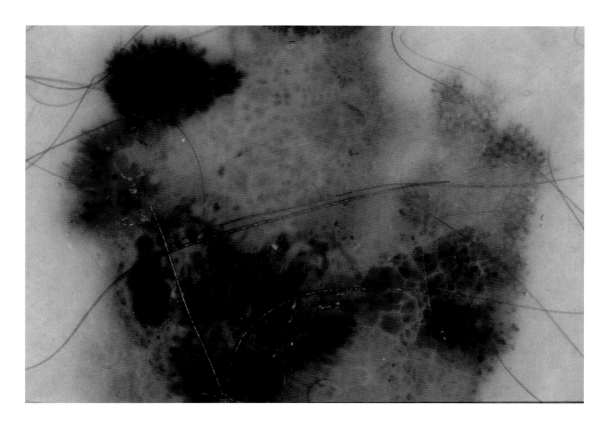

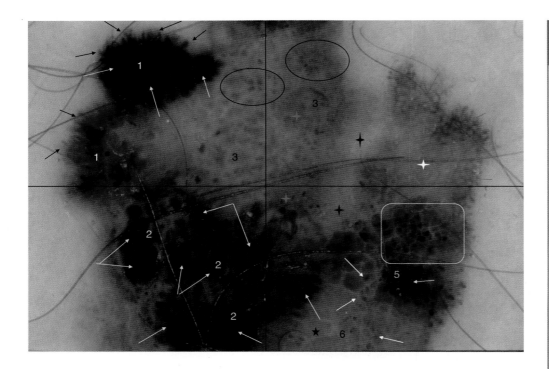

DIAGNOSIS:
Superficial Spreading Melanoma

DERMOSCOPIC CRITERIA

- Asymmetry of color and structure (+)
- Multicomponent global pattern (1,2,3,4,5,6)
- Irregular pigment network (red arrows)
- Irregular dots and globules (yellow box)
- Irregular blotches (yellow arrows)
- Irregular streaks (black arrows)
- White network (white arrows)
- Bluish-white and milky-red colors (red stars)
- Milky-red globules (circles)
- Bony-white color of regression (black stars)
- Hypopigmentation (white star)
- Six colors (black, light/dark brown, blue, white, pink)

DISCUSSION

- This invasive melanoma has it all.
- The melanoma-specific criteria are well-developed and very easy to identify.
- The asymmetry of color and structure is dramatic.
- The multicomponent global pattern has 6 different zones with different sets of criteria.
- There is a focus of pigment network that is only minimally irregular.
- A white network is easy to identify.
- Irregular dots and globules with different sizes and shapes are asymmetrically located.
- Multiple irregular black blotches with different sizes and shapes are asymmetrically located.
- A focus of irregular streaks (defined as being irregular because they are not symmetrically located around the periphery of the lesion) is identified.

- A large area with bluish-white color (melanosis) and subtle pink color filled with milky-red globules (representing neovascularization) is identified.
- The bony-white color of regression in the center of the lesion and 6 vivid colors round off the diagnostic high-risk criteria of this invasive melanoma.

PEARLS

- This is a great case to learn all of the melanoma-specific criteria.
- Take your time to study this lesion, and cement in your mind how the irregular criteria present.
- Diagnosing melanoma may not always be this easy.

CASE 10

HISTORY
This is an "ugly duckling" lesion on the back of a 30-year-old woman. There is no history of dysplastic nevi, but she frequented tanning parlors in college and is thus at increased risk to develop melanoma.

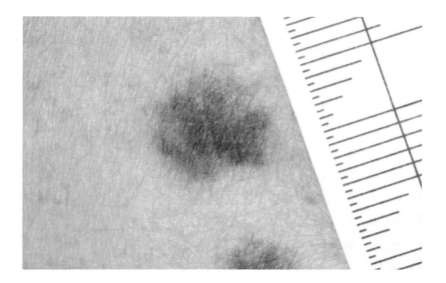

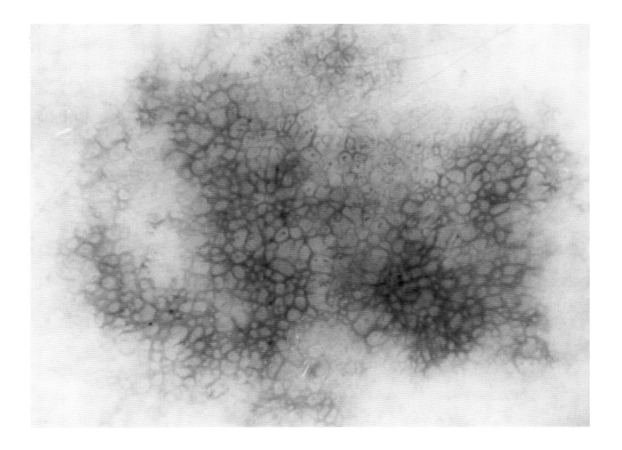

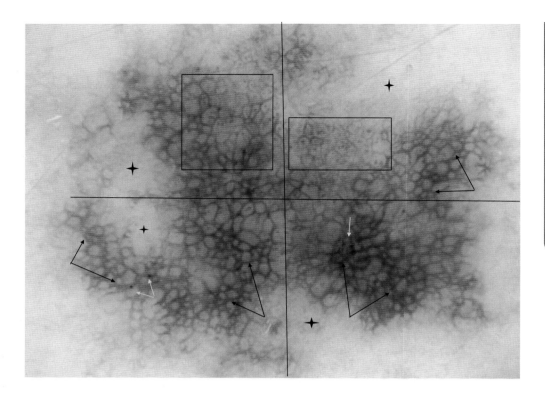

DIAGNOSIS:
Congenital Nevus

DISCUSSION

- An ugly duckling lesion with the ABCD clinical criteria is a red flag for concern, even though at first blush the dermoscopic appearance of this lesion is low-risk.
- Pigment network identifies a melanocytic lesion.
- The global pattern is reticular, because the pigment network fills the lesion.
- A purely reticular global pattern (regular pigment network) without any other significant criteria could be found in benign or malignant (irregular pigment network) melanocytic lesions.
- Debatably, there is a mild asymmetry of color and structure given that the left side of the lesion is not an exact mirror image of the right side and that the upper half is not a mirror image of the lower half.
- In general, interobserver agreement among dermoscopy experts is often not very good when it comes to determining lesional symmetry.
- Light and dark brown regular pigment network fills the lesion.
- Whereas different shades of brown color may be seen in irregular pigment networks, the other features of

irregular pigment network (broadened, thickened, branched with irregular holes) should also be present to conclude irregularity.
- On close inspection, one can see that there are dots in the holes of the pigment network identifying a "target network."
- A target network is a feature of congenital melanocytic nevi.
- There are 2 foci of minimally irregular brown dots and globules, which have no diagnostic significance.
- Areas of normal skin (not to be confused with regression) are also seen in this lesion.

PEARLS

- There are occasions when high-risk clinical features override low-risk dermoscopic features and warrant a histopathologic diagnosis.
- Clinically banal lesions with high-risk dermoscopic features also warrant a histopathologic diagnosis.
- Any clinical and/or dermoscopic ugly duckling lesion should be a red flag for concern and warrants closer attention.

CASE 11

HISTORY
The patient in his 20s has several nevi with very similar clinical and dermoscopic features.

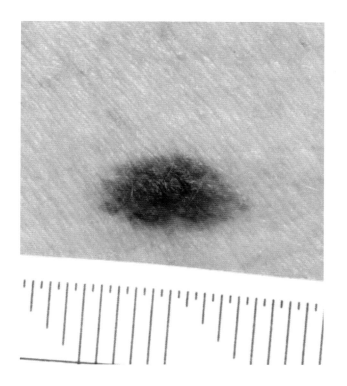

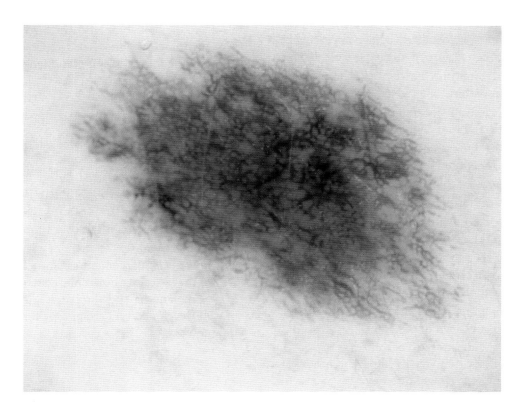

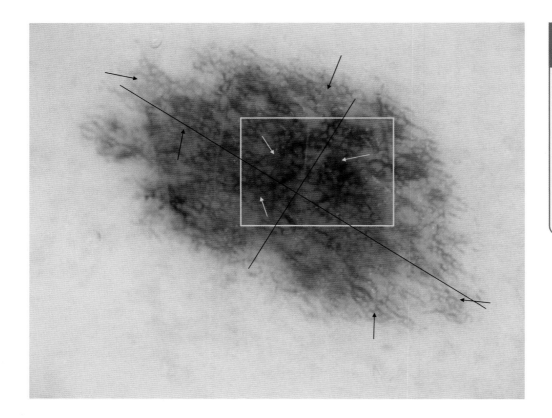

DERMOSCOPIC CRITERIA

- Asymmetry of color and structure (+)
- Reticular global pattern
- Regular pigment network (black arrows)
- Irregular pigment network (box)
- Bluish-white color (yellow arrows)

DIAGNOSIS:
Dysplastic Nevus

DISCUSSION

- This lesion is more malignant than benign appearing but does not have enough features to diagnose a melanoma.
- Pigment network identifies a melanocytic lesion with a reticular global pattern.
- There is a large, centrally located area with irregular pigment network and hints of bluish-white color.
- The network is irregular because the line segments are broadened, thickened, branched, and broken-up.
- In addition, however, a significant portion of the lesion contains regular pigment network.
- The bluish-white color within the focus of irregular network does not fit the definition of a veil or regression.
- That being said, keep in mind that blue and/or white color in any form is often, but not always, associated with high-risk pathology.
- Multifocal hypopigmentation, a common feature of dysplastic nevi, is not seen here.
- A lesion with these dermoscopic features is more worrisome when solitary than if a given patient has several similar-appearing nevi ("signature nevi").

- In general, a provider's experience and confidence level will dictate whether to perform a biopsy for histopathologic diagnosis or to follow the lesion over time to look for evolution of higher-risk clinical or dermoscopic changes.

PEARLS

- Take dermoscopy to the next level by adding digital dermoscopy to your practice.
- Digital images may be used simply for chart documentation or may serve as a useful baseline to be used for side-by-side comparisons of the same lesion at a later date to check for evolution over time.
- Important dermoscopic changes over time include asymmetrical enlargement, asymmetrical changes within the lesion without enlargement, the appearance of new melanoma-specific criteria, the disappearance of well-developed criteria, and/or the appearance of new colors.

CASE 12

HISTORY
A 75-year-old man was not aware of this lesion on his left lower back.

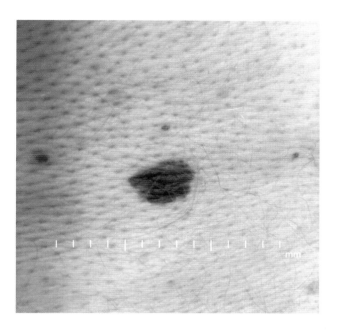

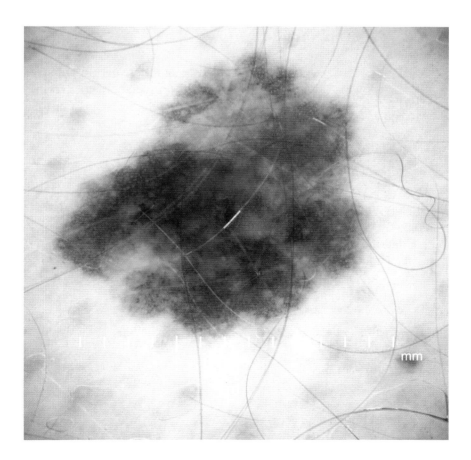

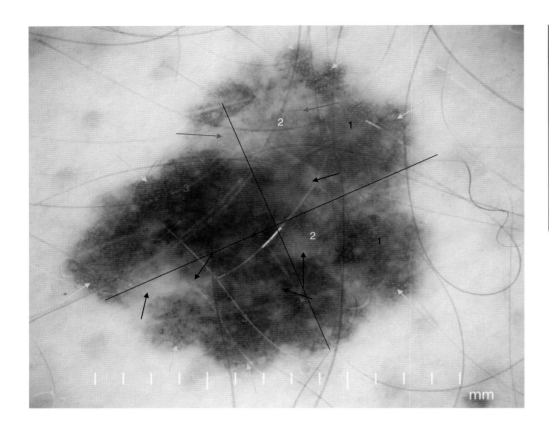

DIAGNOSIS:
Early-Invasive Superficial Spreading Melanoma

DISCUSSION

- At first blush, there is significant asymmetry of color and structure created by irregular coloration.
- This is the first red flag for concern that this could be a melanoma.
- Foci of regular pigment network identify a melanocytic lesion.
- The global pattern is multicomponent. However, the different sections seem to blend into each other.
- A large area of hypopigmentation at the periphery is considered high-risk and can be found in melanoma.
- There is a clear focus of regression with irregular bony-white color and a suggestion of white color throughout out the lesion.
- Hypopigmentation and bony-white color seem to merge in several sections of the lesion.
- In summary, the worrisome features of this clinically banal-looking skin lesion include asymmetry of color and structure, the multicomponent global pattern, irregular light and dark shades of brown, and areas of regression.

- Although these dermoscopic features are not diagnostic for melanoma per se, they are definitely atypical enough to warrant a histopathologic diagnosis posthaste.

PEARLS

- Clinically banal lesions sometimes are surprisingly atypical when examined with dermoscopy—there may be incognito high-risk pathology.
- An important general dermoscopic principle is to examine both banal and clinically atypical skin lesions.
- This thoroughness will increase your chances of finding high-risk melanocytic and high-risk nonmelanocytic lesions.
- Examining low-risk pathology will sharpen your eye for when you encounter high-risk pathology.
- The extra time you spend examining as many lesions as possible could save a life.

CASE 13

HISTORY

The patient in her 50s was born with this nevus on her central upper back.
Her husband noticed that it was changing.

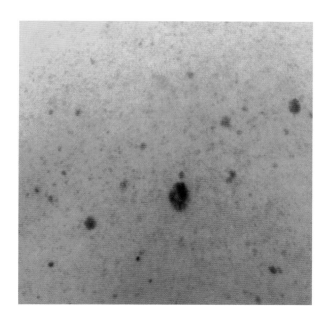

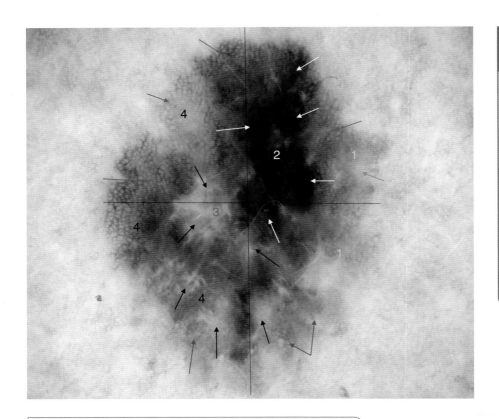

DIAGNOSIS:
Early-Invasive Superficial Spreading Melanoma Arising in a Congenital Nevus

DISCUSSION

- This is a straightforward case with well-developed melanoma-specific criteria.
- Compared with Case 12, the features are much easier to identify.
- Regular pigment network identifies a melanocytic lesion.
- There is significant asymmetry of color and structure with the multicomponent global pattern.
- There are no dots and globules, but rather there is a large, irregular black blotch.
- There are bony-white regression and several areas of hypopigmentation at the periphery.
- There are 5 colors (black, light and dark brown, white, and pink).
- If one looks closely, there seems to be erythema (pink color) over the dark blotch.
- Erythema (representing inflammation) is a nonspecific dermoscopic finding commonly found in benign and malignant melanocytic lesions.
- Typically, erythema blanches away with pressure.

- There are no dermoscopic features associated with a congenital nevus (target network, terminal hairs with perifollicular hypopigmentation).

PEARLS

- There are clinical and dermoscopic clues that may allow you to estimate if you are dealing with a superficial or invasive melanoma.
- A flat or slightly elevated lesion with superficial colors (black and brown) and well-developed, local criteria (network, dots, globules) are associated with an in situ or early-invasive melanoma.
- A nodular lesion with a paucity of local criteria and colors associated with deeper location of pigment (blue and milky-red color) favor a more deeply invasive melanoma.
- The presence of regression is not always associated with a deeper melanoma.
- It is nice to tell a patient that even though they might have a melanoma, based on what you see clinically and with dermoscopy, it does not look like it will be a bad one.

CASE 14

HISTORY
This lesion was located on the upper arm of a 49-year-old man and had been flat for years. It began to itch along with the formation of an area that he thought was a mosquito bite that did not heal.

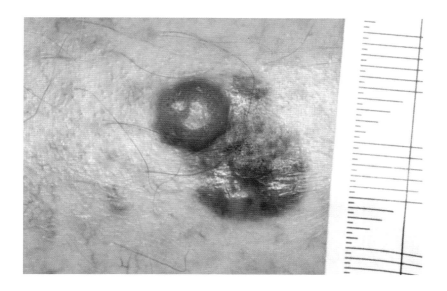

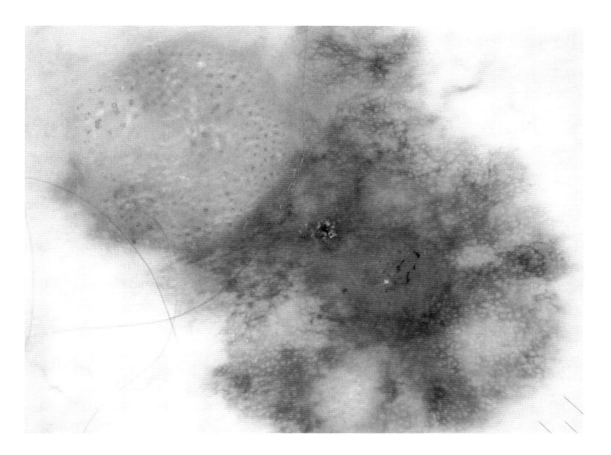

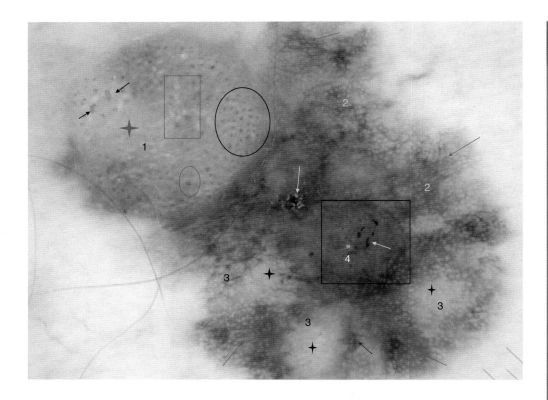

DIAGNOSIS:
Secondary Nodular Melanoma

DISCUSSION

- A regular pigment network scattered throughout identifies a melanocytic lesion.
- There is significant asymmetry of color and structure and a multicomponent global pattern.
- The larger white circular area contains crystalline structures and polymorphous vessels (dotted, hairpin, comma).
- At first blush, the vessels within the white area could be characterized as being pinpoint and glomerular. This would suggest the lesion could be a pigmented Bowen disease. However on closer inspection, irregular hairpin and comma vessels are also seen.
- One can expect the dusky-red nodule seen clinically to appear as a milky-red to pink area by dermoscopy.
- Of note, pressure with instrumentation when taking digital images might blanch away pink color.
- Crystalline structures that fill the white area can only be seen with polarized dermoscopy.
- There is a small round centrally located milky-red area with ulceration and another scabby ulcer adjacent to it.

- Foci of regression (bony-white and gray colors) and 5 colors (light and dark brown, white, gray, pink) are the last melanoma-specific, high-risk criteria in this nodular melanoma.
- It is unlucky that this patient was not seen before the nodule developed, because the dermoscopic features without the nodule might be typical of only in situ or early-invasive melanoma.

PEARLS

- It is important to examine the entire lesion before making a dermoscopic diagnosis.
- Therapeutic decision-making based only on isolated dermoscopic criteria identification can lead to misdiagnosis.
- For example, identifying milia-like cysts and pseudofollicular openings and stopping before an analysis of other criteria could misdiagnose a benign or malignant melanocytic lesion that can have criteria similar to a seborrheic keratosis.

CASE 15

HISTORY

A 42-year-old man was concerned about the appearance of a new dark spot on the lower part of this mole located on his right arm.

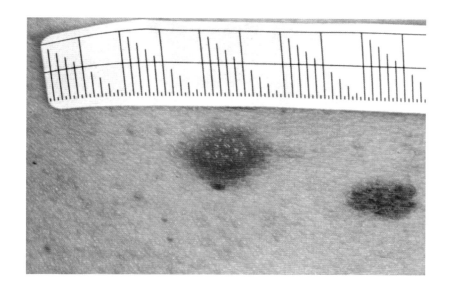

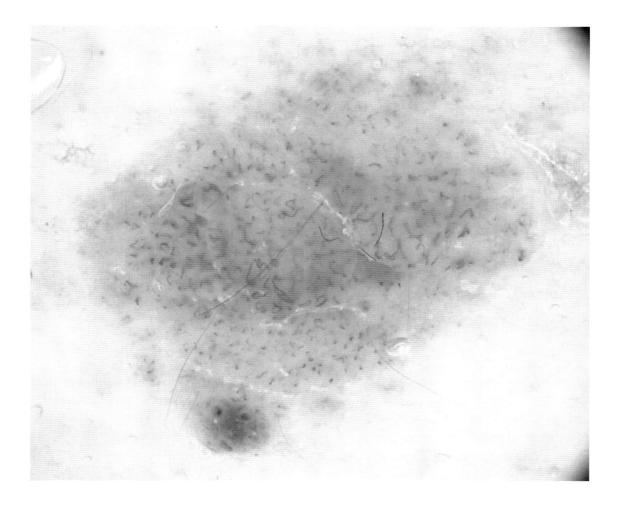

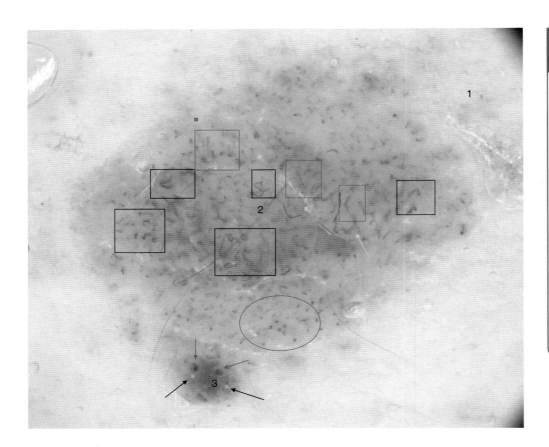

DERMOSCOPIC CRITERIA

- Asymmetry of color and structure
- Multicomponent global pattern (1,2,3)
- Dotted vessels (circle)
- Linear vessels (red boxes)
- Comma vessels (black boxes)
- Hairpin vessel (yellow arrow)
- Pigmented pseudofollicular openings (red arrows)
- Milia-like cysts (black arrows)

DIAGNOSIS:
Collision Lesion Nevus and Seborrheic Keratosis

DISCUSSION

- Clinically, this is a banal-looking compound nevus.
- It is melanocytic by default, because there are no criteria to diagnose a melanocytic lesion, seborrheic keratosis, basal cell carcinoma, dermatofibroma, or hemangioma.
- There is asymmetry of color and structure, the multicomponent global pattern, and milky-red color filled with polymorphous vessels (3 or more different shapes).
- Comma, dotted, linear, and hairpin.
- Melanoma-specific, high-risk criteria (ie, polymorphous vessels, pink color) can be found in low-risk pathology.
- Comma-shaped vessels are associated with compound nevi.
- The new dark spot of concern to the patient is a small seborrheic keratosis with milia-like cysts and pigmented pseudofollicular openings.
- If you had the ability to enlarge the lesion, you could see the shape of the vessels better and would see that there are also incipient ridges of a seborrheic keratosis in the "new dark spot."
- The differential diagnosis of the pigmented pseudofollicular openings would be regular brown globules of a melanocytic lesion.
- A subset of seborrheic keratosis look like this with the predominant vessels being hairpin shaped.

PEARLS

- On-the-spot confident reassurance to the patient that a lesion of concern is low-risk is one of the major benefits of dermoscopy.
- Creating digital dermoscopic images of a lesion, for example with your cell phone, gives you the ability to enlarge the image.
- Enlarging dermoscopic images makes tiny criteria such as the shape of telangiectatic vessels easier to characterize. It also makes visible relatively invisible criteria.
- Always remember while you are improving your dermoscopic skills, "If in doubt, cut it out!"

CASE 16

HISTORY

An 80-year-old man has hypertrophic actinic keratosis on all sun-exposed areas, multiple tumors on his face and trunk with dermoscopic features of basal cell and squamous cell carcinoma, plus this lesion also located on his back.

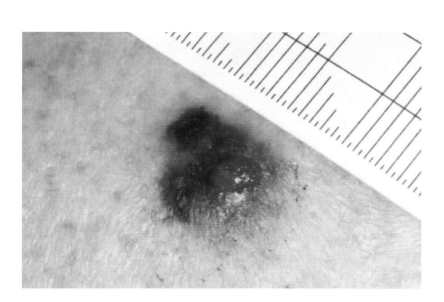

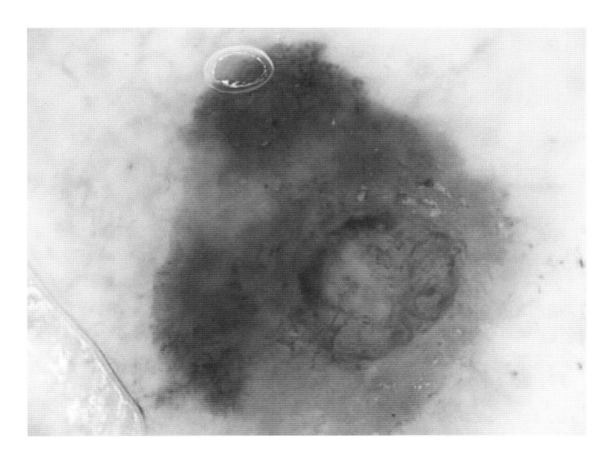

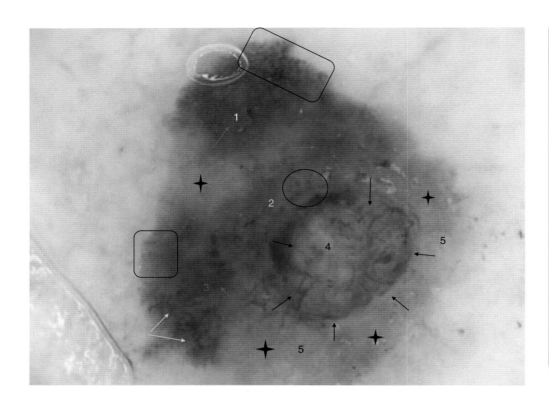

DERMOSCOPIC CRITERIA

- Asymmetry of color and structure
- Multicomponent global pattern (1,2,3,4,5)
- Irregular brown dots and globules (boxes)
- Irregular pigment network (yellow arrows)
- Bluish-white color (red arrows)
- Milky-red nodule (black arrows)
- Milky-red globules (circle)
- Milky-red color (stars)
- Five colors (light/dark brown, blue, white, pink)

DIAGNOSIS:
Invasive Melanoma

DISCUSSION

- Significant findings in this lesion include the following:
  - Irregular brown dots and globules diagnose a melanocytic lesion.
  - Significant asymmetry of color and structure.
  - A questionable focus of irregular pigment network.
  - A milky-red nodule surrounded by milky-red color with milky-red globules.
- Deep blue and bluish-white color do not fit the definition of a veil but nevertheless are also very worrisome features.
- Milky-red and blue colors indicate deep penetration of this melanoma.
- These features are "as bad as it gets" when it comes to dermoscopic features of invasive melanoma.
- Five or 6 colors in a melanocytic lesion should always be a red flag for concern.
- Five separate zones within the lesion making up the multicomponent global pattern.
- Experienced dermoscopists may not always agree on the exact number of separate zones. Different zones represent only one of several dramatic atypical features of this invasive melanoma.

- The final diagnosis does not hinge upon this single determination.
- Deeply invasive melanomas such as this one typically have a paucity of local criteria (network, dots, globules), which are usually located at the periphery of the lesion.
- In summary, brown dots and globules identify a melanocytic lesion. The melanoma-specific criteria include asymmetry of color and structure, multicomponent global pattern, irregular network, irregular dots and globules, milky-red nodule, bluish-white color, and 6 colors in toto.

PEARLS

- Have a checklist of points in mind or written down on what to identify in each lesion, so that you will be consistent in your dermoscopic evaluations.
- Never tell a patient that you are 100% sure they have a melanoma. The worst set of clinical and/or dermoscopic features might not turn out to be melanoma upon histopathologic analysis.

CASE 17

HISTORY
A 62-year-old woman insisted that this lesion on her left upper arm was not there a few months ago.

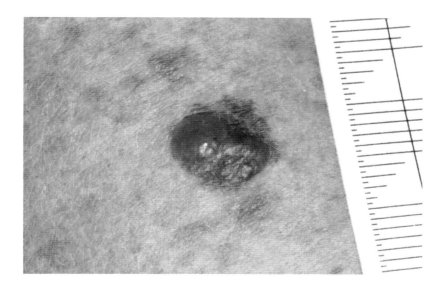

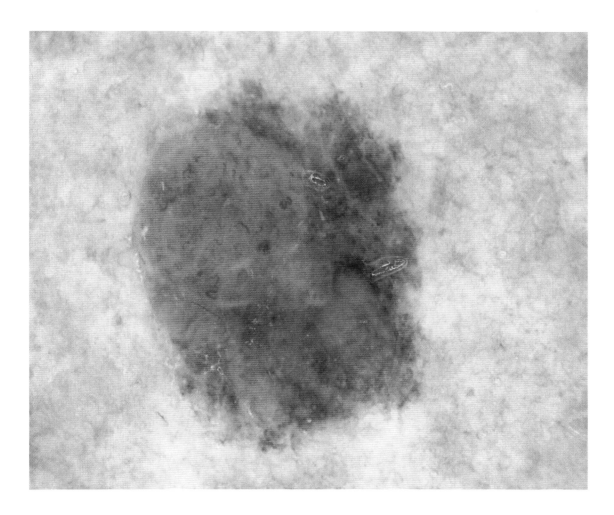

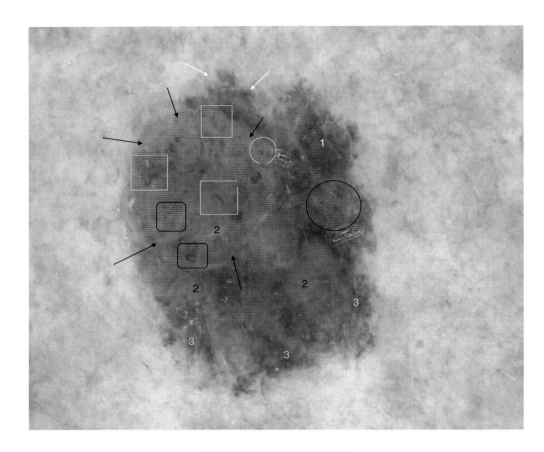

DERMOSCOPIC CRITERIA

- Asymmetry of color and structure
- Multicomponent global pattern (1,2,3)
- Irregular dots and globules (black circle)
- Milky-red nodule (black arrows)
- Comma vessels (black boxes)
- Linear vessels (yellow boxes)
- Dotted vessels (yellow circle)
- Corkscrew vessel (red box)
- Milky-red globules (red circle)

DIAGNOSIS:
Nodular Amelanotic Melanoma

DISCUSSION

- Clinically, we see this nodule as reddish.
- Dermoscopically, we see light and dark brown color and a milky-red nodule with polymorphous vessels.
- In this instance, calmly say to yourself, "This is a nodular amelanotic melanoma," until proven otherwise. Then, excise it posthaste.
- An overview of your organized methodical analysis is "blink first" and make your rapid diagnosis of amelanotic melanoma. Then, "think" to confirm your initial "blink."
- "Blink" is your composite reaction that this could be bad, based on your rapid recognition of the red flags for concern in this lesion.
- "Think" is the subsequent process of taking your time to methodically assess the clinical and dermoscopic features that you see in detail, including the following:
  - Milky-red/pink color, irregular small vessels in a lesion with brown color, and a focus of irregular brown dots and globules—your clues that the lesion is melanocytic.

- Asymmetry of color and structure, a multicomponent global pattern with a milky-red nodule, and flat milky-red color. There are also very subtle milky-red globules that might be overlooked.
- Note the shapes of the telangiectatic vessels:
  - There are comma-shaped, linear, and dotted vessels. There is even a number 3–shaped vessel that might be considered a variation of a corkscrew vessel.

PEARLS

- The "blink and think" approach comes with experience combined with knowledge.
- The novice dermoscopist should "think" more than "blink" to decrease the chance of a misdiagnosis.
- Put in the time to learn as much dermoscopy as you can because the learning curve to becoming a proficient dermoscopist may be steep.

CASE 18

HISTORY
A 50-year-old woman had a lump in her groin and this skin lesion on the same leg.

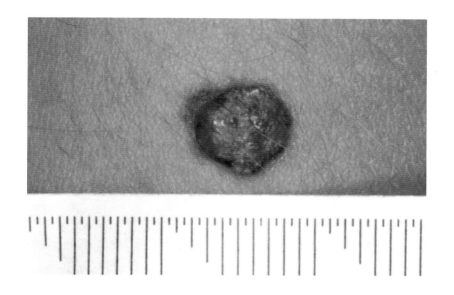

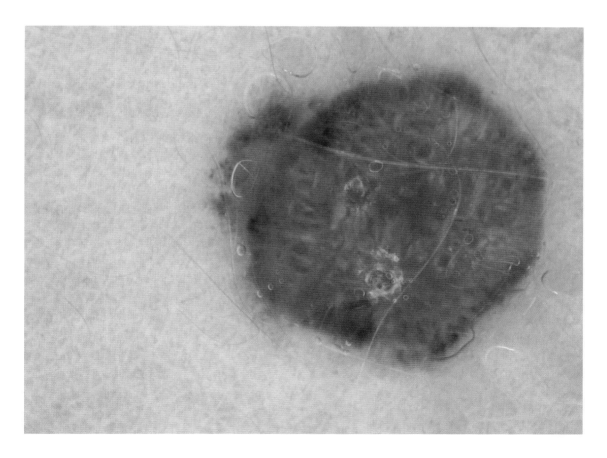

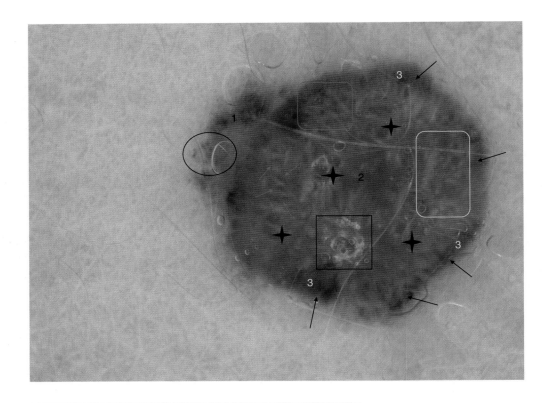

DIAGNOSIS:
Nodular Amelanotic Melanoma

DISCUSSION

- This could be another "blink and think" diagnosis if you know that any milky-red lesion filled with crystalline structures statistically favors the diagnosis of an amelanotic melanoma.
- A focus of irregular brown dots and globules identifies a melanocytic lesion.
- The most worrisome feature of this amelanotic melanoma is the milky-red color filling the lesion with a diffuse distribution of crystalline structures.
- Crystalline structures can be seen in nonmelanocytic benign lesions (such as dermatofibroma) or malignant lesions (such as basal cell carcinoma) as well as in melanocytic benign lesions (such as Spitz nevus) or malignant lesions (such as melanoma).
- When crystalline structures are found in a melanocytic lesion, that favors the diagnosis of a melanoma.
- The size and geometric shape of the crystalline structures vary significantly in this lesion.
- There is no diagnostic significance to the size, shape, or distribution of the crystalline structures.
- Any presentation of crystalline structures should always be a red flag for concern.

- At times, it might be difficult to differentiate a white network from crystalline structures. White network is reticular/netlike, whereas crystalline structures are never reticular/netlike.
- There are very subtle foci of milky-red globules and polymorphous vessels with linear, dotted, and comma shapes. If you could magnify the lesion, the vessels would be easier to see.
- The gray color is an insignificant feature and represents peppering created by an immune response.
- Unfortunately, this patient ended up having a positive sentinel lymph node biopsy.

PEARLS

- A pink lesion clinically or dermoscopically that is not obviously benign should be excised posthaste.
- "When it's pink, stop and think!"
- Digital follow-up of a nodular lesion is contraindicated and could delay the diagnosis of serious pathology.

CASE 19

HISTORY

A patient in his 60s with obvious sun damage came in with a chief complaint of "scaly, nonhealing spots" on his ears. We suggested a total-body skin examination and found this lesion on his left upper back.

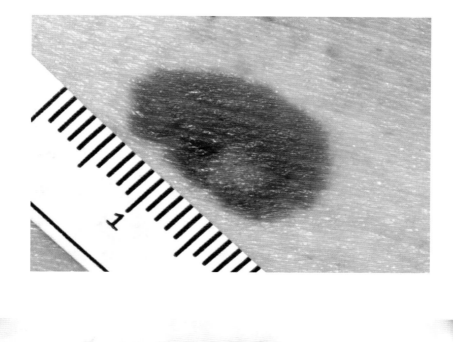

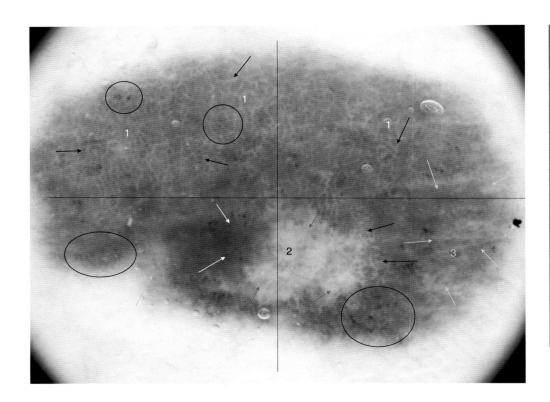

DERMOSCOPIC CRITERIA

- Asymmetry of color and structure (+)
- Multicomponent global pattern (1,2,3)
- Irregular brown dots and globules (circles)
- White network (black arrows)
- Regression (red arrows)
- Melanosis (white arrows)
- Hypopigmentation (yellow arrows)
- Five colors (light/dark brown, pink, white, blue)

DIAGNOSIS:
Superficial Spreading Melanoma

DISCUSSION

- Scattered foci of poorly defined brown dots and globules identify a melanocytic lesion.
- There is obvious asymmetry of color and structure, and the multicomponent global pattern with 3 different zones of criteria.
- Both features should be worrisome to you.
- There is pinkish color filled with white network involving the upper part of the lesion.
- The white network should not be confused with crystalline structures, because the white lines are reticular (netlike).
- Crystalline structures are never reticular (netlike).
- Even the most innocuous presentation of a white network should always be a red flag for concern.
- A white network might be the only clue that the lesion is a melanoma.
- There is also an irregular area with bony-white and pinkish color.
- The white area represents the scarring of regression.
- Within the white area, there is a hint of pink color. By increasing the magnification of the pink color, you can see that this represents telangiectatic vessels that are out of focus.
- Vessels seen with dermoscopy may be in focus or out of focus.
- Vessels on the surface of a lesion typically are in sharp focus, whereas vessels deeper in the lesion typically are out of focus.
- The irregular blue blotch adjacent to the white color represents melanosis, representing heavily pigmented malignant melanocytes located deeper in the dermis.
- Rounding off the list of high-risk criteria are large areas of hypopigmentation at the periphery of the lesion.

PEARLS

- Do not hesitate to offer a total-body skin examination to patients with known risk factors for skin cancer, even if they did not come in for that reason.
- Once in a while you may pick up serious high-risk pathology that the patient would otherwise not be aware of.
- It is very rewarding when this happens, not to mention you might save a life.

CASE 20

HISTORY
This was found on the right calf of a 47-year-old woman.

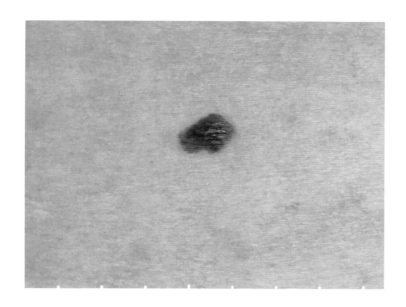

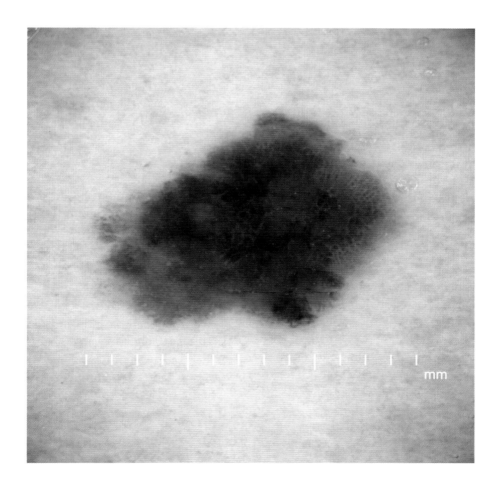

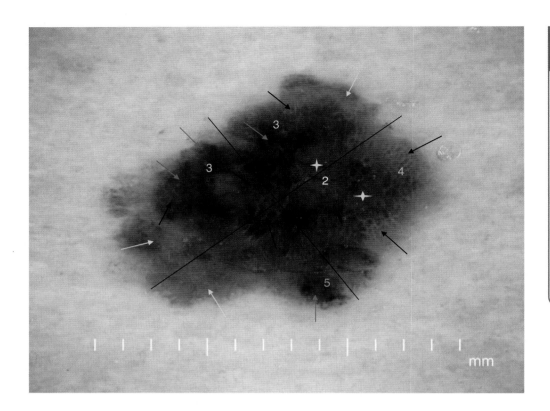

DERMOSCOPIC CRITERIA

- Asymmetry of color and structure (+)
- Multicomponent global pattern (1,2,3,4,5)
- White network (black arrows)
- Bluish-white veil (stars)
- Irregular dark blotches (red arrows)
- Hypopigmentation (yellow arrows)
- Five colors (black light/dark brown, blue white)

DIAGNOSIS:

Superficial Spreading Melanoma

DISCUSSION

- This lesion is melanocytic by default. Namely, there are no criteria to diagnose a melanocytic lesion, a seborrheic keratosis, a basal cell carcinoma, a hemangioma, or a dermatofibroma. The lesion is categorized as melanocytic in order not to miss a potential melanoma, as was found in this case.
- There is asymmetry of color and structure. The left half of the lesion is not a mirror image of the right half. The top half of the lesion is not a mirror image of the lower half.
- It is debatable how many different zones of criteria are present in this lesion. Nevertheless, it has a high-risk multicomponent global pattern.
- There are definite areas of white network. Compared with Case 19, the white network is much less prominent yet is clearly seen throughout the lesion.
- The veil with bluish-white color is well-developed and easy to identify.

- Irregular dark blotches and irregular hypopigmentation are seen at the periphery.
- In some areas the white network is a component of the veil, irregular dark blotches, and hypopigmentation.
- Finally, there are 5 colors.
- In summary, this is a melanocytic lesion with well-developed, melanoma-specific criteria: asymmetry of color and structure, multicomponent global pattern, white network, bluish-white veil, irregular dark blotches, irregular peripheral hypopigmentation, and 6 colors.

PEARLS

- The criteria identification and analysis in this case should be straightforward.
- If there is any confusion, it may be a good time to review Chapter 2, "Comprehensive Dermoscopy Criteria Review."

CASE 21

HISTORY
The wife of a 34-year-old man was concerned about this solitary lesion on her husband's upper back.

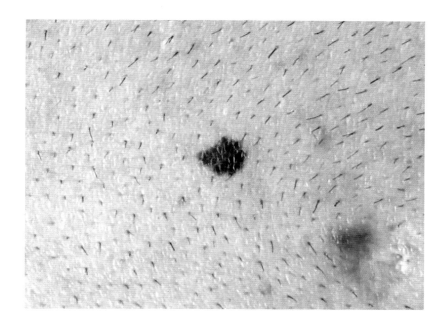

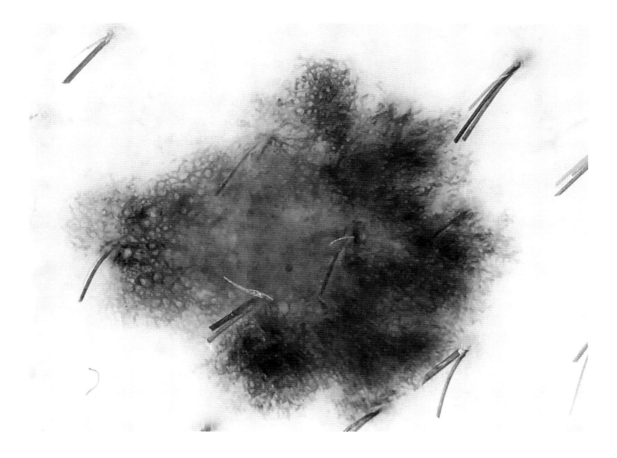

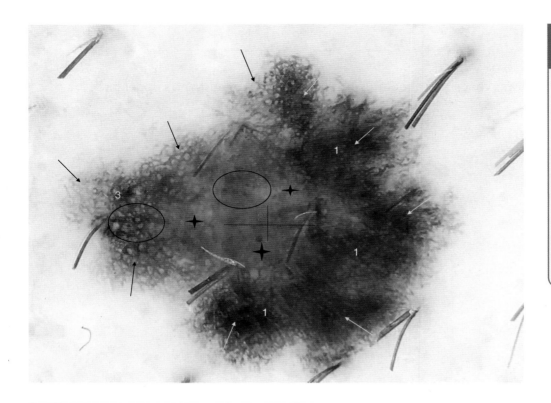

DIAGNOSIS:
Dysplastic Nevus

DISCUSSION

- A solitary pigmented skin lesion on the back of an adult male with some features of the ABCDE criteria are a red flag for concern.
- At first blush, the dermoscopic appearance is more malignant looking than benign looking, but not clearly malignant.
- Pigment network and foci of brown dots and globules identify a melanocytic lesion.
- Globally, there are asymmetry of color and structure and the multicomponent global pattern with 3 zones of different criteria.
- Novice dermoscopists might consider the pigment network to be irregular; however, it is in the regular range. The line segments are the same color and thickness and the holes are uniform.
- There are 2 foci of irregular brown dots and globules. These are minor, but useful, features to diagnose this dysplastic nevus.
- The most striking features are the areas of irregular hyper- and hypopigmentation that fill the lesion. They both have a smudged appearance.

- This smudged appearance is a common feature of dysplastic nevi.
- The hyperpigmentation could also be described as an irregular blotch.
- It is a good sign that there are no other high-risk criteria to favor a diagnosis of a melanoma (eg, more colors, irregular streaks, regression, polymorphous vessels).
- Irregular pigment network, multifocal hypopigmentation, and hyperpigmentation are all common features of dysplastic nevi.

PEARLS

- Encourage your patients to do periodic skin self-examinations.
- Recommend that your patient's partner check the back and scalp, which obviously are difficult areas to self-examine.
- In practice, "Anything new or changing, any color, anywhere," is your mantra. Skin cancers may or may not look like those depicted in brochures, but regardless, it is up to us to find them.

CASE 22

HISTORY

A 67-year-old woman was curious about this changing dark spot on her right lower back and mentioned it to her dermatologist at her yearly skin examination.

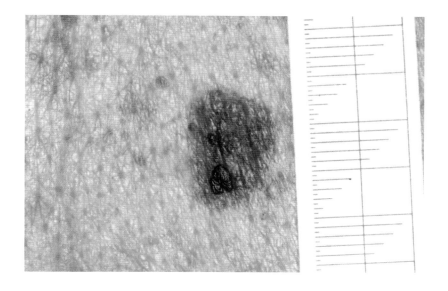

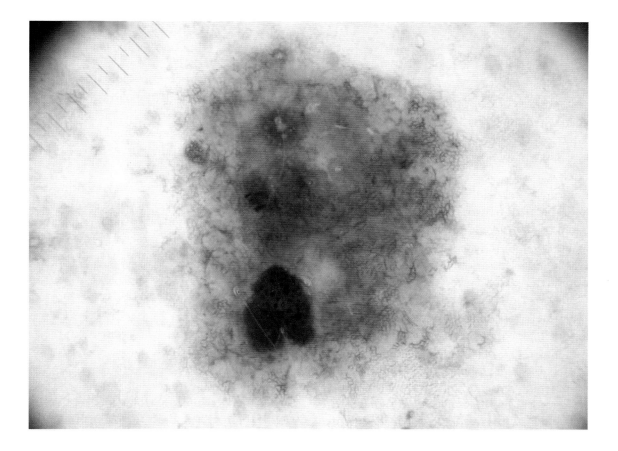

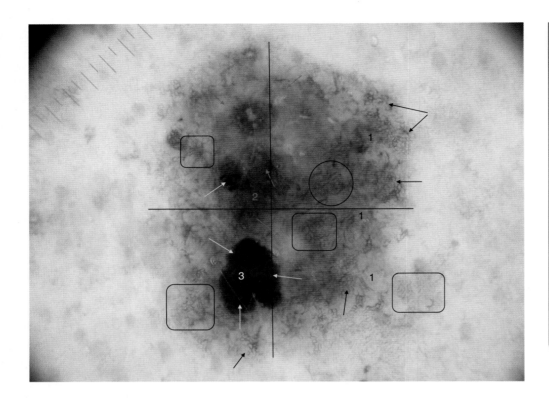

DIAGNOSIS:
Early-Invasive Superficial Spreading Melanoma Arising in an In Situ Melanoma

DISCUSSION

- The clinical impression that this could be a melanoma is confirmed when the lesion is examined with dermoscopy.
- Black, blue, pink, and white colors are high-risk clues in a "blink."
- The lesion is melanocytic, filled with foci of regular and irregular pigment network with different shades of brown and broken-up and branched line segments.
- It is debatable whether the focus of irregular dots and globules really represents broken-up line segments of irregular pigment network; a very minor point in the context of the other high-risk criteria.
- There is asymmetry of color and structure and the multicomponent global pattern.
- The prominent irregular black blotch is filled with irregular black dots and globules. It should not be confused with pigmented pseudofollicular openings of a seborrheic keratosis. For the novice dermoscopist, this confusion could lead to a misdiagnosis of a pigmented seborrheic keratosis.

- There are 2 distinct regression areas.
- In the upper section, the regression area is composed of bony-white scarring, blue melanosis, fine gray peppering, and a suggestion of pink color.
- In the lower half of the lesion, there is a focus of purely bony-white color.
- In summary, pigment network identifies a melanocytic lesion. There are asymmetry of color and structure, multicomponent global pattern, regular and irregular pigment network, irregular brown and black dots and globules, irregular blotches, regression areas, and 7 colors. Seven colors!

PEARLS

- Words to live by, to always remember these important high-risk dermoscopic clues:
  - If there's pink, stop and think!
  - If there's blue, they might sue!
  - If there's white, control your fright!
  - If there's black, don't turn your back!

CASE 23

HISTORY

A stranger at Surfrider Beach in Malibu, California, saw this lesion on the lower leg of a surfer and suggested he show it to a dermatologist as soon as possible.

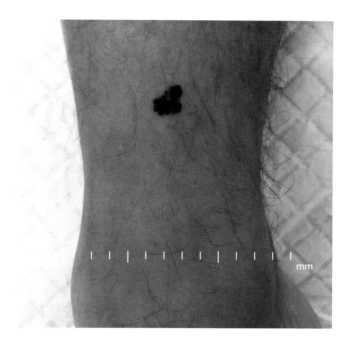

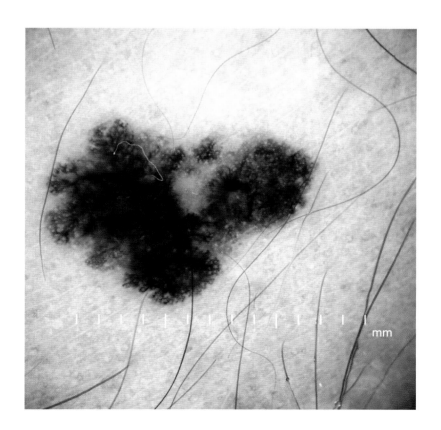

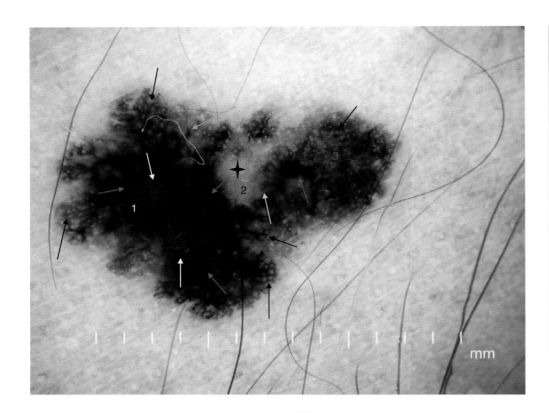

DIAGNOSIS:
Early-invasive Superficial Spreading Melanoma

DISCUSSION

- Irregular pigment network identifies a melanocytic lesion.
- The global pattern could be characterized as multicomponent (3 zones) or reticular homogeneous (reticular network and homogeneous color).
- There is asymmetry of color and structure.
- The irregular black blotches are well-developed.
- A subtle bluish-white veil contains crystalline structures.
- We have to focus our attention to see a few foci of irregular streaks at the periphery of the lesion.
- The area of light color does not represent the bony-white color of regression. Rather, it is identical to the surrounding skin and thus represents normal skin within an irregularly shaped lesion.

- In summary, pigment network identifies a melanocytic lesion. There are irregular pigment network, irregular streaks, irregular blotches, bluish-white veil, and crystalline structures.
- With these facts in mind, the presence of a flat lesion with colors associated with pigment high up in the skin (black and brown) and the presence of significant pigment network within the lesion, one could estimate that this is an in situ or early-invasive melanoma.

PEARLS

- This could be considered an ethical dilemma: If we see a suspicious skin lesion on another person, should we bring it to that person's attention?
- We recommend pointing out potentially high-risk lesions to a friend or stranger, but we do not recommend handing them your business card!

CASE 24

HISTORY
The patient's family doctor was concerned about this dark mole on the shoulder of a 44-year-old woman.

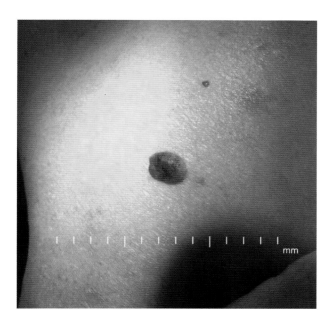

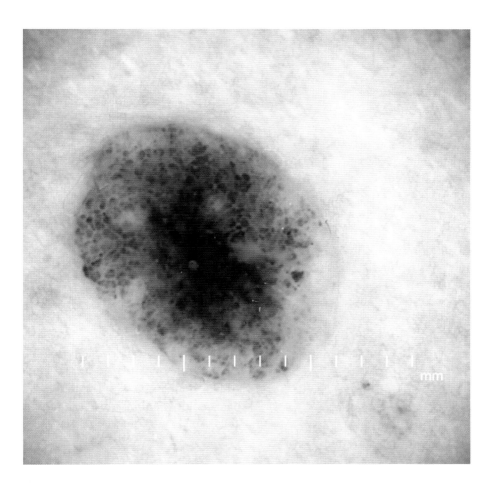

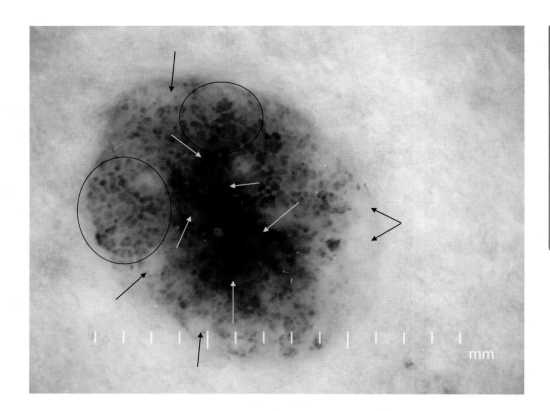

- Asymmetry of color and structure
- Cobblestone global pattern
- Regular brown dots and globules (circles)
- Irregular blotch (yellow arrows)
- Islands of normal skin (black arrows)

DIAGNOSIS:

Irritated Congenital Nevus

DISCUSSION

- Brown dots and globules identify a melanocytic lesion.
- This is the cobblestone global pattern, a variation of the globular pattern in which a nevus is filled with regular/uniform brown dots and globules. The dots and globules of the cobblestone pattern are larger and angulated, giving the appearance of a cobblestone street.
- The global pattern could also be characterized as being homogeneous (black blotch)-globular (dots and globules).
- The cobblestone global pattern here also possesses a centrally located irregular black blotch, characterized by its irregular borders. This irregular black blotch should be a red flag for concern in a "blink."
- The globular or cobblestone global patterns in most cases are associated with benign nevi. In fact, they are the most common patterns seen in the pediatric population.
- Irregular brown dots and globules forming a cobblestone pattern may also be seen in melanoma.
- The differential diagnosis of this centrally located irregular black blotch includes transepidermal

elimination of pigment, foci of atypical melanocytes, and irritation.

- The foci of white color are identical to the white color in the surrounding skin and represent normal skin within the lesion, not regression.
- A combined nevus has features of a nevus with brown and blue color. Black color indicates that pigmentation is at the upper levels of the skin and is not a feature of combined nevi.
- A globular or cobblestone pattern with regular brown dots and globules does not need intervention. However, this lesion with the irregular black blotch requires a histopathologic diagnosis posthaste.

PEARLS

- Always keep this general dermoscopic rule in mind: for any given criteria you identify in a lesion, you have to determine whether they are regular or irregular, good or bad, low-risk or high-risk.
- Black color should always be a red flag for concern but does not always translate to high-risk pathology.

CASE 25

HISTORY
This is one of several nevi on the back of a 22-year-old woman.

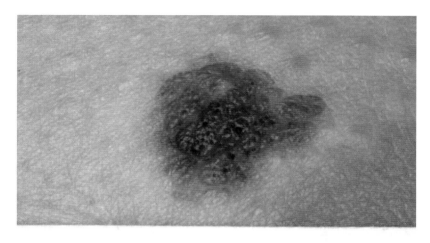

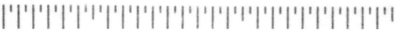

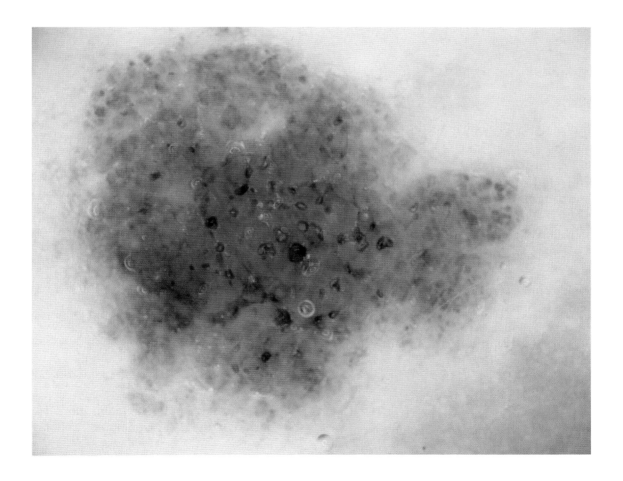

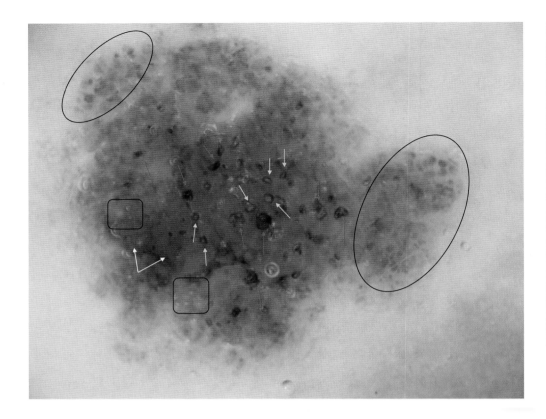

DERMOSCOPIC CRITERIA

- Asymmetry of color and structure
- Globular/cobblestone global pattern
- Regular brown dots and globules (circles)
- Pigmented pseudofollicular openings (red arrows)
- Nonpigmented pseudofollicular openings (yellow arrows)
- Milia-like cysts (boxes)
- Grayish blotch (white arrows)

DIAGNOSIS:
Nevus

DISCUSSION

- Regular brown dots and globules identify a melanocytic lesion.
- The nevus demonstrates features of both the globular pattern with regular brown dots and globules and the cobblestone pattern with larger angulated brown dots and globules.
- This combination of criteria is commonly encountered.
- The dots and globules are not as well-developed as in the previous case.
- A prominent feature is the presence of pigmented and nonpigmented pseudofollicular openings.
- Pseudofollicular openings represent invaginations of the epidermis filled with keratin, similar to comedones seen in patients with acne. Oxidized sebum creates the pigmentation.
- Pseudofollicular openings are considered primary criteria used to diagnose seborrheic keratosis. Nevertheless, they may also be present in benign as well as malignant melanocytic lesions.
- At times it is difficult to differentiate pigmented pseudofollicular opening from brown dots and globules

of a melanocytic lesion (dermoscopic differential diagnosis).
- In addition, there are a few milia-like cysts. These are also considered primary criteria used to diagnose seborrheic keratosis that can be seen in melanocytic lesions.
- There is a small grayish blotch that represents a focus of inflammation.
- This lesion does not need to be excised, and you can confidently reassure the patient that it represents a benign nevus.

PEARLS

- The wobble sign technique may aid in differentiating a seborrheic keratosis from a compound nevus. To perform this technique, place the glass plate of your dermatoscope over the lesion in question and gently move it from side to side.
  - A seborrheic keratosis remains more fixed to the surface of the skin and does not wobble (– wobble sign)
  - A compound nevus is more pliable or rubbery and will easily move from side to side (+ wobble sign)

CASE 26

HISTORY
A 25-year-old woman with a history of dysplastic nevi and tanning bed use was found to have this lesion on her upper back.

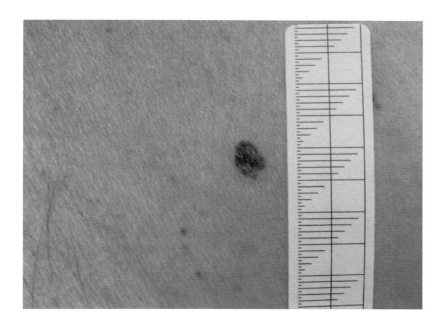

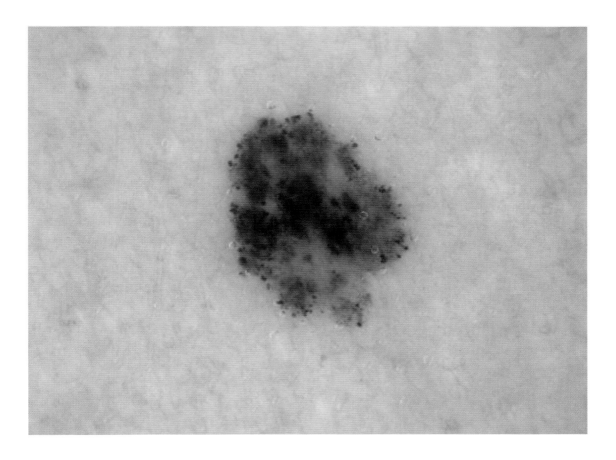

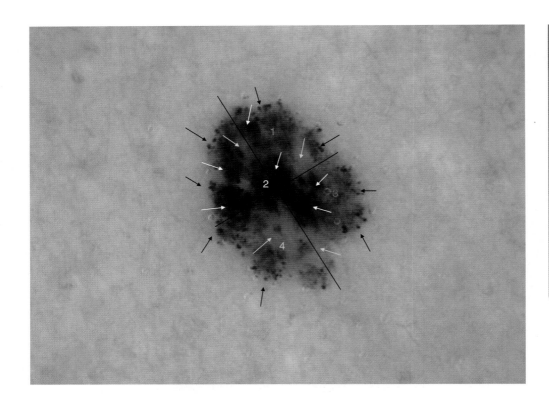

DIAGNOSIS:
Dysplastic Nevus

DISCUSSION

- Brown dots and globules identify a melanocytic lesion.
- There is asymmetry of color and structure with the multicomponent global pattern.
- The dots and globules are deemed irregular because of their differing sizes and shapes and their haphazard distribution at the periphery of the lesion.
- Peripheral brown dots and globules may be seen in actively changing nevi, Spitz nevi with the starburst pattern (ie, dots, globules, and/or streaks at the periphery), and in melanoma.
- Irregular black blotches fill most of this lesion.
- There are foci of hypopigmentation with a grayish tinge and faint erythema. Both of these features represent an inflammatory response in this dysplastic nevus.
- The lesion looks more malignant than benign, bordering on an in situ or early-invasive melanoma. Indeed, the diagnosis of a dysplastic nevus is not a good dermoscopic-pathologic correlation.

- In summary, brown dots and globules identify a melanocytic lesion. There are asymmetry of color and structure, multicomponent global pattern, irregular dots and globules, irregular blotches, and 5 colors.

PEARLS

- It is essential that there always be a good dermoscopic-pathologic correlation.
- Examples of bad dermoscopic-pathologic correlation:
  - You see criteria suggestive of Bowen disease, yet the biopsy reports only an actinic keratosis.
  - The pathology shows in situ melanoma, yet you see more atypical features of invasive melanoma not revealed in the pathology report.
- Be proactive and discuss your concerns with your pathologist.
- Additional sections or second opinions might be in order.
- There are times when the area in question should be rebiopsied.

CASE 27

HISTORY
This is the only pigmented lesion on the thigh of a 22-year-old man. It started itching a few weeks ago.

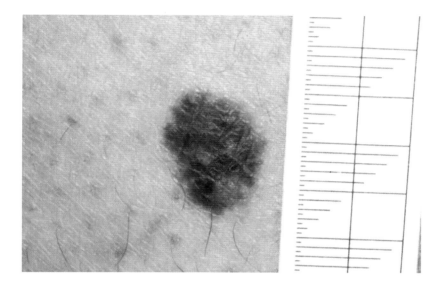

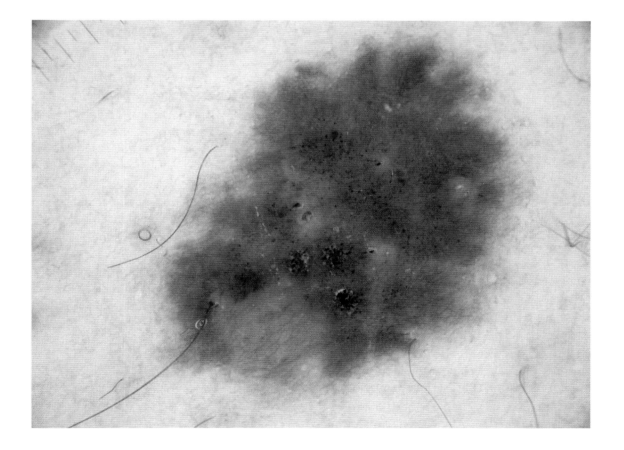

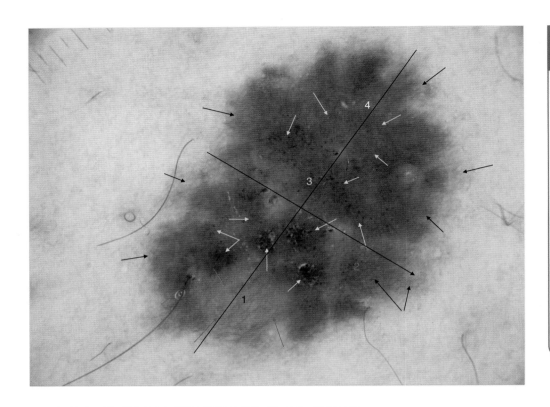

DIAGNOSIS:
Irritated Congenital Nevus

DISCUSSION

- There are subtle features in this lesion that will need your focused attention to evaluate.
- Regular pigment network identifies a melanocytic lesion.
- There are asymmetry of color and structure and the multicomponent global pattern.
- There are centrally located, irregular black dots and globules. At first blush one might think that these could represent pigment fragments located high up in the epidermis, which may or may not hail from malignant melanocytes.
- Foci of irregular black dots and globules seen at the periphery of a lesion are often associated with melanomas.
- Upon close inspection, there is also grayish-white color associated with the black dots and globules. This could represent regression (fibrosis and peppering).
- This assessment makes sense in the context of the histopathologic diagnosis of an irritated congenital nevus and given the patient's report of itching.
- An example of a good dermoscopic-pathologic correlation.

- In the lower section is a large area of hypopigmentation filled with regular pigment network.
- Diffuse light and dark brown color with a smudged appearance is a feature often seen in dysplastic nevi, but it may also be seen in inflamed nevi.
- In summary, pigment network identifies a melanocytic lesion. There is asymmetry of color and structure, the multicomponent global pattern, areas of peppering, hypopigmentation, smudging of light and dark brown color, and 5 colors in total.
- A positive feature is the absence of other criteria associated with melanoma, such as no irregular streaks, no irregular blotches, no milky-red color, no polymorphous vessels, to mention only a few.

PEARLS

- There are times when the significance of global features and local criteria will not be clear. At such times, your dermoscopic differential diagnostic skills will need to kick in.
- Do what you have to do to become as knowledgeable as possible. Your patients' lives depend on your dermoscopic skills.

CASE 28

HISTORY

A 62-year-old man with many light and dark seborrheic keratoses on his trunk and extremities performed periodic skin self-examinations because he has a history of nonmelanoma skin cancer. He did not notice this lesion located on his left shoulder that was brought to his attention by his dermatologist.

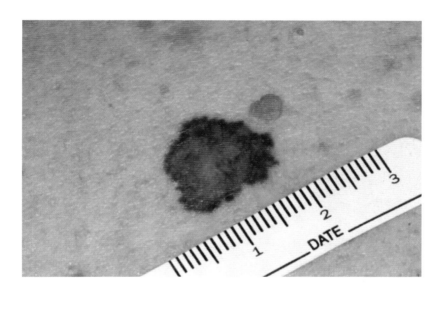

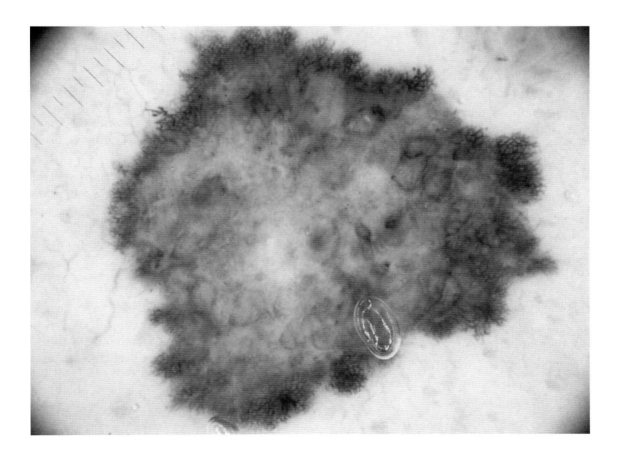

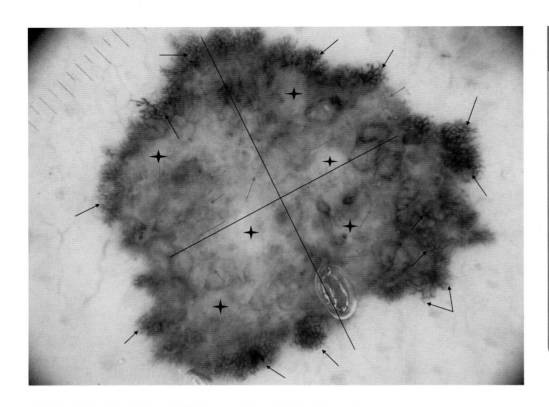

DERMOSCOPIC CRITERIA

- Asymmetry of color and structure (+)
- Homogeneous-reticular global pattern
- Irregular pigment network (black arrows)
- Irregular streaks (yellow arrows)
- Regression (stars)
- Gray color with peppering (red arrows)
- Milky-red/pink color (within the regression area)
- Five colors (light/dark brown, gray, white, pink)

DIAGNOSIS:
Superficial Spreading Melanoma

DISCUSSION

- Irregular pigment network at all points along the periphery identifies a melanocytic lesion.
- There is a good comparison between regular pigment network seen at the periphery in the previous case (fine, uniform light lines) and irregular pigment network (dark, thickened, branched, and broken up line segments) seen at the periphery in this case.
- There is asymmetry of color and structure.
- The global pattern could be considered reticular-homogeneous or multicomponent.
- Reticular-homogeneous because pigment network and whitish color are the main features filling the lesion.
- More dramatic than the irregular pigment network is the regression that fills the lesion.
- It is composed of bony-white and subtle milky-red/pink color plus gray peppering.
- White color represents scarring.
- Gray peppering represents melanophages and free melanin in the papillary dermis.

- The pinkish/milky-red color could represent neovascularization or inflammation.
- There are foci of irregular streaks (representing the radial growth phase of melanoma).
- Streaks may be found by themselves, attached to pigment network (as is the case here), or protruding from dark blotches.
- Note that there are no criteria to suggest this could be a seborrheic keratosis, such as milia-like cysts, pseudofollicular openings, fissures and ridges, fat fingers, and/or hairpin vessels.

PEARLS

- Seborrheic keratoses and melanoma can share one or more similar dermoscopic criteria.
- Be sure to examine carefully your patients with many seborrheic keratoses so that you do not miss a melanoma masquerading as a seborrheic keratosis.

CASE 29

HISTORY
This was found on the upper central back of a 62-year-old man at a free skin cancer screening.

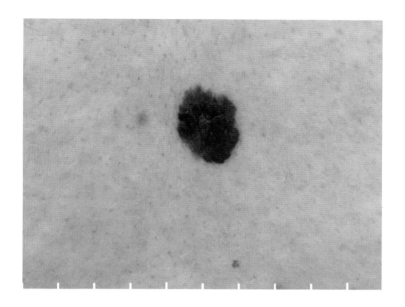

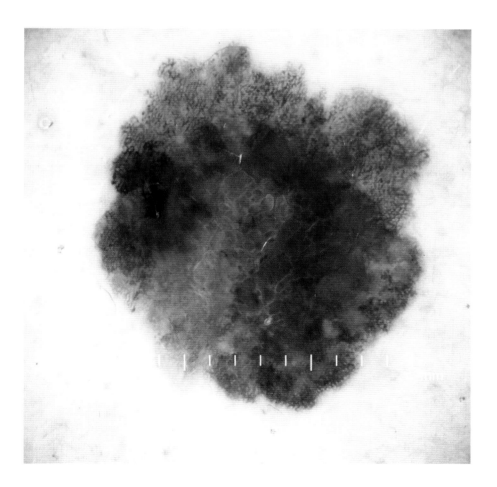

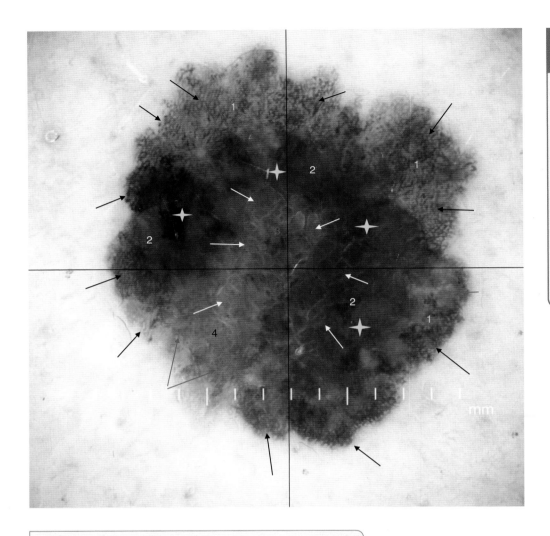

DIAGNOSIS:
Superficial Spreading Melanoma

DISCUSSION

- This is yet another melanoma with irregular pigment network surrounding the lesion at the periphery.
- There is significant asymmetry of color and structure with the multicomponent global pattern that has the following 4 different zones:
  - Zone 1 is composed of irregular pigment network and hypopigmentation.
  - Zone 2 is composed of an irregular blotch created by dark brown and black color.
  - Zone 3 is centrally located, formed by white network and some gray color.
  - Zone 4 is composed of a large area of hypopigmentation with barely perceptible regular pigment network.
- This is a dramatic example of how much color and structure you can see with dermoscopy that cannot be seen with the naked eye or even with the standard (nondermoscopic) magnification used by some clinicians.
- In summary, this early-invasive superficial spreading melanoma has the following criteria: asymmetry of color and structure, the multicomponent global pattern, irregular pigment network, an irregular blotch, white network, hypopigmentation, and peppering.

PEARLS

- This is another great case to study carefully to cement in your mind how irregular, melanoma-specific, high-risk criteria can look.
- Remember to always define the criteria you see in a given lesion as regular or irregular when making your dermoscopic analysis.

CASE 30

HISTORY
A 77-year-old man with years of excessive sun exposure has solar lentigines on all sun-exposed areas. This spot on his left forearm has been expanding slowly over the past several years.

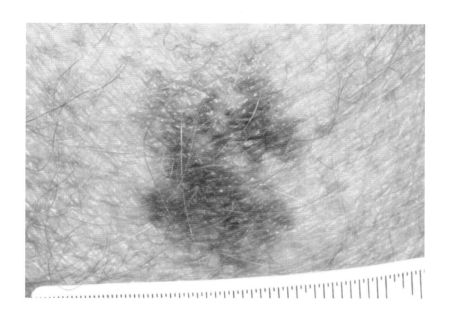

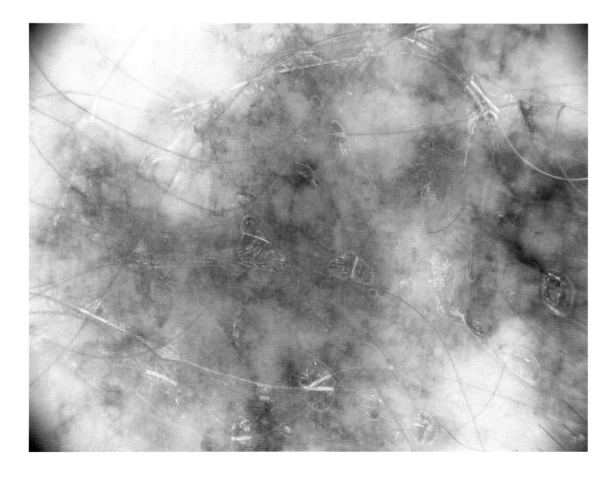

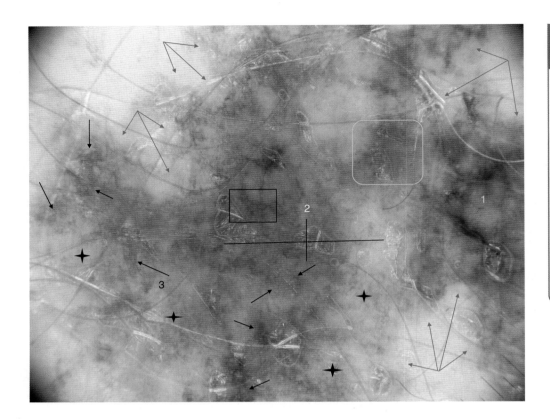

DIAGNOSIS:
In Situ Lentiginous Melanoma

DISCUSSION

- Foci of regular to slightly irregular pigment network found throughout diagnose a melanocytic lesion.
- There is asymmetry of color and structure with the multicomponent global pattern.
- Moth-eaten borders (concave and sharply demarcated borders) and hypopigmentation are also identified.
- The fingerprint pattern associated with a solar lentigo with parallel line segments is missing.
- The absence of the fingerprint pattern in a lesion that you think could be a solar lentigo should be a red flag for concern, especially in a slowly enlarging lesion.
- The focus of gray color represents inflammation. This is a common yet nonspecific feature seen in both benign and malignant lesions.
- Characteristics favoring diagnosis of a lentiginous melanoma include patient age over 40 to 60 years; growth that starts as a small tan macule and grows slowly over years; located on sun-exposed skin of the arms, legs, or trunk; and may or may not demonstrate the ABCDE clinical criteria.
- The differential diagnosis includes solar lentigo and flat (macular) seborrheic keratosis.
- One should use the same criteria to diagnose as with other melanomas.

PEARLS

- This subset of melanomas involving sun-exposed skin could easily be missed because of the following:
  - Low index of suspicion
  - Typically subtle clinical and dermoscopic features
- At times we may not be sure if a lesion is high-risk, but our "gut" feeling is that something is not right, which sounds our alarm.
- Negative gut feelings should never be ignored, and in most cases they warrant a histopathologic diagnosis.

CASE 31

HISTORY
A pediatrician referred a 4-year-old girl to diagnose this new black lesion on her right thigh.

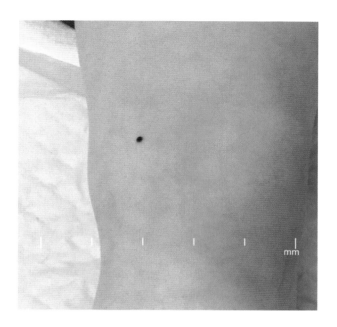

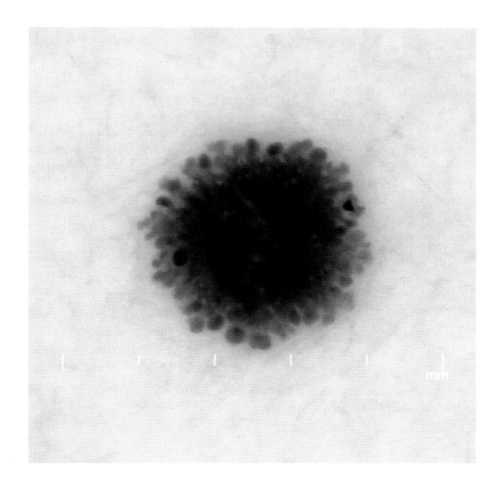

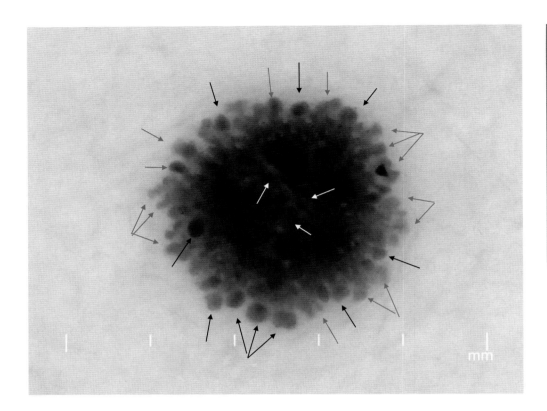

DIAGNOSIS:
Spitz Nevus

DISCUSSION

- This is the classic starburst pattern of a Spitz nevus.
- This pattern may have regular dots, globules, and/or streaks symmetrically located at all points along the periphery.
- The center of the lesion may have light brown color, a regular dark blotch, white network, or blue color.
- Indeed, there is a suggestion of a white network in the center of this lesion.
- The starburst pattern is the most common pattern seen in Spitz nevi. However, there are 5 other patterns that you might encounter:
  - Globular, which is filled with regular brown dots and globules. The only clue that it might be a Spitz nevus is the presence of some blue color within the lesion.
  - Homogeneous, which simply has shades of brown color, and the diagnosis of a Spitz nevus is usually a surprise.
  - Vascular, which is typically a pink papule that has pink/milky-red color and may have polymorphous

vessels. A very important point not to be overlooked is that the vascular pattern in the pediatric population may be indistinguishable from amelanotic melanoma.
- Black pigment network is the rarest presentation and is composed, not surprisingly, of just a prominent black pigment network. Similar to an ink spot lentigo.
- Nonspecific pattern, which itself may share any number of melanoma-specific criteria.

PEARLS

- Any lesion with features suggestive of a Spitz nevus is referred to as being *spitzoid*.
- Spitzoid melanomas can and do develop in the pediatric population, contrary to popular belief.
- Any atypical feature such as irregular streaks or irregular blotches should raise a red flag for concern.
- Finally, beware! Melanoma can have a *symmetrical* starburst pattern.

CASE 32

HISTORY

A 67-year-old Haitian man with Fitzpatrick skin Type 4 came in to treat some warts. A total-body skin examination was offered to the patient, and this lesion was found on his buttock.

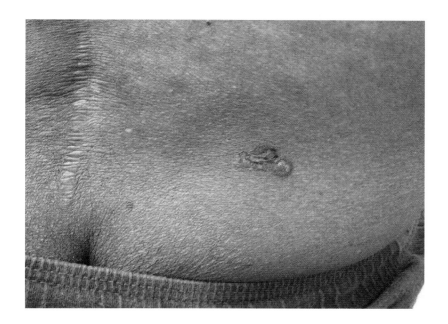

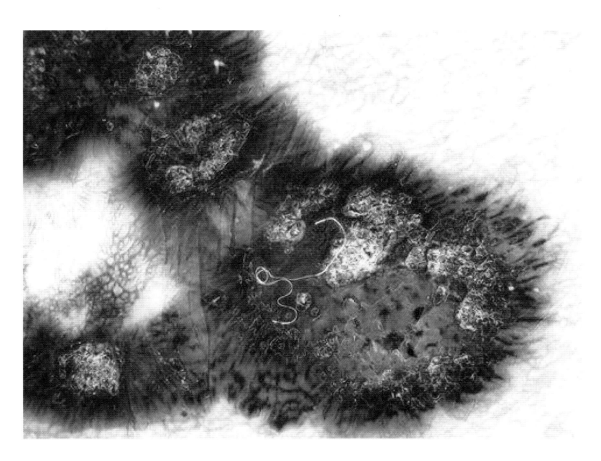

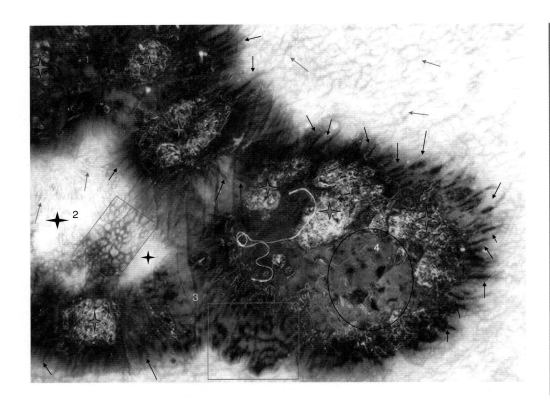

DERMOSCOPIC CRITERIA

- Asymmetry of color and structure
- Multicomponent global pattern (1,2,3,4)
- Irregular pigment network (boxes)
- Irregular streaks (black arrows)
- Irregular dots and globules (circle)
- Hyperkeratosis (red stars)
- Normal skin (black stars)
- Pigment network in surrounding skin (red arrows)
- Six colors (black, light/dark brown, gray, white, blue)

DIAGNOSIS:
In Situ Melanoma

DISCUSSION

- The intense dark blue color filling the lesion was a complete surprise and a red flag for concern, considering we thought clinically that it was a seborrheic keratosis. "If there's blue, they might sue!"
- Irregular streaks make this a spitzoid lesion.
- Any feature in a lesion that makes you think of a Spitz nevus should then be categorized as spitzoid.
- To review, streaks are defined as *regular* if they are roughly symmetrically located around the lesion. Streaks not symmetrically located around the lesion are defined as *irregular*. The shape of the streaks themselves is *not* the determining factor.
- There is asymmetry of color and structure and the multicomponent global pattern.
- There are 2 foci of irregular pigment network: one has a brown color and is easy to identify, whereas the other has black broken-up line segments. Whether the latter focus is a true network is debatable.

- There is also a focus of what looks like irregular black dots and globules.
- Hyperkeratosis and 6 colors round off the criteria of this in situ, seborrheic, keratosis-like melanoma.
- Of note, there is an irregular pigment network in the uninvolved skin surrounding the lesion. This network is not unusual to see in darker-skinned persons.

PEARLS

- Any acquired spitzoid lesion in an adult is always a red flag for concern and deserves a histopathologic diagnosis posthaste.
- The incidence of melanoma is increasing in nonwhite Latino, African American, and African Caribbean populations.
- Dermoscopy is helpful for all Fitzpatrick skin types.

CASE 33

HISTORY

While performing a routine yearly skin examination, this lesion was found on the upper inner arm of a 40-year-old woman.

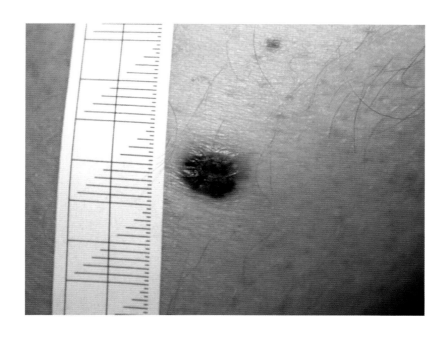

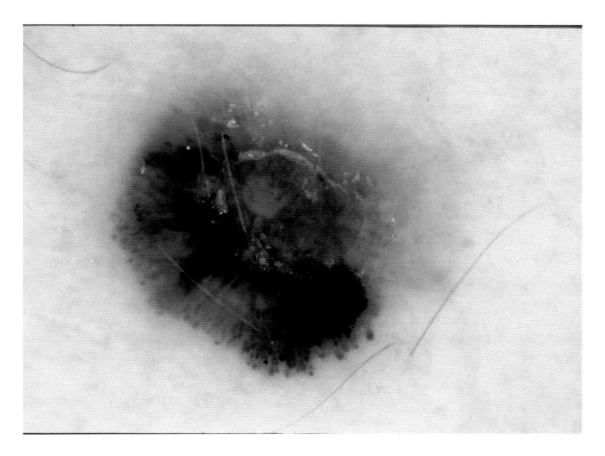

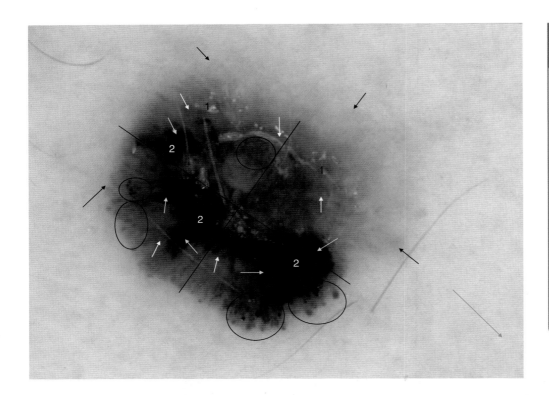

DERMOSCOPIC CRITERIA

- Asymmetry of color and structure (+)
- Multicomponent global pattern (1,2,3)
- Irregular dots and globules (circles)
- Irregular blotch (yellow arrows)
- Bluish-white veil (white arrows)
- Peripheral erythema (black arrows)
- Six colors (black, light/dark brown, blue, white, pink)

DIAGNOSIS:
Invasive Spitzoid Melanoma

DISCUSSION

- Irregular brown dots and globules identify a melanocytic lesion.
- There are asymmetry of color and structure and a multicomponent global pattern.
- There are an irregular black blotch and a bluish-white veil, which fill large parts of the lesion.
- Finally, there are irregular dots, globules, and possibly a few irregular streaks asymmetrically located at the periphery.
- With the foci of peripherally located irregular dots, globules, and streaks, we diagnose a highly irregular spitzoid pattern.
- Invasive spitzoid melanoma is at the top of our differential diagnostic list, and for that reason wide local excision of this lesion is the most appropriate next step.
- Spitzoid dermoscopic patterns do not always translate into spitzoid features histopathologically, and spitzoid histopathology does not always correspond with spitzoid dermoscopic features—in other words, there may be poor dermoscopic-pathologic correlation when confronted with spitzoid features.
- In summary, dots and globules identify a melanocytic lesion. There is asymmetry of color and structure, an atypical spitzoid global pattern with an irregular black blotch, bluish-white veil, peripheral erythema, a few streaks, and 6 colors.

PEARLS

- Both regular and irregular spitzoid patterns are always a red flag for concern, regardless of the age group.
- Following a symmetrical spitzoid pattern in a child as many dermoscopy "experts" do could be a fatal mistake.

CASE 34

HISTORY
This was found on the shoulder of a 77-year-old man.

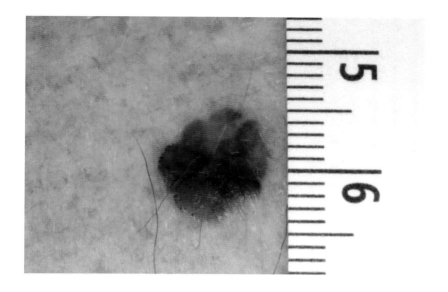

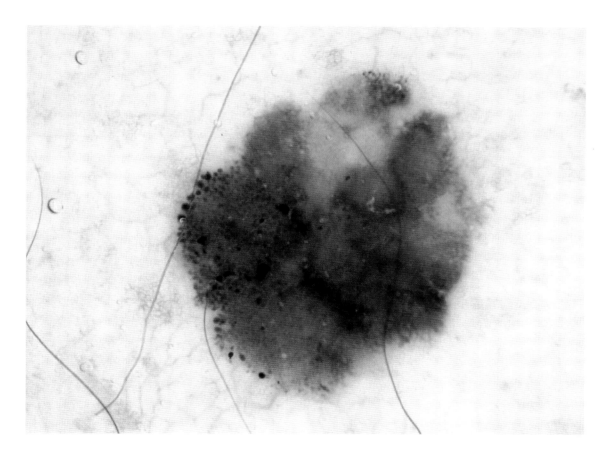

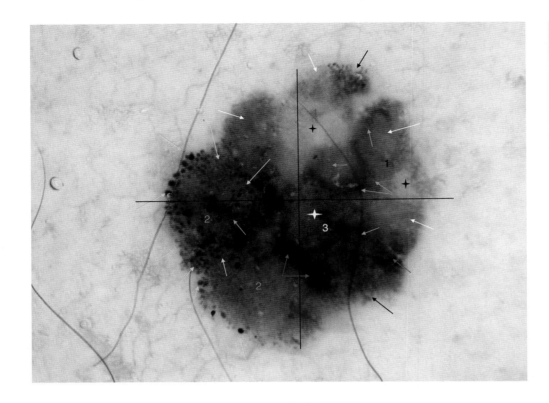

DIAGNOSIS:
Superficial Spreading Melanoma

DISCUSSION

- Irregular dots and globules and irregular pigment network diagnose a melanocytic lesion.
- Even though the dots and globules are seen at the periphery of the lesion, they also additionally fill a large portion of the lesion elsewhere. Thus, the pattern is not deemed to be spitzoid.
- There is dramatic asymmetry of color and structure with the multicomponent global pattern made up of 3 zones.
  - Zone 1 contains hypopigmentation, regression, and irregular pigment network. Significant gray peppering is seen within the regression area and other areas of the lesion.
  - Zone 2 is made up of irregular brown dots and globules, peppering, and diffuse erythema.
  - Zone 3 is made up of irregular black blotches, bluish-white veil, peppering, irregular network, and erythema.
- Of note, our delineation of the zones and what they contain is up for debate, because the criteria blend into each other. Nevertheless, it is obviously high-risk and supports a diagnosis of invasive melanoma.
- The extent of the bluish-white veil is not as well-developed as it was in our previous case.
- The pink color represents inflammation and blanches away with pressure from instrumentation.
- In summary, this superficial spreading melanoma has dramatic and well-developed melanoma-specific criteria, including asymmetry of color and structure, a multicomponent global pattern, irregular pigment network, irregular dots and globules, irregular black blotches, bluish-white veil, regression, hypopigmentation, and 7 colors.

PEARLS

- You might encounter well-developed regression areas with bony-white color and well-developed bluish-white veil. However, many times you will not.
- Remember, white and/or blue color in any form should always be a red flag for concern.

CASE 35

HISTORY

A 70-year-old woman was referred by her gynecologist to evaluate this changing pigmented skin lesion located on her right upper thigh.

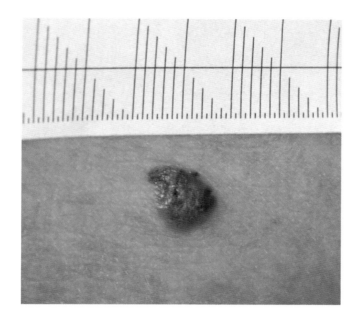

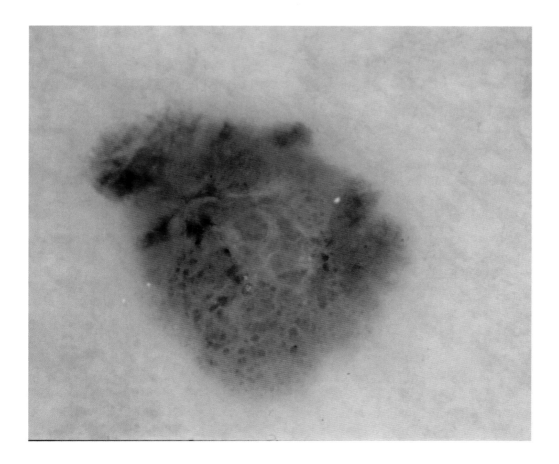

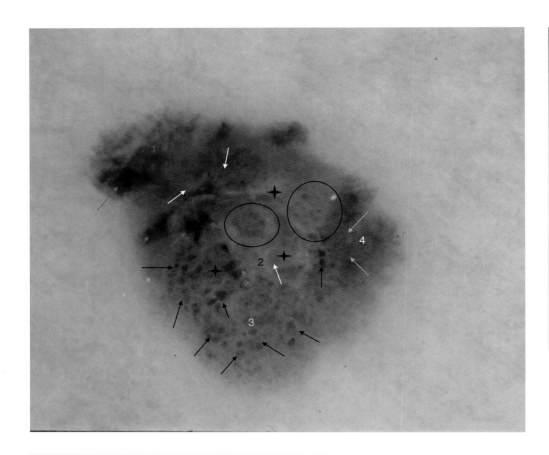

DERMOSCOPIC CRITERIA

- Asymmetry of color and structure
- Multicomponent global pattern (1,2,3,4)
- Irregular brown dots and globules (black arrows)
- Irregular blotches (red arrows)
- Milky-red color (stars)
- Milky-red globules (circles)
- Bluish-white color (white arrows)
- Irregular gray blotch (green arrows)

DIAGNOSIS:
Nodular Melanoma

DISCUSSION

- Irregular brown dots and globules reminiscent of the globular pattern diagnose a melanocytic lesion. This makes us think this nodular melanoma arose in a nevus.
- By contrast, meta-analyses have shown that the majority of melanomas actually arise de novo.
- There is asymmetry of color and structure and a multicomponent global pattern with 4 zones.
- The centrally located milky-red area with milky-red globules is a very important feature that suggests this is a deeply invasive melanoma.
- Adjacent to the milky-red area are nonimpressive irregular black blotches and a focus of gray color that represents peppering.
- This is a good case to compare the *in-focus* irregular brown dots and globules (nests of atypical melanocytes) to the *out-of-focus* milky-red globules (neovascularization).
- There is a poorly defined focus of bluish-white color that does not fit the definition of the veil.

- The preoperative dermoscopic analysis favors the diagnosis of invasive superficial spreading melanoma. The histopathologic diagnosis of nodular melanoma was therefore unexpected.
- To wit, nodular melanoma typically has a paucity of well-developed local criteria (ie, the dots and globules) and more intense areas of blue, black, pink color and polymorphous vessels.
- Foci of local criteria are usually found at the periphery of nodular melanomas.

PEARLS

- It is important to differentiate the well-demarcated, sharply *in-focus* vascular spaces (lacunae) and fibrous septae of a benign vascular lesion from the *out-of-focus* irregular milky-red globules and color of a deeply invasive melanoma.
- Be aware that melanoma and cutaneous metastatic melanoma may be hemangioma-like.
- Always remember, "If in doubt, cut it out!"

CASE 36

HISTORY

A 27-year-old man with a history of melanoma on his back presented at your office with multiple similar-looking lesions not only in his melanoma scar but all over his back.

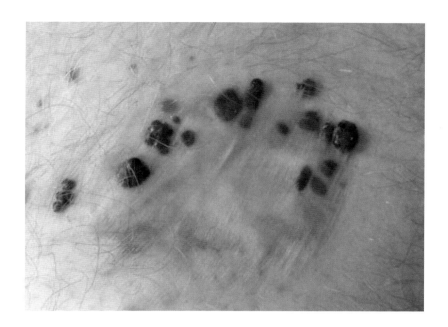

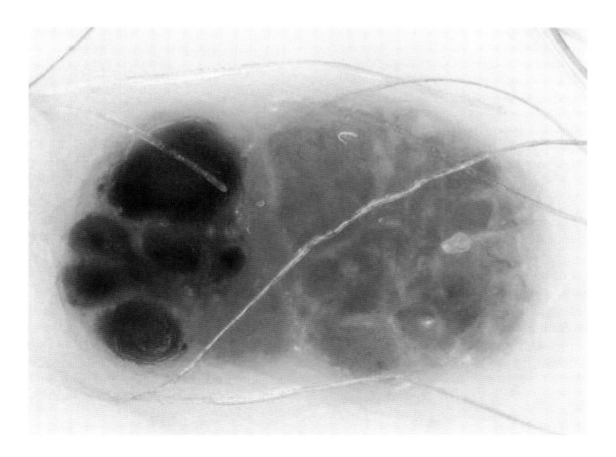

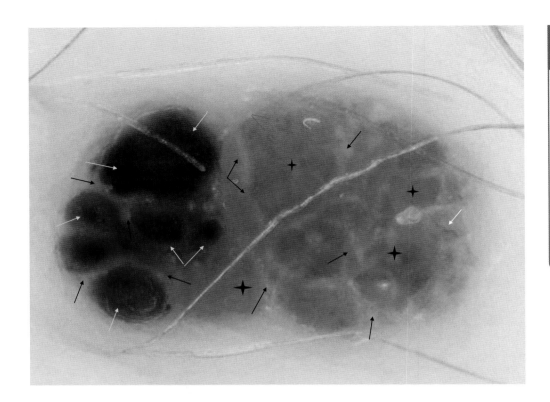

DERMOSCOPIC CRITERIA

- Asymmetry of color and structure
- Lacunae-like roundish blotches (yellow arrows)
- Diffuse orange-brown color (stars)
- Furrows (black arrows)
- Irregular hairpin vessels (red arrows)
- Serpentine vessel (white arrow)

DIAGNOSIS:
Cutaneous Metastatic Melanoma

DISCUSSION

- In a "blink" before you lay your dermatoscope on this unfortunate young man, you know this is not good.
- At first blush the left side of the lesion has well-demarcated roundish purplish-black lacunae-like areas and the right side of the lesion has a peculiar orange-brown color.
- Orange color is seen in granulomatous lesions.
- Could this be a collision tumor such as a hemangioma with possibly an amelanotic melanoma? (Collision tumors are defined as 2 or more different pathologies that can be adjacent to one another or one within the other.)
- On closer inspection, there are 2 irregular hairpin vessels and one serpentine vessel in the light area.
- The white lines appear to be furrows as one would see in a papillomatous nevus or seborrheic keratosis.
- The white lines also look like fibrous septae that can be seen in hemangiomas (dermoscopic differential diagnosis).
- Of note, the multiple lesions on his back all appear similar clinically and dermoscopically.

- A biopsy confirmed our clinical impression of cutaneous metastatic melanoma.
- This is an example of a relatively rare hemangioma-like cutaneous metastatic melanoma.
- The history of a previous melanoma in the area of cutaneous metastatic melanoma is usually more helpful to make the diagnosis than what you see with dermoscopy.
- The dermoscopic features of cutaneous metastatic melanoma can range from A to Z with any combination of criteria that are known to us.
- A patient can have monomorphous lesions as is the case here or a heterogeneous combination of pigmented and amelanotic lesions.

PEARLS

- Be aware that there are seborrheic keratosis–like melanomas, basal cell–like melanomas, hemangioma-like melanomas, dermatofibroma-like melanomas and more.
- Be aware that collision tumors can have combinations of benign-benign (eg, nevus and hemangioma) or benign-malignant pathologies (eg, seborrheic keratosis and basal cell carcinoma).

CASE 37

HISTORY
This was a curious lesion on the back of a 20-year-old woman.

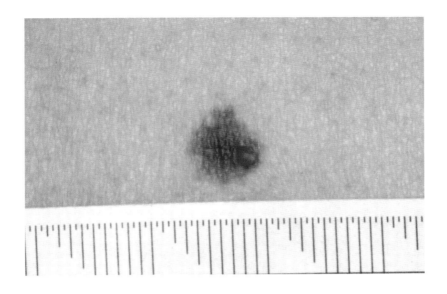

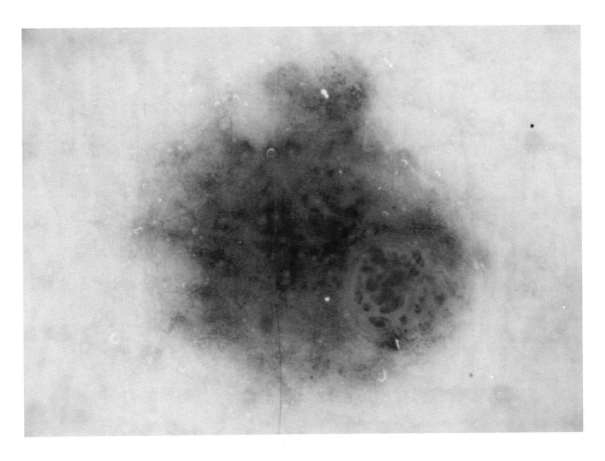

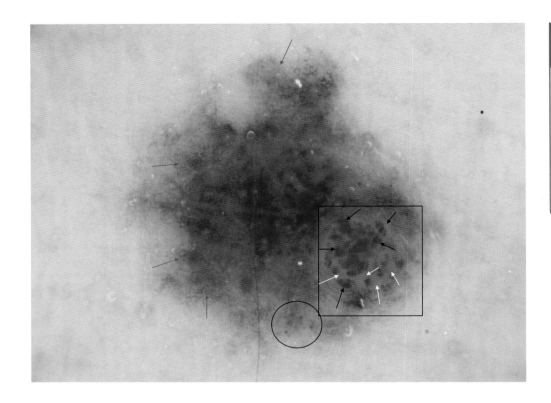

DIAGNOSIS:
Collision Tumor Junctional Nevus and Hemangioma

DISCUSSION

- There are by nature 2 components in this collision tumor: a junctional nevus and a hemangioma.
- The junctional nevus is composed of regular pigment network, a focus of tiny regular brown dots and globules, and a central area of darker brown color. Light and dark brown colors are commonly found in benign nevi.
- The hemangioma is classic with well-demarcated vascular spaces (lacunae) and fibrous septae.
- There are no atypical features compared with the previous case of hemangioma-like metastatic melanoma.
- This is an easy, low-risk case to diagnose.
- If the patient was concerned, you could reassure him or her that there is no problem with this pigmented skin lesion.

- The most common tumors found in collision are seborrheic keratoses, melanocytic nevi, hemangiomas, basal cell carcinomas, in situ and invasive squamous cell carcinomas, and in situ or invasive melanomas, whether pigmented or amelanotic.
- And, any combination is possible.
- Triple collision tumors exist, but are not common.

PEARLS

- As a general rule, identify the criteria in a collision tumor and determine if they are regular or irregular, just as you would do with a noncollision tumor.
- If there is any suggestion of high-risk pathology, make a histopathologic diagnosis posthaste.

CASE 38

HISTORY

This seborrheic keratosis-like lesion was found on the back of an 80-year-old man. The patient was not aware of its presence.

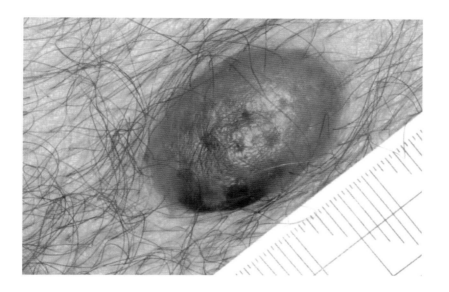

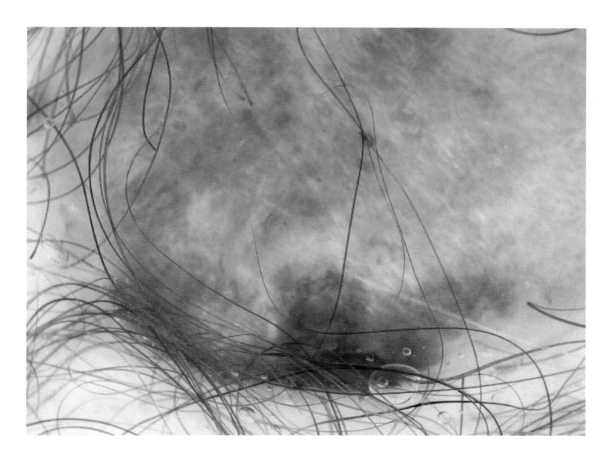

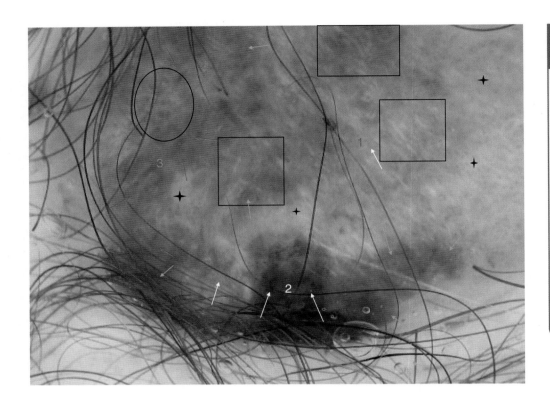

DIAGNOSIS:
Nodular Melanoma

DISCUSSION

- It is important to examine with dermoscopy even banal-looking lesions to avoid missing incognito melanomas.
- Clinically this looks like a seborrheic keratosis, but there are no dermoscopic criteria to make that diagnosis—your first red flag for concern.
- A focus of light brown irregular globules diagnoses a melanocytic lesion.
- If you missed those globules, then this should be considered to be melanocytic by default.
- Blue color and crystalline structures are your second set of clues that this could be a melanoma.
- Pink/milky-red color is another high-risk clue: "If there's pink, stop and think!"
- Diffuse bony-white color suggestive of regression fills the lesion. "If there's white, control your fright!"
- Patchy light and dark brown color are also identified. Brown color, even though it is nonspecific, also favors a melanocytic lesion.
- This 11-mm nodular melanoma with an artist's palette of high-risk colors and its paucity of local criteria give you enough clues to warrant a histopathologic diagnosis posthaste.
- In summary, there is no good clinico-dermoscopic correlation, because clinically, but not dermoscopically, it looks like a seborrheic keratosis. There are asymmetry of color and structure; multicomponent global pattern; bluish-white color suggestive of melanosis; bony-white color suggestive of regression; irregular brown globules; crystalline structures, which in a melanocytic lesion favor the diagnosis of a melanoma; and milky-red color.
- There is nothing good in this hidden nodular lesion.

PEARLS

- You should always seek a good clinico-dermoscopic–pathologic correlation.
- There will be times when you will only have dermoscopic clues and not concrete features to help make a diagnosis. This holds true especially for amelanotic, desmoplastic, and nodular melanomas.

CASE 39

HISTORY

This was one of 4 suspicious pinkish lesions on the arms of an 84-year-old retired physician.

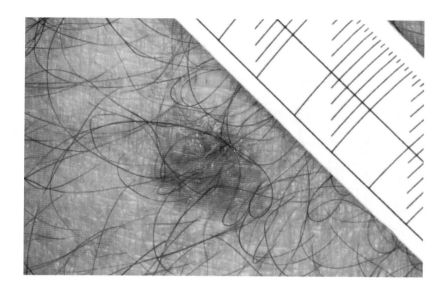

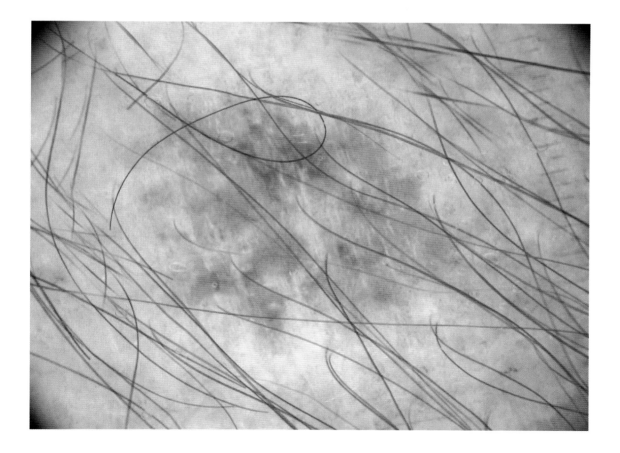

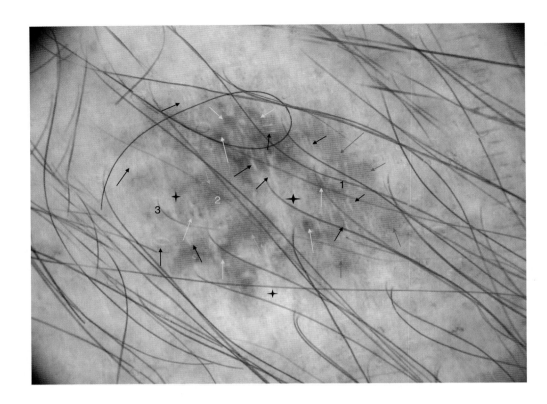

DERMOSCOPIC CRITERIA

- Asymmetry of color and structure
- Multicomponent global pattern (1,2,3)
- Bony-white color (stars)
- Peppering (yellow arrows)
- Milky-red/pink color with polymorphous vessels (red arrows)
- Crystalline structures (black arrows)
- Irregular hypopigmentation (green arrows)

DIAGNOSIS:
Superficial spreading Melanoma

DISCUSSION

- Pink color is nonspecific and can define melanocytic, nonmelanocytic, benign, malignant, or even inflammatory lesions.
- Small pink lesions on sun-exposed skin in the older population typically can be basal or squamous cell carcinoma or melanoma (amelanotic). Statistically, however, amelanotic melanoma is less common.
- The type of vessels identified is a very important clue and guides the dermoscopic diagnosis.
- Arborizing vessels suggest a basal cell carcinoma.
- Pinpoint/glomerular vessels point to the diagnosis of Bowen disease.
- Polymorphous vessels suggest melanoma.
- The combination of milky-red/pink color and polymorphous vessels is even more suggestive of melanoma.
- This lesion is melanocytic by default, and there are many clues to suggest this is a melanoma.
  - Bony-white color with peppering and crystalline structures.
  - Milky-red/pink color with polymorphous vessels (the tiny vessels are not clearly seen at this magnification).

- With the negative feature of the absence of vessels associated with basal or squamous cell carcinoma and the potentially high-risk criteria, melanoma should now be at the top of your differential diagnostic list.
- The previous case with similar criteria was a nodule, and deep invasion was expected. This lesion was slightly elevated, and the diagnosis of early-invasive melanoma is a logical dermoscopic-pathologic correlation.
- A flat lesion is better than a slightly-raised lesion, and nodules are potentially the most invasive when it comes to melanomas.

PEARLS

- The sensitivity and specificity of a dermoscopic diagnosis is much better in pigmented versus pink lesions.
- Dermoscopy is not as helpful for pink lesions.
- Any clinical and/or dermoscopic pink lesion should always be a red flag for concern. "If it's pink, stop and think!"
- Beware! Pink/amelanotic melanoma can be featureless with dermoscopy!

CASE 40

HISTORY
A 69-year-old woman was referred to you by her primary care provider because the patient was concerned about this lesion on her lower leg.

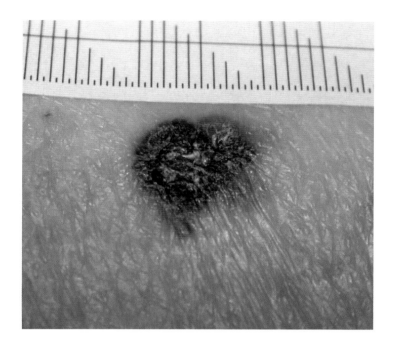

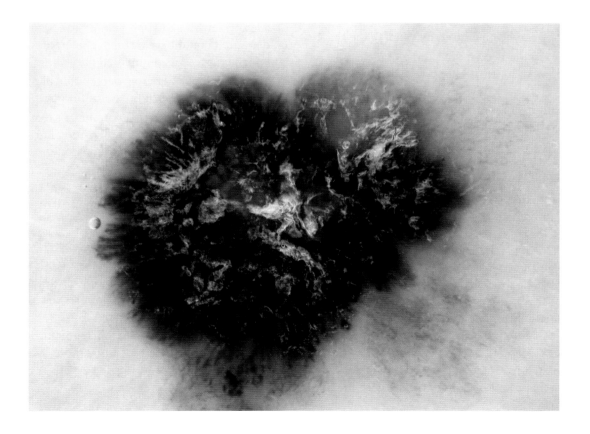

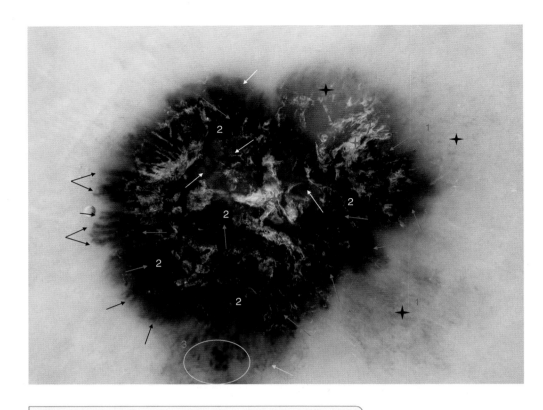

DIAGNOSIS:
Secondary Nodular Melanoma

DISCUSSION

- This should be easy to analyze at this point in the chapter.
- A focus of irregular brown dots and globules and irregular pigment network diagnose a melanocytic lesion.
- There is significant asymmetry of color and structure. The left half of the lesion is not a mirror image of the right half, nor is the upper half a mirror image of the lower half.
- There are 3 zones in this multicomponent global pattern:
  - Zone 1 is made up of peripheral irregular hypopigmentation with a suggestion of fine regular pigment network.
  - Zone 2 is the most dramatic feature and is made up of an irregular, very black blotch with well-developed foci of irregular streaks and hyperkeratosis.
  - Zone 3 at the bottom of the lesion is a small area of hypopigmentation that contains a focus of irregular brown dots and globules and a focus of irregular pigment network.
- The black blotch is irregular, because it demonstrates an irregular shape and irregular borders with foci of hyperkeratosis.

- A regular black blotch of a benign nevus could also fill a lesion, in which case it would have a uniform border and it could have a shiny appearance. (The black lamella represents pigmented parakeratosis.)
- There is a focus of barely perceptible bluish-white color that does not fit the definition of the veil.
- A common theme is that you may or may not see a classic veil, and that's OK because blue and or/white color in any presentation should be considered high-risk.
- In this case the bluish-white color is of minor significance compared with the dramatic irregular black blotch.

PEARLS

- Black color in a flat lesion with well-developed local criteria (eg, network, dots, globules) favors an in situ or early-invasive melanoma.
- Black color with a paucity of irregular criteria at the border favors the diagnosis of a more deeply invasive melanoma.

CASE 41

HISTORY

This innocuous-looking spot on the posterior upper arm of an 82-year-old man catches your eye while you are doing a total-body skin examination, and you decide to examine it further with dermoscopy.

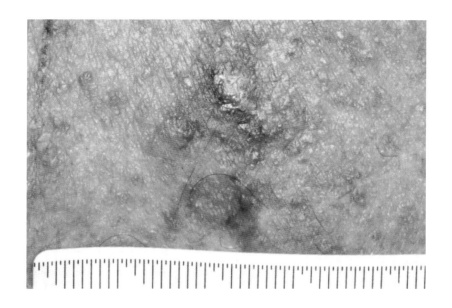

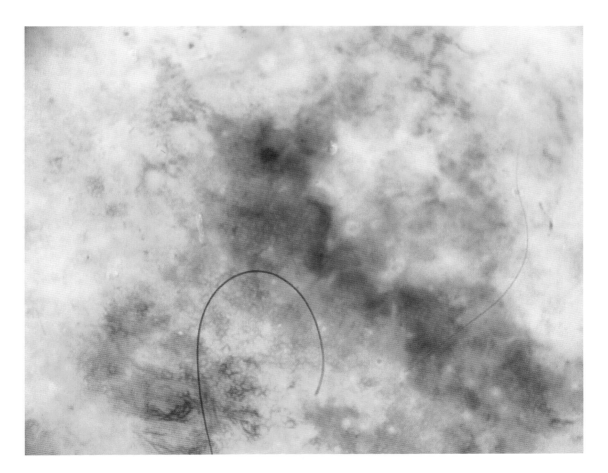

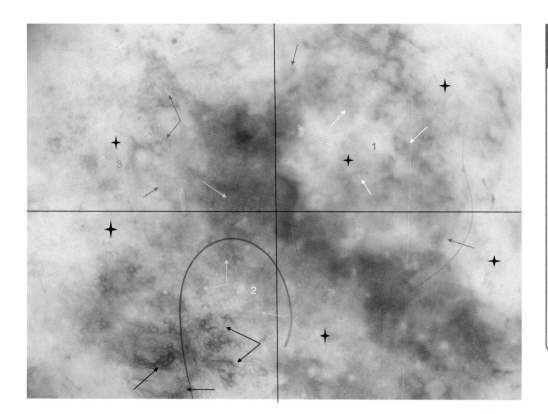

DERMOSCOPIC CRITERIA

- Asymmetry of color and structure (+)
- Multicomponent global pattern (1,2,3)
- Irregular pigment network (black arrows)
- Regular pigment network (yellow arrows)
- Regression (stars)
- Gray peppering (red arrows)
- Blue melanosis (white arrows)
- Five colors (light/dark brown, white, gray, blue)

DIAGNOSIS:
Regressive Melanoma

DISCUSSION

- Regular and irregular pigment network diagnoses a melanocytic lesion.
- Large areas of irregular white, gray, and blue colors offer important clues that this could be a regressive melanoma.
- Now look for more melanoma-specific criteria.
  - There is asymmetry of color and structure—the left half of the lesion is not the mirror image of the right half, and the upper half is not the mirror image of the lower half.
  - There is the multicomponent global pattern with 3 different zones.
  - Inter-observer agreement might not be 100% on the exact number of zones. This is a minor point in the context of the overall analysis of this lesion.
  - The regression area is made up of diffuse bony-white color with foci of gray and blue color.
  - Gray represents peppering and blue represents melanosis.
  - Peppering might be the only criterion left in a regressive melanoma.

- Peppering has a dermoscopic differential diagnosis that includes postinflammatory hyperpigmentation and the chronic stage of a lichen planus–like keratosis.
- Of note, regression in most cases will be made of up white and gray color. Blue color is encountered less frequently.
- The clinical and dermoscopic appearance of melanoma can be dramatic as seen in the previous case or understated as in this case of invasive regressive melanoma.

PEARLS

- A Wood's lamp examination can help visualize regressive melanoma.
- A focused, unrushed cutaneous examination with a good eye, a high index of suspicion, and, most important, dermoscopic knowledge, helps find potentially high-risk lesions that have subtle clinical and/or dermoscopic features.
- "One cannot see what one does not know," Johann Von Goethe.

CASE 42

HISTORY

An 80-year-old African American woman came in specifically to check this lesion on the bottom of her left foot that has been present for 2 years.

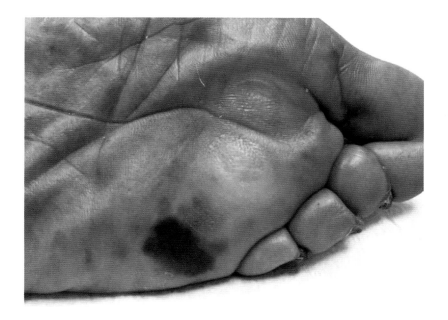

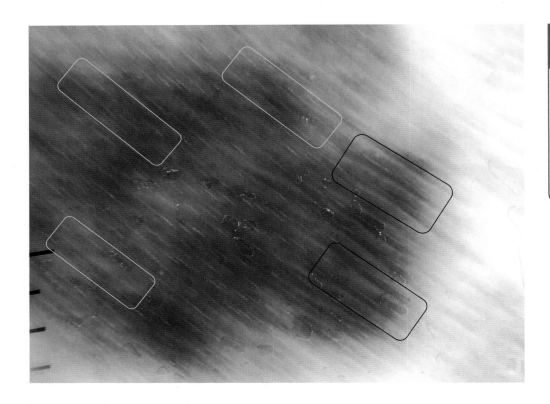

DIAGNOSIS:
In Situ Acral lentiginous Melanoma

DISCUSSION

- With this very irregular pigmented lesion on the plantar surface of an African American person, you know that this is a melanoma, and you expect to see the parallel-ridge pattern associated with acral melanoma.
- The periphery of the lesion has a well-developed parallel-ridge pattern with light thinner furrows that surround dark brown thicker ridges.
- The rest of the lesion has a less well-developed parallel-ridge pattern with very thin, broken up white lines representing furrows outlining linear hyperpigmented ridges.
- The "string of pearls" that are always found in the ridges are not seen in this case.
- To our surprise, a skin biopsy did not diagnose in situ acral melanoma.
- This was not a good clinical-dermoscopic-pathologic correlation.
- The pathology was reviewed by the dermatopathologist, and it was confirmed that the biopsy did not diagnose melanoma.
- A repeat sampling biopsy also did not demonstrate melanoma.
- Despite the repeat pathology results, clinically and dermoscopically with a classic malignant parallel-ridge pattern, the patient was nevertheless referred to a Mohs surgeon for excision.
- The final excisional pathology finding did reach the level of in situ acral lentiginous melanoma.

PEARLS

- This case points out that there will be times when the dermatopathologist will have difficulty making the diagnosis of acral melanoma.
- This might translate into the surgeon being hesitant to do a wide excision when the pathology is not diagnostic.
- With a well-developed malignant parallel-ridge pattern and an equivocal pathology report, your dermoscopy helps you to reassure the surgeon that the lesion is atypical and that he or she should proceed with excision to rule out melanoma.

CASE 43

HISTORY

A 32-year-old man was aware of this lesion on the bottom of his right foot. As far as he knows, it has never changed. But he admits he rarely checks it.

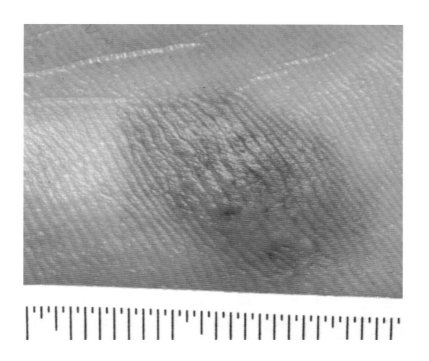

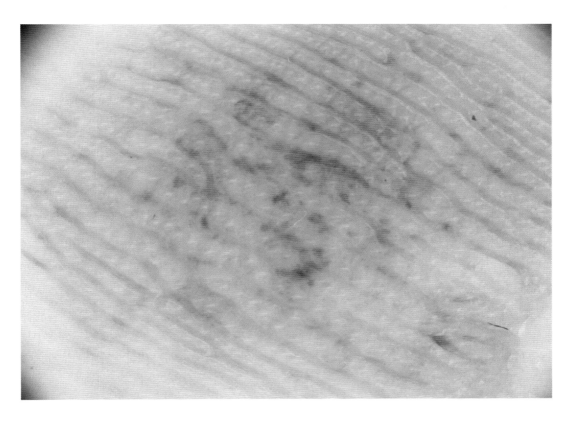

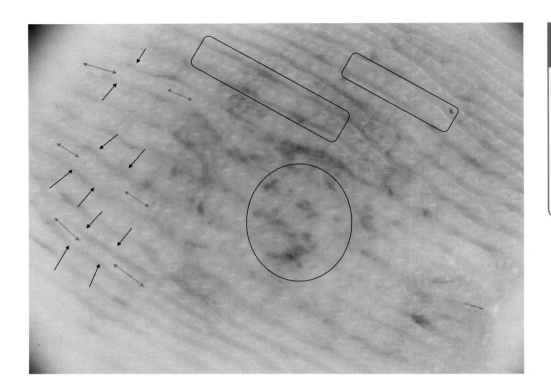

DERMOSCOPIC CRITERIA

- Parallel-furrow pattern
- Pigmented thin furrows (black arrows)
- Thicker light ridges (red arrows)
- Acrosyringia/"string of pearls" (rectangles)
- Peppering (circle)

DIAGNOSIS:
Acral Nevus

DISCUSSION

- This is a banal-appearing acral nevus with the classic benign parallel-furrow pattern (contrast to the parallel-ridge pattern of the previous malignant acral lesion).
- The parallel-furrow pattern is the most common benign acral pattern you will encounter.
- The parallel thin brown lines represent pigment in the furrows ("furrows are fine").
- The pigmentation of the furrows borders the thicker light ridges that are filled with acrosyringia.
- Acrosyringia represent intraepidermal eccrine sweat ducts, and they are always in the ridges.
- Typically, they are linear monomorphous white dots that are said to resemble a string of pearls.
- Acrosyringia may or may not be present in an acral melanotic lesion, and they can also be found in normal surrounding skin.
- However, an irregular, nonlinear presentation of acrosyringia should be a red flag for concern and can be seen in irritated nevi and in melanoma.

- The centrally located grayish color represents peppering, which represents a localized inflammatory reaction. Inflammation may be expected, because the plantar surface of the foot is constantly traumatized during routine walking.
- With this clinical and dermoscopic presentation, a histopathologic diagnosis is not indicated, and the patient can be reassured that it is a benign nevus. He should also be instructed to make his feet be part of his monthly total-body self-examinations.

PEARLS

- There are times when you will not be able to determine if pigmentation is in the furrows of a benign lesion or in the ridges of a melanoma.
- Search for the string of pearls, because it will always be in the ridges.
- The presence of this string of pearls might be the only way to differentiate a benign parallel-furrow pattern from a malignant parallel-ridge pattern.
- And remember, "If in doubt, cut it out!"

CASE 44

HISTORY

A 25-year-old man was not concerned about this mole on the bottom of his right foot.

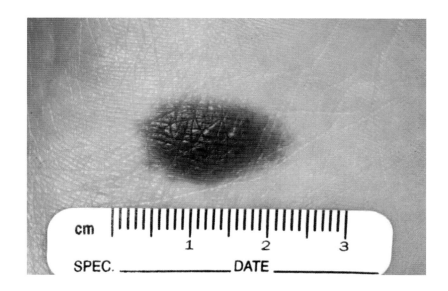

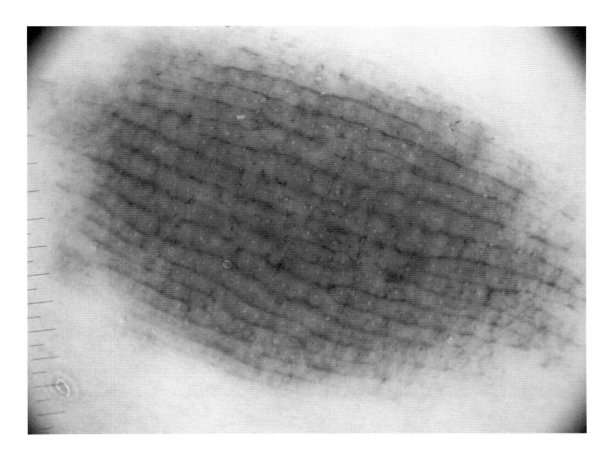

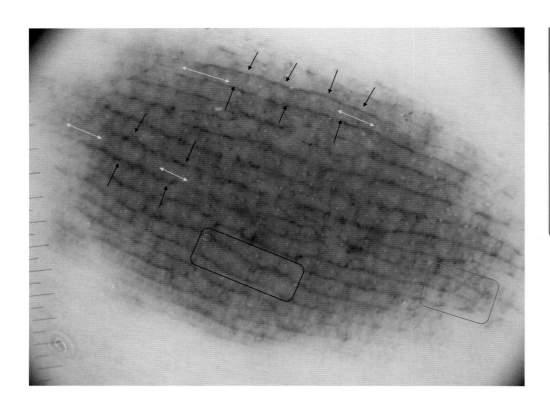

DIAGNOSIS:
Acral Nevus

DISCUSSION

- Clinically the nevus has no atypical features, but the dermoscopic picture appears less straightforward.
- Linear dark brown color is seen in all of the furrows that border thicker ridges.
- The ridges have acrosyringia, some areas have bluish color, and some areas tannish color.
- The bluish color is a red flag for concern. However, this does not always translate into high-risk pathology—it could simply represent inflammation.
- In this case, the bluish color represents pigmentation located deeper in the dermis, similar to what might be seen in a combined or blue nevus (the Tyndall effect).
- The tan color in the ridges represents background pigmentation of the nevus. However, pigmentation in the parallel-ridge pattern is not always dark brown; it could be tan.
- There is no asymmetry of color or structure; a positive finding.
- The disposition of this lesion would depend on the dermoscopist's experience.

- An experienced dermoscopist will likely diagnose a benign acral nevus and follow it over time to look for changes in the form of baseline clinical and dermoscopic images to be used for comparison at follow-up visit(s).
- A novice dermoscopist seeing bluish color and pigmentation in the ridges might be worried and want to make a histopathologic diagnosis (optimal for the patient) by taking a less invasive, incisional biopsy and not by wide excision to rule out melanoma.

PEARLS

- Acral lesions can be difficult to diagnose, often having conflicting dermoscopic features.
- With experience, your confidence will grow, and lesions that may have looked worrisome in the past but turned out to be low-risk will look less worrisome when seen again.
- The dermoscopy learning curve is steep, but not insurmountable.

CASE 45

HISTORY

A 33-year-old runner came in because this mole on the side of her foot had been itching.

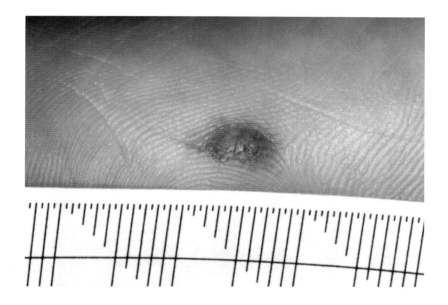

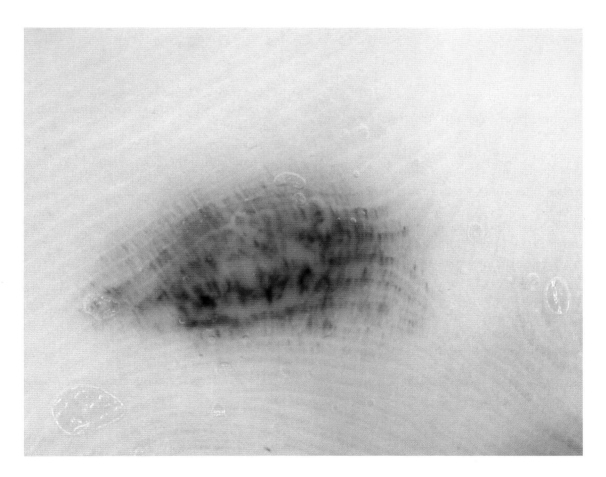

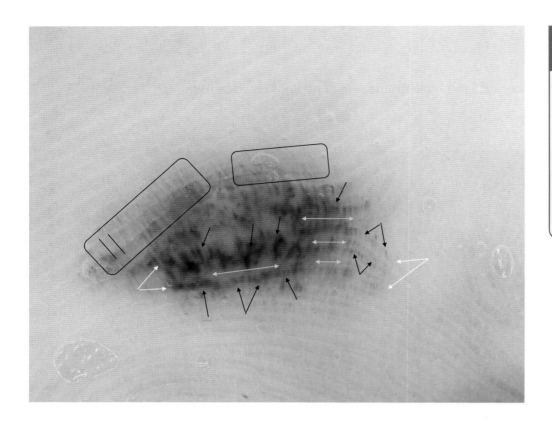

DERMOSCOPIC CRITERIA

- Parallel-furrow pattern (white arrows)
- Fibrillar pattern (rectangles)
- Dots and globules in furrows (black arrows)
- Ridges (yellow arrows)
- Gray peppering (green arrows)

DIAGNOSIS:
Irritated Acral Nevus

DISCUSSION

- There is asymmetry of color and structure, a red flag for concern.
- There are 2 benign acral patterns in this nevus.
- There are fibrillar pattern with very fine, tan oblique lines at the periphery of the lesion and the parallel-furrow pattern.
- In this case, the parallel-furrow pattern is made up of regular and irregular brown dots and globules.
- There are several variations that can create the parallel-furrow pattern.
  - A more common pattern, which has uniform brown parallel lines in the thin skin furrows.
  - Less frequently, one may see a single or double row of lines and/or dots and globules in the furrows.
- In many cases, the lines, dots, and globules are broken up and irregular in their shape and color.

- There is also a focus of gray color representing peppering, an inflammatory reaction secondary to the trauma of running.
- Even though a biopsy is indicated, you can reassure the patient that there is a very little chance that this will be a melanoma as there is no suggestion of the malignant parallel-ridge pattern in any portion of this lesion.

PEARLS

- In general, asymmetry of color and structure at any location is always a red flag for concern.
- A lesion with an unusual benign pattern or more than one benign acral pattern should also be a red flag for concern.
- The parallel-ridge pattern is not the only pattern you can see in acral melanomas.

CASE 46

HISTORY
A 48-year-old woman is concerned about these spots. They will not go away and she is getting more for no reason.

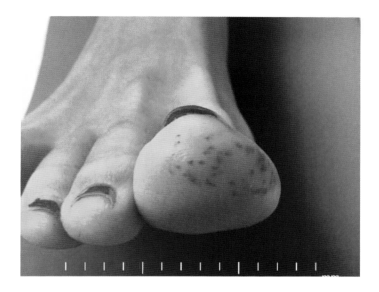

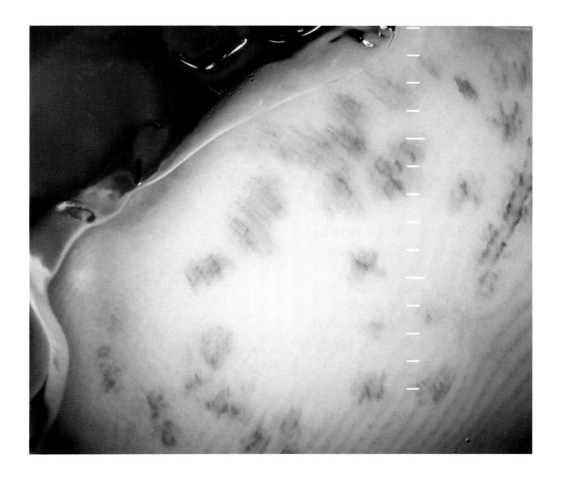

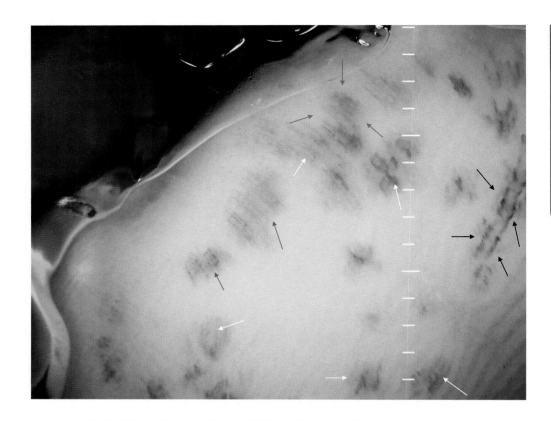

DIAGNOSIS:
In Situ Multicentric Acral Melanoma

DISCUSSION

- The history and clinical appearance of irregular tan macules on the toe is unusual and worrisome.
- The dermoscopic picture is also worrisome with asymmetry of color and structure and what appear to be varying benign acral patterns.
- On close inspection there is one focus of parallel-furrow pattern.
- There appear to be a few foci of the fibrillar pattern.
- We would have to stretch our imagination to discern a focus of the parallel-ridge pattern.
- There are also multiple irregular tan blotches.
- A biopsy was performed and was read as a junctional nevus. Given a poor dermoscopic-pathologic correlation, another biopsy was performed, and the diagnosis of in situ melanoma was made.
- This is a very unusual case of multicentric acral melanoma.
- The area was excised and grafted, and the patient is doing well with no recurrence.

- A lesion with multiple benign acral patterns could be a melanoma.
- A plausible theory here is that there are not enough atypical cells to create the parallel-ridge pattern associated with acral melanoma.
- Sampling error should be taken into account when the dermoscopic-pathologic correlation is poor, and repeat biopsy may be critical to making the correct diagnosis as was the case here.

PEARLS

- Maintain a high index of suspicion with acral lesions, because the clinical and dermoscopic findings may not be clear-cut. If you cannot be sure a lesion is benign, do not hesitate to take one or more than one biopsy for histopathologic diagnosis.
- A good dermoscopic-pathologic correlation is essential.

CASE 47

HISTORY

These nevi were found on the bottom of the right foot in a 50-year-old woman during a routine total-body skin examination.

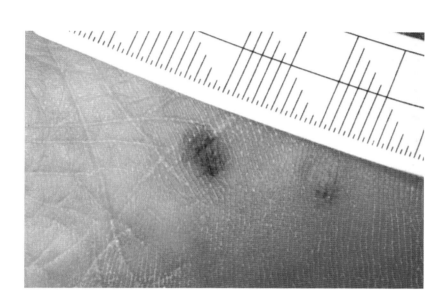

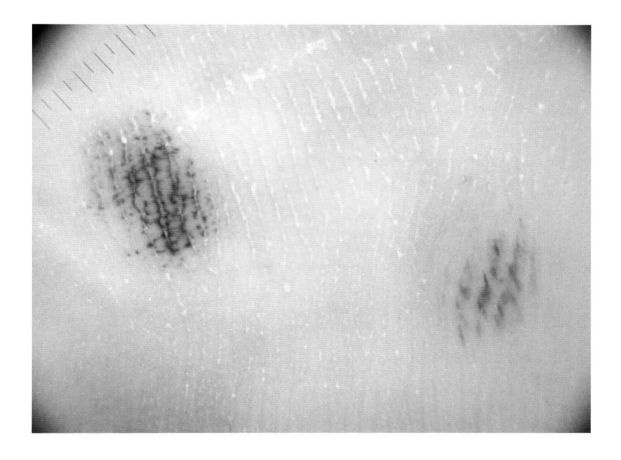

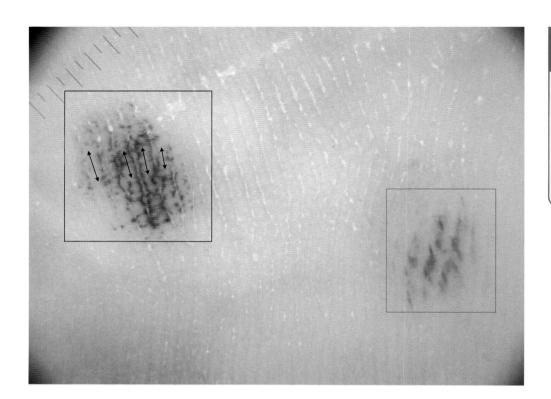

DIAGNOSIS:
Acral Nevi

DISCUSSION

- This is a typical scenario compared with the previous case—finding innocuous-looking nevi on the plantar surface of the feet.
- This patient has the benign fibrillar pattern with oblique fine lines and the benign double-line variant of the parallel-furrow pattern. Histopathologic diagnosis is not indicated.
- The double-line variant is made up of 2 fine brown lines forming the borders of the furrows.
- The parallel-furrow pattern can have a single or double line in the furrows with or without brown dots and globules.
- A review of the common acral patterns is in the following order:
  - The parallel-furrow pattern shows pigmented lines in the typically thin skin furrows. This is the most common benign acral pattern.
  - The lattice-like pattern with fine linear pigmentation in the furrows and fine lines running perpendicular to the furrows gives the appearance of a lattice or ladder.
  - The fibrillar pattern shows fine lines running obliquely.
- The parallel-ridge pattern is associated with melanoma with pigmentation in the ridges. The ridges may or may not contain acrosyringia (string of pearls).
- The parallel-ridge pattern is not diagnostic of melanoma. Rather, it may also be seen in skin hemorrhage or in hemangiomas with red or purple lacunae seen in the ridges.
- Amelanotic acral melanoma could appear to be a hemangioma. The irregular distribution of lacunae is a clue that the "hemangioma" is really a melanoma.
- The parallel-ridge pattern can also be seen diffusely on acral surface in darker-skinned people.

PEARLS

- There are also benign acral patterns without parallel lines. There can be homogeneous brown color with or without pigment network and/or dots and globules.
- Advanced acral melanoma can further have any of the features of invasive melanoma seen at other body sites.

CASE 48

HISTORY
Bleeding was the reason for the consultation on this acral lesion in a 68-year-old man.

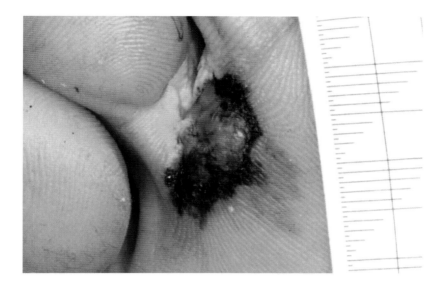

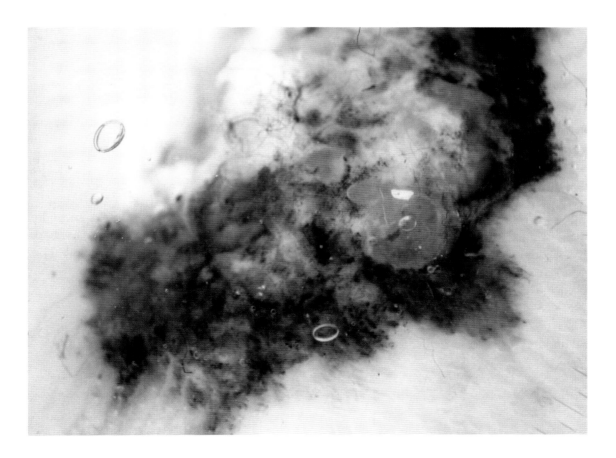

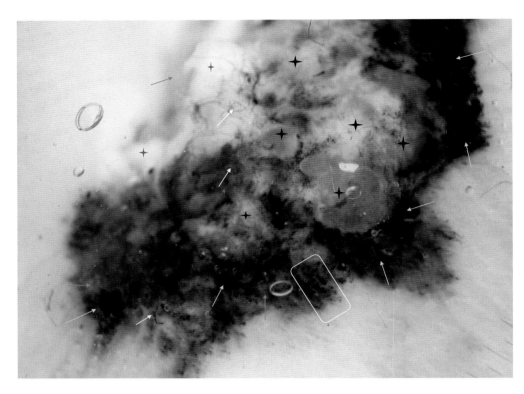

DERMOSCOPIC CRITERIA

- Asymmetry of color and structure
- Multicomponent global pattern
- Remnants of the parallel-furrow pattern (white rectangle)
- Irregular black blotches (yellow arrows)
- Milky-red nodule (black stars)
- Bony-white color (red stars)
- Bluish-white color (blue arrows)
- Blue thread from a sock (white arrows)
- Six colors (black, light/dark brown, pink, white, blue)

DIAGNOSIS:
Invasive Acral Melanoma

DISCUSSION

- Clinically, this is an obvious and very, very ugly acral melanoma.
- A focus of the parallel-furrow pattern with dots in the furrows confirms this is a melanocytic lesion.
- This could also be considered to be melanocytic by default.
- A large milky-red nodule and very irregular jet-black blotches help you make a "blink" diagnosis that this is an invasive melanoma.
- Clinically, radiating from the bulk of the tumor is flat, irregular brown color. The parallel-ridge pattern is not seen.
- There are cases of nail apparatus melanoma or other acral tumors that contain remnants of the

parallel-ridge pattern radiating from the more serious and potentially nonspecific components of the lesion.
- There is nothing more that you need to know about this deeply invasive acral melanoma. It should be excised posthaste.

PEARLS

- In contrast to this lesion, you will encounter invasive acral melanomas that are not this easy to diagnose.
- The only clue to their seriousness might be focal remnants of the parallel-ridge pattern.
- Keep an eye out for subtle clues.

CASE 49

HISTORY
A 47-year-old man has a nonhealing area on the bottom of his left foot.

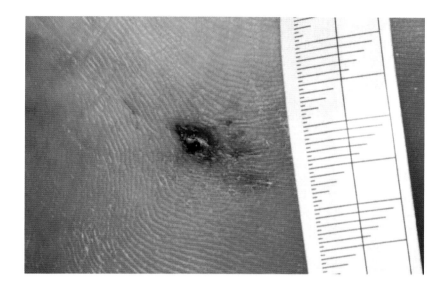

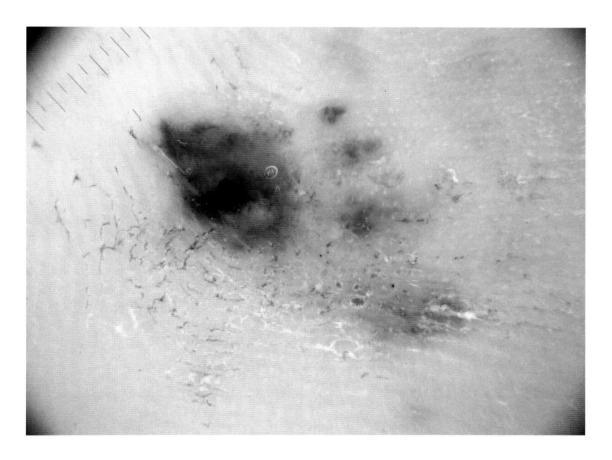

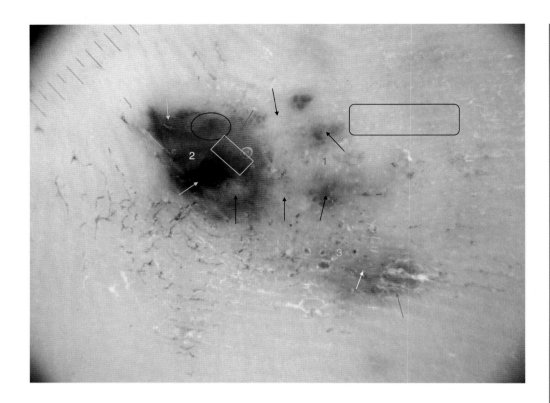

DIAGNOSIS:
Invasive Acral Melanoma

DISCUSSION

- Clinically, it looks like hemorrhage. Unfortunately, the purple color and criteria (ie, blood pebbles) associated with hemorrhage are not seen.
- "If there's white, control your fright." Melanoma?
- "If there's blue, they might sue." Melanoma?
- "If there's pink, stop and think." Melanoma?
- "If there's black, don't turn your back." Melanoma?
- There are no features to suggest this is not a melanoma.
- This is a melanocytic lesion by default.
- There is asymmetry of color and structure, and the multicomponent global pattern—decidedly high-risk.
- An irregular blackish-gray blotch, milky-red/pink color with a few milky-red globules, and bluish-white color blend into each other—high-risk.

- There is a focus of 3 linear black globules, possibly reflecting the last remnants of a parallel pattern. This could be the criterion for diagnosis of a melanocytic lesion.
- An irregular brownish-gray area does not add much compared with the other high-risk colors.
- A nonhealing area with high-risk colors is melanoma until proven otherwise.

PEARLS

- One high-risk color in any presentation, whether white, blue, pink, or black, in a clinically equivocal acral lesion is all you need to warrant a histopathologic diagnosis.
- Invasive acral melanoma can be feature-poor if not entirely featureless.

CASE 50

HISTORY

A podiatrist found this lesion on the plantar surface of the foot of a 57-year-old woman. He wisely referred her to you because he was not sure if it needed a biopsy.

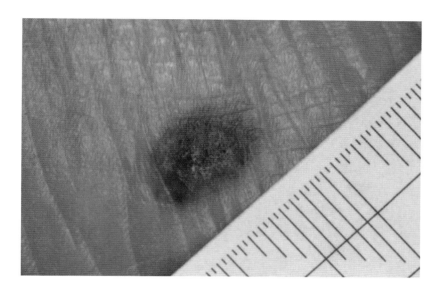

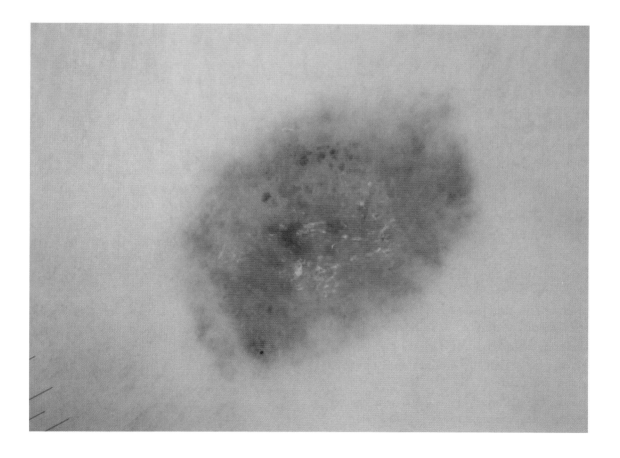

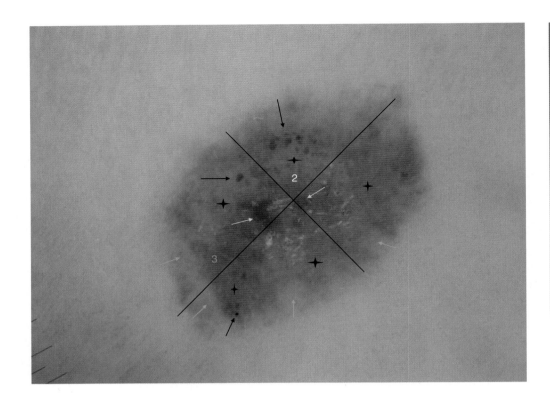

DERMOSCOPIC CRITERIA

- Asymmetry of color and structure (+)
- Multicomponent global pattern (1,2,3)
- Irregular brown dots and globules (black arrows)
- Hypopigmentation (stars)
- Purple blotches (yellow arrows)
- Normal skin within the lesion (green arrows)
- Hyperkeratosis (red arrows)

DIAGNOSIS:
Invasive Acral Melanoma

DISCUSSION

- There is no clue to suggest that this is a Level IV, 1.6-mm acral lentiginous melanoma. It looks like a dysplastic nevus at most.
- There are no parallel patterns associated with benign or malignant pathology.
- There are a few irregular brown dots and globules that diagnose a melanocytic lesion.
- There is mild asymmetry of color and structure and an unimpressive multicomponent global pattern.
- A focus of purple color suggests hemorrhage.
- Hemorrhage can often be found in acral and nail apparatus melanomas caused by trauma.
- Hypopigmentation could raise a red flag for concern that could easily be overlooked as being insignificant.
- It is not the bony-white color of regression.
- Hyperkeratosis seen clinically should not be confused with crystalline structures.
- Crystalline structures found in a melanocytic lesion are more often found in melanoma.
- Normal skin within the lesion and at the periphery should not be confused with regression.

- So that's it—no high-risk colors, no high-risk local criteria. No gut feeling that this could be high-risk acral lesion.
- This represents melanoma incognito: a lesion that clinically and with dermoscopy does not have the features highly suggestive of a melanoma.
- Compared with the previous 2 cases with significant clinical and dermoscopic clues to diagnose acral melanoma, this lesion looks quite low-risk.
- The indications to make a histopathologic diagnosis were features of a dysplastic nevus (ie, asymmetry of color and structure, irregular dots and globules, multifocal hypopigmentation) at a "special" site (plantar foot).
- Think about it: When was the last time you diagnosed a dysplastic nevus on the plantar surfaces of the feet?

PEARLS

- Melanoma incognito is out there—beware!
- Clinically and dermoscopically melanoma can mimic benign lesions.

CASE 51

HISTORY

A colleague e-mails you this lesion that he discovered on the plantar surface of a 50-year-old woman for your expert opinion. He is hesitant to excise it before he gets your analysis.

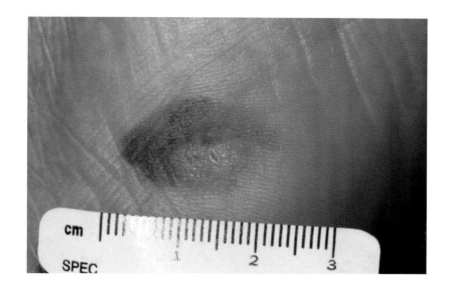

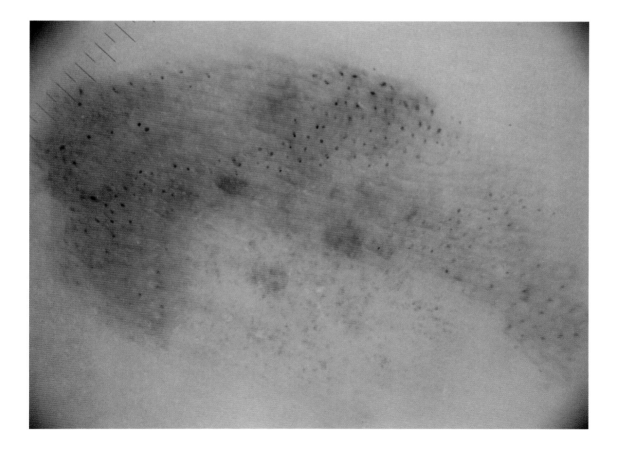

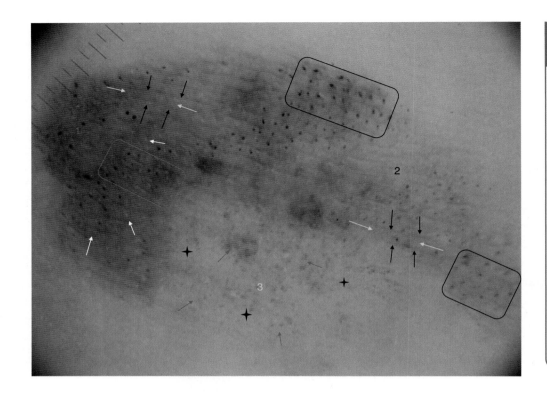

DIAGNOSIS:
Invasive Acral Melanoma

DISCUSSION

- Even for an experienced dermoscopist this lesion is hard to describe, which, in and of itself is your first red flag for concern.
- There is a large milky-red area with milky-red globules, your second red flag for concern.
- There are foci of what appear to be the parallel-furrow pattern, yet there are irregular brown dots and globules in the ridges where the white acrosyringia should be—another red flag for concern.
- The left side of the lesion demonstrates the parallel-ridge pattern. The furrows can be seen with pigmentation in the spaces that represent the ridges.
- The white string of pearls, the acrosyringia, is seen in the ridges along with some irregular brown dots and globules.
- In summary, we see clinically what appears to be a pink area of regression. Dermoscopically, we see asymmetry of color and structure, the multicomponent global pattern with an unusual benign parallel-furrow pattern that contains irregular brown dots and globules. There is also suggestion of a malignant parallel-ridge pattern with pigmentation and acrosyringia in the ridges. The dermoscopic differential diagnosis of the whitish area is a milky-red area with milky-red globules versus regression with polymorphous vessels. Both are high-risk features.
- You can confidently convey to your colleague that there are many atypical features and a histopathologic diagnosis should be made posthaste.

PEARLS

- If you have to think too much about a lesion, that is a sign that a histopathologic diagnosis is in order.
- You should tell your patients, "If we have to think too much about a lesion, then we should biopsy it." This usually receives a positive response.

CASE 52

HISTORY
A 17-year-old girl has had this pigmentation on her fifth finger for 2 years. The color seems to be changing; there is no history of trauma.

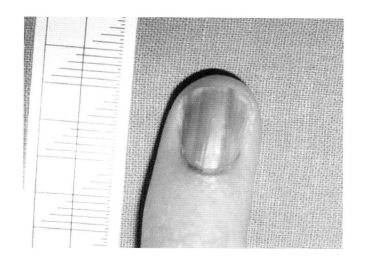

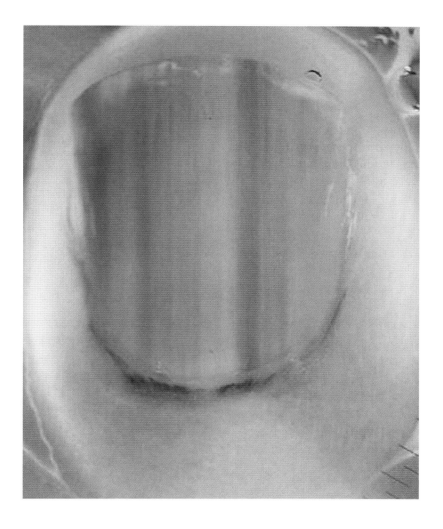

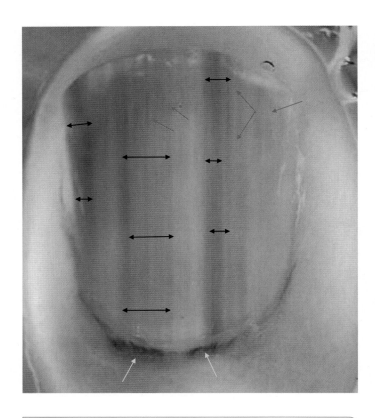

DERMOSCOPIC CRITERIA

- Irregular pigmented bands (black arrows)
- Loss of parallelism (red arrows)
- Hutchinson sign (yellow arrows)

DIAGNOSIS:
Nail Apparatus Melanoma

DISCUSSION

- In a white patient, multiple pigmented bands (melanonychia), especially if they involve only a single nail, are a red flag for concern, and nail apparatus melanoma should be on your mind.
- Any changing lesion without suggestion of a benign cause such as trauma or other inflammation is a major red flag for concern.
- Most cases of nail apparatus melanoma arise between the fifth through seventh decades. However young people, as is the case here, can get nail apparatus melanoma. Even children may be affected.
- Nail apparatus melanoma can develop on any finger.
- Although this patient is young, the history and clinical and dermoscopic features are worrisome.
- The bands are irregular with variable thickness, irregular spacing, and loss of parallelism. These are the classic features of irregular bands associated with melanoma.
- Malignant melanocytes produce pigment irregularly, which presents as broken-up line segments. This is referred to as *loss of parallelism*.

- There is also variegated color (light/dark brown, gray)—a red flag for concern.
- The presence of pigmentation on the proximal cuticle, referred to as the *Hutchinson sign*, is a feature that may or may not be seen in nail apparatus melanoma.
- In summary, this is a classic example of nail apparatus melanoma—single nail involvement with all of the dermoscopic features associated with melanoma. Bands with irregular thickness, spacing, loss of parallelism, and variegated colors plus the Hutchinson sign.

PEARLS

- Here are the ABCDEs of nail apparatus melanoma:
  - A (Age, commonly between the fifth and seventh decades)
  - B (Irregular bands)
  - C (Changing bands)
  - D (Digits especially the first toe or fingernail)
  - E (Extension onto the cuticle; Hutchinson sign)
  - Pigmented or nonpigmented nail dystrophy that does not improve with expected therapy could be a melanoma!

CASE 53

HISTORY
A 63-year-old woman got her finger caught in her car door a few years ago. The discoloration that she was told was blood still has not gone away. Instead, the color is getting darker and spreading onto her finger.

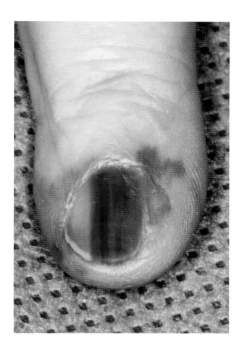

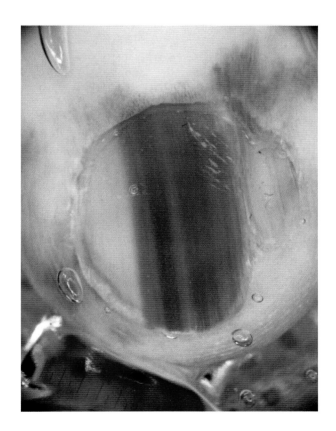

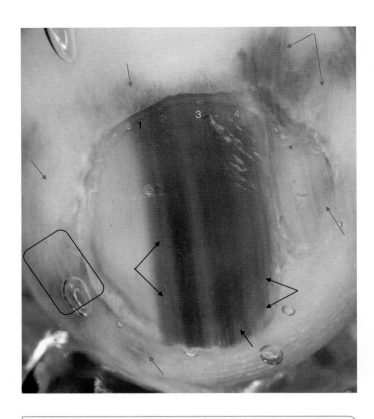

DERMOSCOPIC CRITERIA

- Irregular pigmented bands (1,2,3,4)
- Loss of parallelism (black arrows)
- Hutchinson sign (red arrows)
- Parallel-ridge pattern (rectangle)

DIAGNOSIS:
Nail Apparatus Melanoma

DISCUSSION

- Clinically, this is an obvious melanoma.
- The bands are irregular because there are different shades of brown color, the widths vary irregularly, and there are areas of loss of parallelism.
- Compared with the previous case, the spread of pigment onto the finger (positive Hutchinson sign) is dramatic.
- In addition, there is one focus of the parallel-ridge pattern.
- It has thin, light furrows with pigment in the thicker ridges.
- This is a good finding, because it makes your life easier in making the diagnosis.
- It is not necessary to do a nail matrix biopsy if you can identify the parallel-ridge pattern on the surrounding skin. Biopsy of this area alone should confirm the diagnosis.
- A history of trauma is commonly associated with nail apparatus melanoma.

PEARLS

- Do not forget to examine the skin surrounding the nail for pigmentation. If you find pigmentation and it contains the parallel-ridge pattern you can do a biopsy there, thus avoiding the more technical and invasive nail matrix biopsy.
- Even if you do not see the parallel-ridge pattern, still biopsy any skin pigmentation. It might also make the diagnosis.

CASE 54

HISTORY
An 11-year-old girl presented with a changing nail discoloration on her right second toe nail.

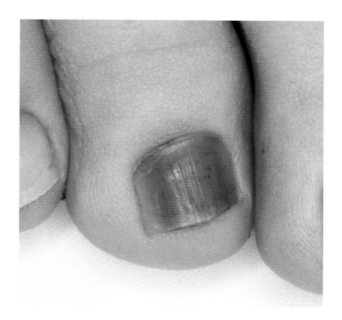

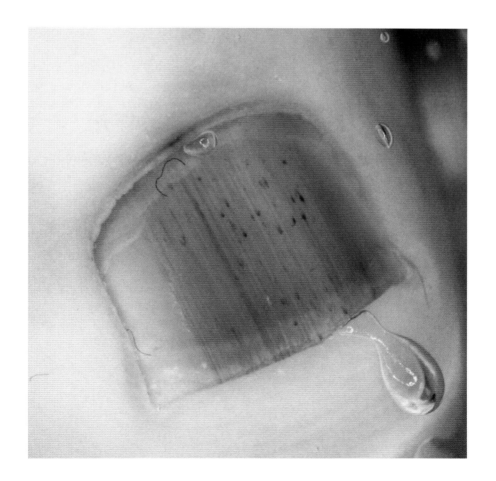

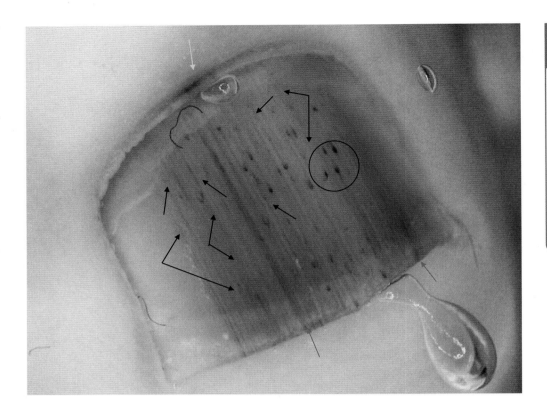

DERMOSCOPIC CRITERIA

- Irregular pigmented bands (red arrows)
- Loss of parallelism (black arrows)
- Hutchinson sign (yellow arrow)
- Irregular dots and globules (circle)
- Three colors (light/dark brown, gray)

DIAGNOSIS:
In Situ Melanoma

DISCUSSION

- The majority of the lesion consists of loss of parallelism. The defining feature of this sign is the presence of irregular and broken-up line segments, which reflect the irregular amounts of melanin produced by malignant melanocytes.
- This is a major red flag for concern.
- Indeed, the loss of parallelism here fills the entire lesion, which is both unusual and very worrisome. More so given that the patient is only 11 years old.
- Irregular brown dots and globules are another unusual high-risk feature.
- A differential diagnosis could be hemorrhage, if the color were purple. However, the dots and globules are brown and not purple.
- Furthermore, such low-risk dermoscopic features as regular longitudinal line segments with respect to color, spacing, thickness, and parallelism are not seen here.

- Only one thin brown band is clearly identified.
- There is a minimal amount of pigment on the cuticle (Hutchinson sign), which is not an important feature compared with the other high-risk criteria in the lesion.
- A nail matrix biopsy is indicated posthaste.

PEARLS

- If there are high-risk dermoscopic features, do not let the young age of a patient with melanonychia decrease your index of suspicion for potential high-risk pathology.
- Learn the low-risk and high-risk features of nail apparatus pigmentation.
- "If in doubt, cut it out!" Unfortunately, in a pediatric patient, you will certainly have your work "cut out" for you!

CASE 55

HISTORY

A 50-year-old woman has been treating this discoloration on her right first toe as a nail fungus with over-the-counter antifungal cream for a year. It will not clear.

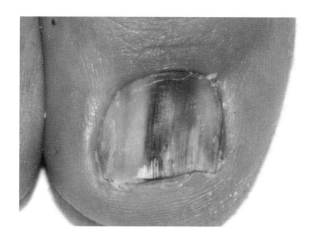

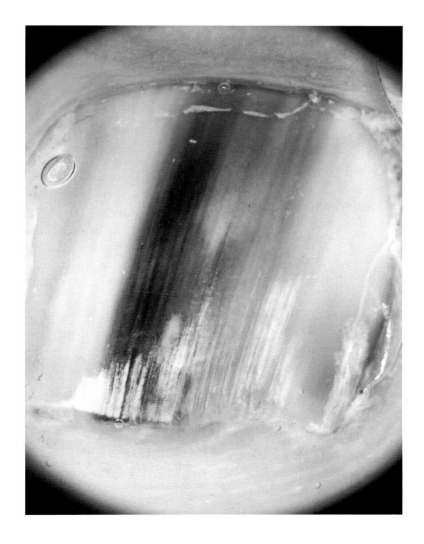

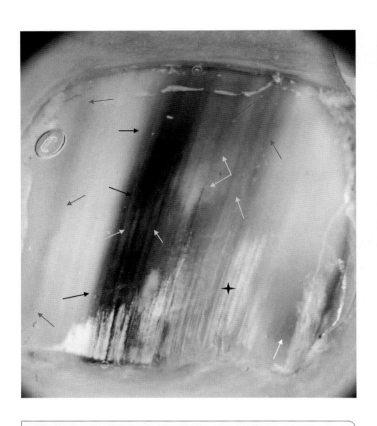

DIAGNOSIS:

In Situ Melanoma

DISCUSSION

- This case is a no-brainer, or is it?
- Irregular yellow color of a tinea. Throw in a little green color of pseudomonas.
- The clinical picture of a nail with tinea and bacterial colors makes sense. It is not getting better with over-the-counter antifungals. That is usually the case.
- But what about the irregular blackish-white band? Here is where your dermoscopic differential diagnosis comes into play.
- It could be associated with nail apparatus melanoma or a dark band created by dematiaceous fungus.
- Fungal melanonychia is relatively rare and may be caused by dematiaceous or nondematiaceous fungi, both of which may produce melanin.
- *Trichophyton rubrum* is one of the most frequently isolated organisms from fungal melanonychia.
- There are clues, however, that the dark band is associated with melanoma: borders are very straight, it is wider at the base, and there is loss of parallelism.
- In contrast, the pigmented bands of fungal infection are wider distally and taper proximally, consistent

with distal-to-proximal spread of infection. The opposite is true of the pigmented bands associated with melanoma.

- Because there is a question of nail apparatus melanoma, a nail matrix biopsy is indicated.
- The confounding feature of this case of in situ acral lentiginous melanoma is the simultaneous presence of a tinea infection. Yellow and green colors are a red herring (no pun intended) that are *not* typically associated with nail apparatus melanomas. Always keep an open mind.

PEARLS

- "If there's black, don't turn your back," in any clinical scenario.
- If you are not reasonably sure you are not dealing with a nail apparatus melanoma, biopsy the lesion posthaste.
- The breakdown of tissue that often accompanies melanoma can be a portal of entry for microorganisms.
- So, don't be fooled by tinea or bacteria that can be associated with nail apparatus melanoma.

CASE 56

HISTORY
A 58-year-old female cosmetic patient of yours is upset because she cannot apply nail polish to cover her discolored big toe nail.

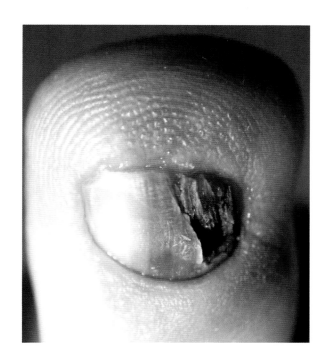

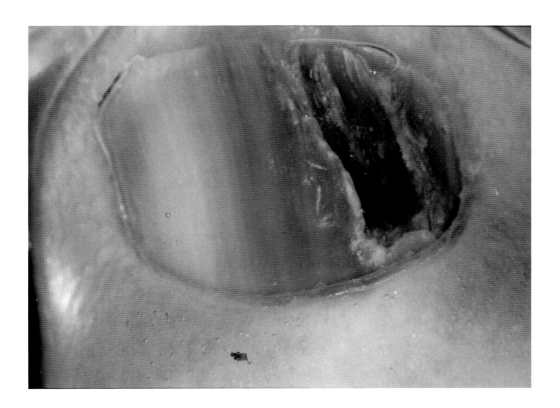

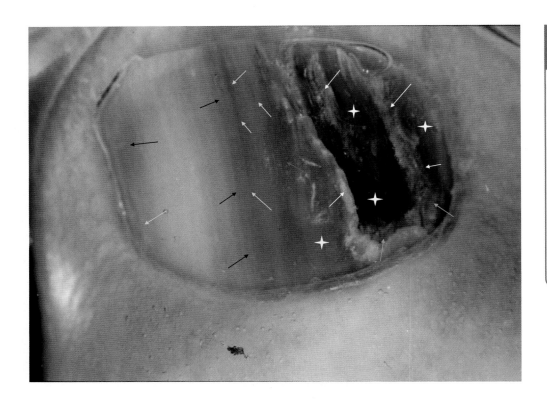

DERMOSCOPIC CRITERIA

- Irregular brownish bands (black arrows)
- Loss of parallelism (yellow arrows)
- Dark homogeneous brown color (stars)
- Nail plate destruction (white arrows)
- Bluish-white color (blue arrows)
- Purplish color (red arrows)

DIAGNOSIS:
Invasive Melanoma

DISCUSSION

- No wonder the patient is having trouble putting nail polish on her toenail—she has nail plate destruction from her invasive, destructive melanoma.
- Poorly defined, irregular bands with loss of parallelism—melanoma!
- Nail plate destruction over a dark blotch of pigmentation—invasive, destructive melanoma.
- The bluish-white color does not add anything to help make the diagnosis.
- If you look carefully, there is the purplish color of blood centrally, which is created by a malignant destructive process.
- The absence of the Hutchinson sign does not rule out melanoma.
- Nail plate destruction is an important clue to suggest a malignant diagnosis (eg, squamous cell carcinoma,

melanoma) in a nonpigmented or pink nail apparatus tumor.
- Amelanotic nail apparatus melanoma, the antithesis of this case, is not rare and could be devoid of any pigmentation. In such a case, making the correct diagnosis is often a challenge.

PEARLS

- You might not have the opportunity to diagnose a case like this if you do not perform a total-body skin examination, including the tops and bottoms of the feet.
- If your patients are wearing nail polish, ask them if they have any discoloration in their toenails. They might say yes.
- Have nail polish remover handy so you can thoroughly examine your patients even if they use nail polish.

CASE 57

HISTORY
This was discovered on a 87-year-old man living in a nursing home.

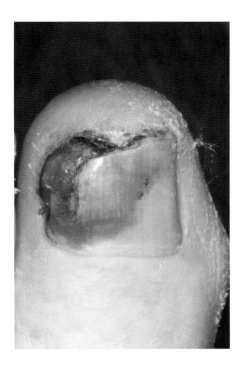

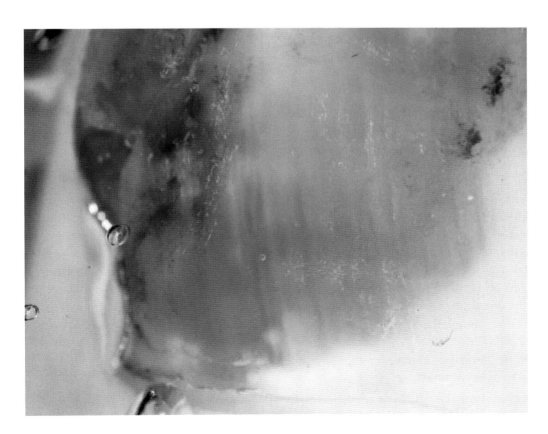

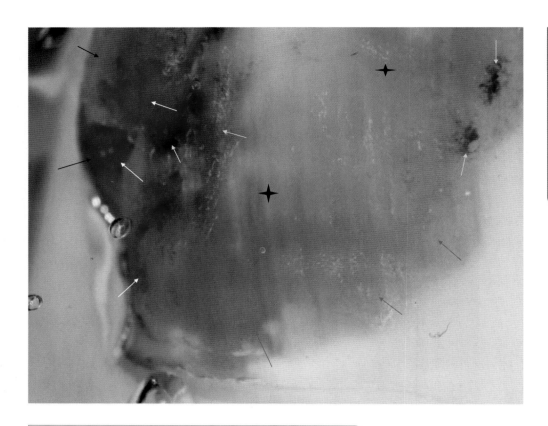

DERMOSCOPIC CRITERIA

- Bluish-white color (stars)
- Milky-red nodule (black arrows)
- Ulceration (white arrows)
- Milky-red/pink color (red arrows)
- Scabs (yellow arrows)

DIAGNOSIS:
Nodular Amelanotic Melanoma

DISCUSSION

- There is an ulcerated amelanotic nodule with nail plate destruction.
- The clinical differential diagnosis includes pyogenic granuloma, squamous cell carcinoma, and amelanotic melanoma.
- Pyogenic granuloma typically has a milky-red pink color, with or without bleeding, and there may be a white collarette of scale. This does not look like a pyogenic granuloma.
- There are no dermoscopic clues to diagnose a squamous cell carcinoma, such as irregular hairpin vessels, irregular bony-white circles, and larger irregular bony-white scaly areas.
- The bluish-white and milky-red/pink colors are clues that point in the direction of a melanoma.
- Nail apparatus nodular amelanotic melanoma is typically devoid of pigmented bands.
- In situ amelanotic lesions could have pink longitudinal bands referred to as erythronychia.

- Up to 50% of nail apparatus melanomas are amelanotic, a sobering statistic.
- In a "blink," it is obvious that a histopathologic diagnosis is indicated posthaste.
- This case is the antithesis of the last case of pigmented destructive nail apparatus melanoma in which the dermoscopic features are clearly present.

PEARLS

- Amelanotic melanoma in any location is the great masquerader and should always be included in the differential diagnosis of a pyogenic granuloma or pink Spitz nevus.
- Avoid contaminating your dermatoscope from bleeding lesions by using a noncontact technique.
- Polyethylene food wrap film barrier (eg, Saran wrap) could be used as an interface between ulcerated or bleeding lesions and your dermatoscope to avoid contamination.

CASE 58

HISTORY
According to the patient, this lesion literally came out of nowhere within a 4-month period. There was no history of trauma or any preexisting genital problem.

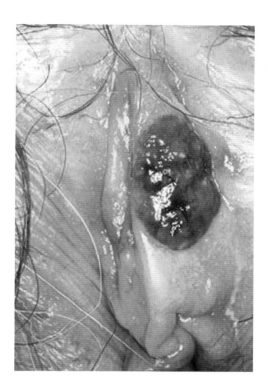

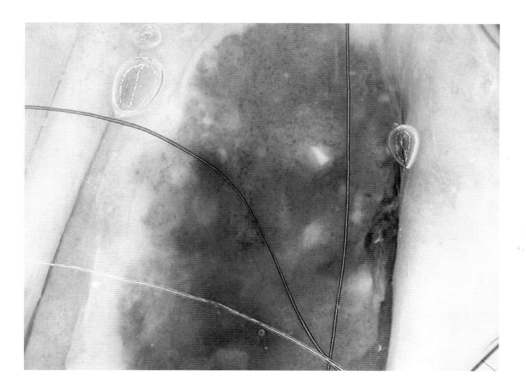

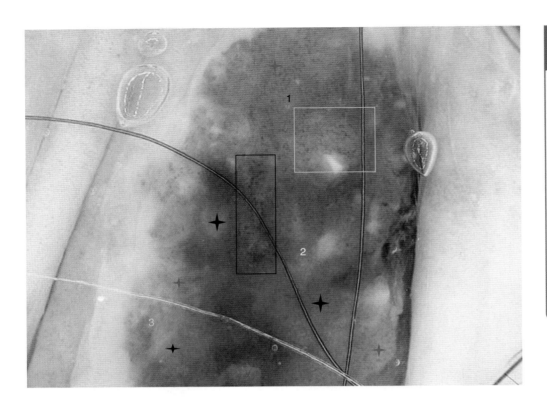

DERMOSCOPIC CRITERIA

- Asymmetry of color and structure
- Multicomponent global pattern (1,2,3,4)
- Bluish-white color (black stars)
- Milky-red/pink color (red stars)
- Polymorphous vessels (fill the lesion)
- Dotted vessels (black rectangle)
- Dotted, comma and linear vessels (yellow box)

DIAGNOSIS:
Invasive Genital Melanoma

DISCUSSION

- "Blink"—invasive melanoma.
- Interestingly, similar colors as seen in the last case of amelanotic nail apparatus melanoma.
- This is a melanocytic lesion by default.
- There is asymmetry of color and structure, and the multicomponent global pattern with 3 to 4 zones.
- Irregular bluish-white color fills the lesion—melanoma.
- Milky-red/pink color with polymorphous vessels—melanoma.
- The polymorphous vessels include dotted, comma, and linear-shaped vessels.
- A minor point in the context of the palette of high-risk melanoma-associated colors is that there are no benign patterns (eg, globular, parallel, ring-like) associated with benign genital mucosal lesions anywhere to be found in this invasive genital mucosal melanoma.

- Benign genital mucosal lesions are rarely encountered; rarer still, malignant ones.
- The combination of blue, gray, or white color with structureless zones has been shown to be the strongest discriminator between benign and malignant mucosal lesions.
- Benign genital mucosal lesions will be presented in the next chapter.

PEARLS

- Avoid contaminating your dermatoscope with mucosal lesions by using a noncontact technique.
- Polyethylene food wrap film barrier (eg, Saran wrap) could be used as an interface between the genital mucosa and your dermatoscope to avoid contamination.

CHAPTER 4

Benign and Malignant Nonmelanocytic Lesions

General Instructions

- For each case, there is a short history along with a clinical and an unmarked dermoscopic image.
- Study the unmarked dermoscopic image and try to identify the global and local dermoscopic features.
- Make your diagnosis.
- Next, turn the page and the dermoscopic image will be presented again, this time marked with all the salient dermoscopic findings.
- On the same page you will also find the diagnosis along with a detailed discussion and a few pearls for your review.

CASE 1

HISTORY

A 76-year-old woman has a slowly growing lesion on her left cheek.

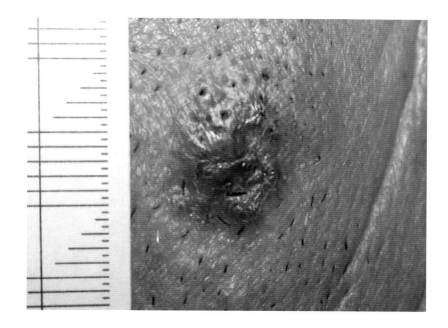

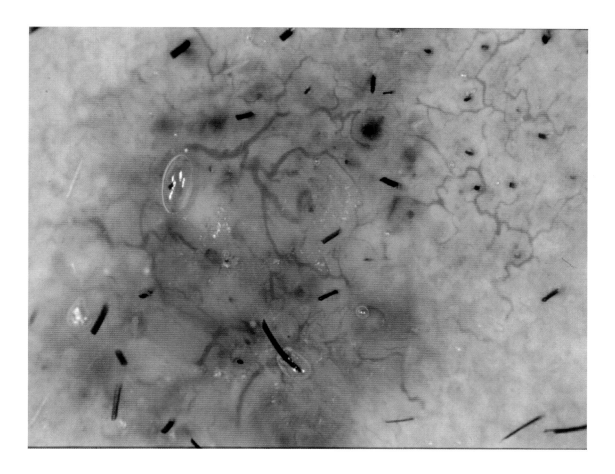

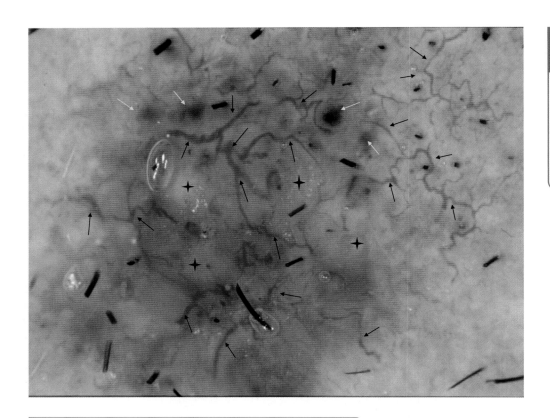

DIAGNOSIS:
Pigmented Basal Cell Carcinoma

DISCUSSION

- This is a classic pigmented basal cell carcinoma. As such, it has in-focus, thick- and thin-walled, arborizing (tree-like branching) vessels that fill the lesion, along with spotty pigmentation.
- For the expert dermoscopist, this is a "blink" diagnosis.
  - However, arborizing vessels are highly suggestive of basal cell carcinoma, they may also be seen in melanoma, nevi, neurofibromas, sebaceous gland hyperplasia, Merkel cell carcinoma, scar tissue and on sun damaged skin.
  - More concerning here is the bluish-white color, which itself is frequently seen in melanoma and thus presents a red flag for concern. Remember, "If there's blue, they might sue!"
- Thus, for the novice dermoscopist, it is best to follow the 2-step algorithm to evaluate this lesion.
  - First, determine if the lesion is melanocytic. Here, there are no criteria associated with a melanocytic lesion (eg, pigment network, brown dots and globules, homogeneous blue color).
  - Knowing the lesion is not melanocytic, next determine if there are other criteria present to indicate a seborrheic keratosis, basal cell carcinoma, hemangioma, or dermatofibroma.

- There are no criteria for a seborrheic keratosis (milia-like cysts, pseudofollicular openings, fissures and ridges, "fat fingers," hairpin vessels).
- There are no criteria for a hemangioma (lacunae, fibrous septae).
- There are no criteria for a dermatofibroma (central white patch, peripheral pigment network).
- There are, however, the classic criteria for a pigmented basal cell carcinoma, including the in-focus arborizing vessels and pigmentation.
  - Of note, pigmentation in basal cell carcinoma may present in a myriad of ways. In this case, the pigmentation presents as a few bluish-white and blackish-gray globules; ovoid nests.

PEARLS

- There are many dermoscopic presentations of basal cell carcinoma.
- There will be times when the differentiation of a basal cell carcinoma from a melanoma is problematic.
- An important clue to remember in such situations is that you will never see pigment network in a basal cell carcinoma.

CASE 2

HISTORY

This pigmented lesion was found on the face of an 80-year-old woman during a routine total-body skin examination.

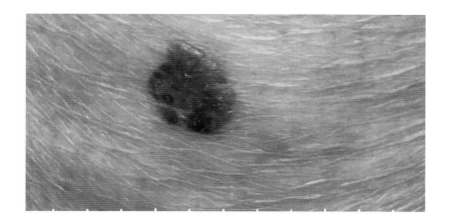

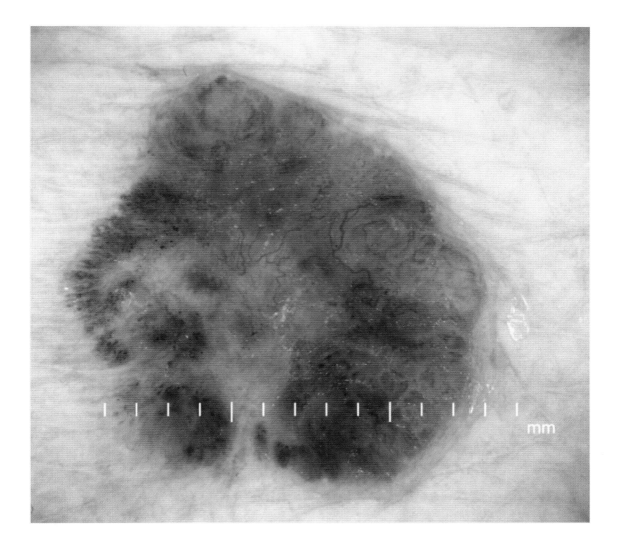

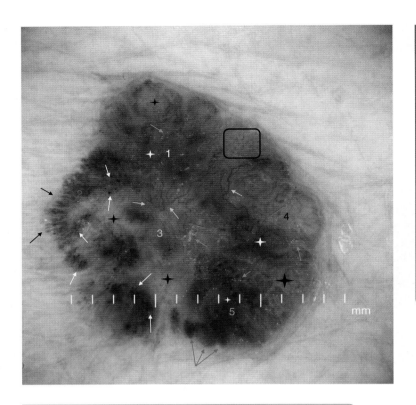

DERMOSCOPIC CRITERIA

- Asymmetry of color and structure
- Multicomponent global pattern (1,2,3,4,5)
- Arborizing vessels (yellow arrows)
- Serpentine vessels (red arrows)
- Dotted and linear vessels (box)
- Bluish-white color (white stars)
- Milky-red color (black stars)
- Tiny black and brown dots and globules (white arrows)
- Irregular streaks (black arrows)
- Leaf-like area (green arrows)
- Six colors (black, brown, gray, blue, white, milky-red)
- White dots are reflection artifact (blue arrows)

DIAGNOSIS:
Pigmented Basal Cell Carcinoma

DISCUSSION

- There is a lot going on in this lesion that looks high-risk. Is this a melanoma or a pigmented basal cell carcinoma?
  - There are foci of brown dots and globules that could diagnose a melanocytic lesion. However, brown dots and globules may also be seen in a pigmented basal cell carcinoma.
    - Thus, we have a dermoscopic differential diagnosis.
  - There is asymmetry of color and structure, plus the multicomponent global pattern. Both may be seen in a basal cell carcinoma or a melanoma. Therefore, they are nonspecific findings.
  - Bluish-white and milky-red colors are high-risk colors—nonspecific.
  - There are polymorphous vessels with arborizing, serpentine, dotted, and linear shapes—nonspecific.
    - Arborizing vessels are not the only vessels found in basal cell carcinoma.
  - A focus of irregular brown streak-like structures—nonspecific.
  - Peripheral foci of tiny black dots and globules—nonspecific.
  - Possibly the only criterion specific for a basal cell carcinoma is a focus of leaf-like structure composed of bulbous extensions forming a leaf-like pattern.

  - This is a common descriptor, which is often hard to visualize and whose value is doubted by some dermoscopists.
  - The presence of 6 colors is very high-risk, but also nonspecific.
- So there you have it. A pigmented skin lesion filled with nonspecific, high-risk criteria. It is essential to be knowledgeable so that you are able to think in terms of dermoscopic differential diagnosis.
- The difficulty in making a specific diagnosis makes clear as day the need for a histopathologic diagnosis posthaste.
- In reality, the experienced dermoscopist will not have trouble diagnosing a pigmented basal cell carcinoma. He or she will see arborizing and serpentine vessels, tiny specks of black pigment, and 1 well-developed leaf-like structure.

PEARLS

- Dermoscopy helps you plan your surgical approach to make a diagnosis, whether incisional or excisional.
  - In most cases excisional to rule out melanoma and incisional to rule out nonmelanoma skin cancer such as basal cell carcinoma.
- Unfortunately, we all have to eat humble pie at times in our career, no matter how many years we have put in.
- Dermoscopy is not a perfect science, and expectations should be measured accordingly.

CASE 3

HISTORY
This was found on the face of a 92-year-old man.

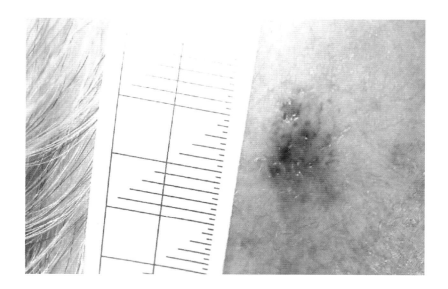

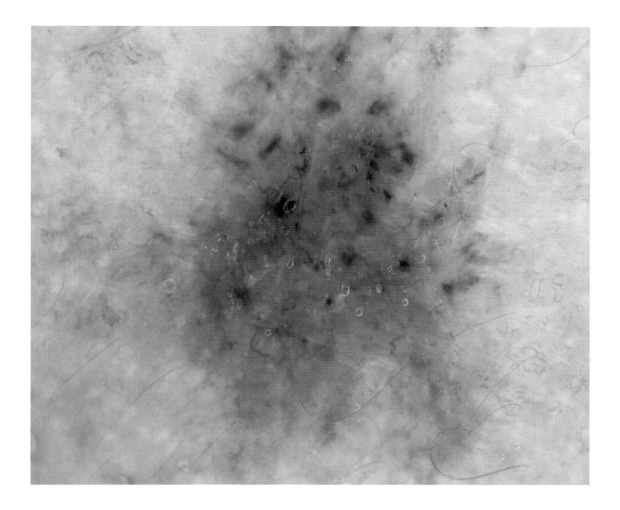

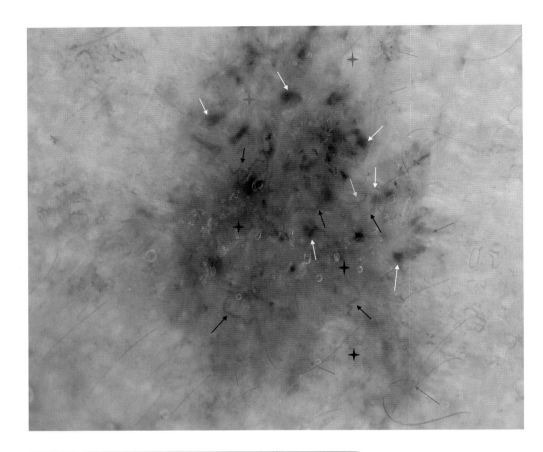

DIAGNOSIS:
Pigmented Basal Cell Carcinoma

DISCUSSION

- There are no criteria to diagnose a melanocytic lesion, seborrheic keratosis, hemangioma, or dermatofibroma.
- Serpentine blood vessels and blue ovoid nests of pigment are classic criteria that help to diagnose this pigmented basal cell carcinoma.
- There is also 1 tiny centrally located arborizing vessel.
- There are also a few foci of gray blotches and minute stippling (tiny dots) of brown color. Both of these features support the diagnosis.
  - Brown stippling of pigment is a common feature that is not seen in melanocytic lesions. It can help point you in the right direction when there is a basal cell, whether or not there are telltale arborizing vessels.
- Asymmetry of color and structure and the multicomponent global pattern are both high-risk, yet nonspecific, global patterns that may be seen in benign and malignant melanocytic, and nonmelanocytic lesions.

- Milky-red and bony-white colors are also nonspecific and may be seen in melanoma and basal cell carcinoma.
- Basal cell carcinoma may or may not have arborizing vessels or pigmentation.
- There are innumerable presentations of pigment in basal cell carcinoma. Some are thought to be specific in support of the diagnosis.
  - Blue ovoid nests, leaf-like structures, and blue-gray globules.

PEARLS

- Learn how to recognize serpentine vessels.
  - They might be your only clue to help make the diagnosis of questionable basal cell carcinomas.
- Another clue in feature-poor basal cell carcinomas may be the presence of spoke-wheel structures.

CASE 4

HISTORY
This pink lesion was found on the right upper back of a 35-year-old man while doing a total-body skin examination.

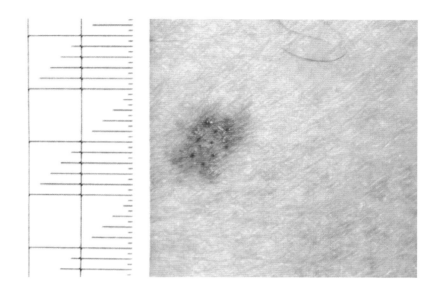

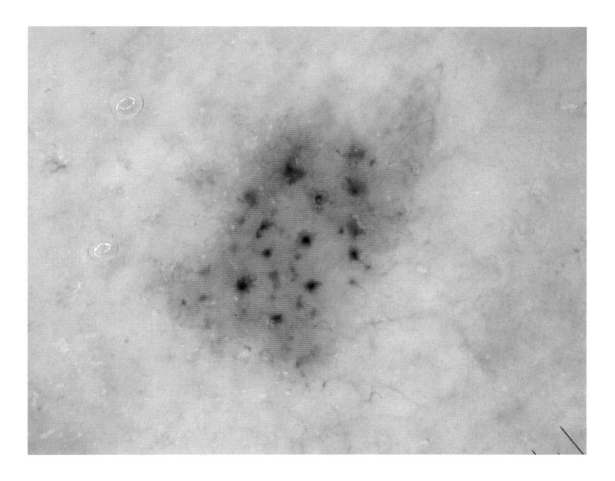

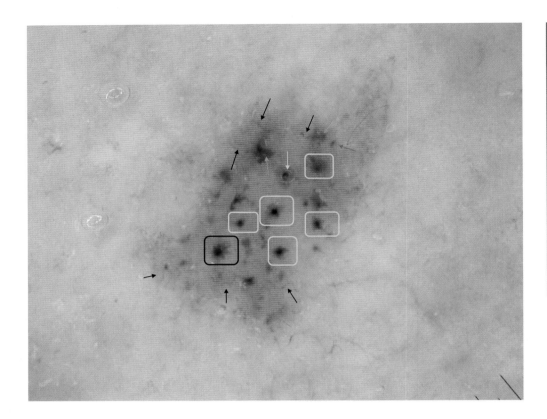

**DERMOSCOPIC
CRITERIA**

- Well-developed spoke-wheel structure (black box)
- Poorly developed spoke-wheel structures (yellow boxes)
- Serpentine vessels (black arrows)
- Superficial ulceration (yellow arrow)
- Blue globule (red arrow)
- Gray blotches (blue arrows)

DIAGNOSIS:
Pigmented Basal Cell Carcinoma

DISCUSSION

- The lesion is filled with spoke-wheel structures.
  - One spoke-wheel structure is well-developed with a series of lines radiating from the central hub. Even though the "spokes" do not completely surround the hub, they are considered well-developed because they are easy to recognize.
    - Spoke-wheel structures are well-circumscribed brown-to-gray projections that radiate out from a dark brown central hub.
    - Sometimes, radial projections are not visible, and instead one sees a concentric globule consisting of a round structure with a central darker hub. These are described as *poorly developed*. This lesion has many poorly developed spoke-wheel structures.
    - Spoke-wheel structures are highly suggestive, if not diagnostic, of basal cell carcinoma.
    - Histopathologically, they correspond to the nests of basal cell carcinoma emanating from the undersurface of the epidermis.
- Even though this lesion does not have the arborizing vessels associated with basal cell carcinoma, there are many serpentine vessels that support the diagnosis.

Serpentine vessels are commonly found in basal cell carcinoma.
- A few gray blotches and 1 blue globule are the pigments that classify this as a pigmented basal cell carcinoma.
- One focus of superficial ulceration also supports the diagnosis, because superficial ulceration is commonly found in superficial basal cell carcinoma.
- In summary, the criteria that diagnose a pigmented basal cell carcinoma include spoke-wheel structures, serpentine vessels, blue and gray color, plus a small superficial ulceration.

PEARLS

- Note that this constellation of features reveals an uncommon, yet not rare, presentation of basal cell carcinoma.
- We often have to use our imagination to identify spoke-wheel structures.
- Have a high index of suspicion, because these structures might be the only clue to diagnose a basal cell carcinoma.

CASE 5

HISTORY
This was found on the mid back of a 73-year-old man with a history of excessive sun exposure.

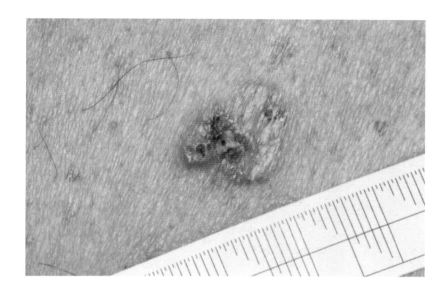

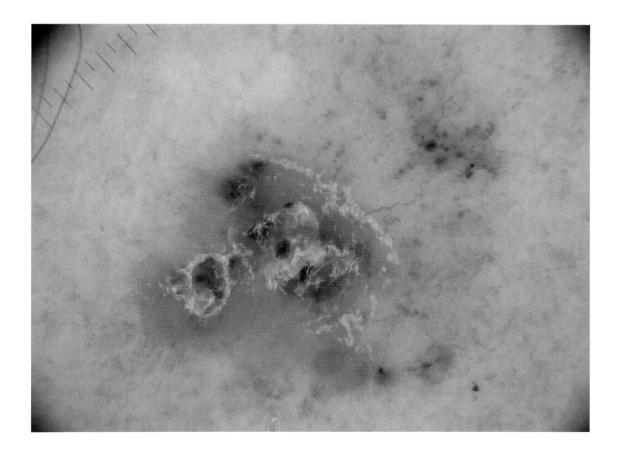

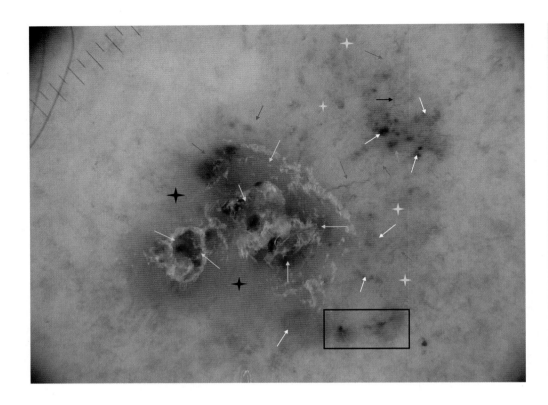

DERMOSCOPIC CRITERIA

- Asymmetry of color and structure
- Multicomponent global pattern
- Arborizing vessels (black arrow)
- Serpentine vessels (red arrows)
- Ulceration (yellow arrows)
- Blue dots and globules (blue arrows)
- Gray dots, globules, blotches (white arrows)
- Spoke-wheel structures (box)
- Milky-red/pink color (black stars)
- Brownish-white color (yellow stars)

DIAGNOSIS:
Pigmented Basal Cell Carcinoma

DISCUSSION

- As compared with the previous case of an uncommon presentation of pigmented basal cell carcinoma, this is a very common presentation.
- The diagnostic criteria include a thin-walled arborizing vessel, serpentine vessels, blue dots and globules, grayish dots, globules and blotches, and a large scaly ulceration.
- Ulceration is very common in basal cell carcinoma and is often an important clue to suggest the diagnosis.
- There are also 2 poorly developed spoke-wheel structures at the lower border of the lesion.
- Nonspecific criteria include asymmetry of color and structure, multicomponent global pattern, and milky-red/pink and brownish-white colors.
- It is not always necessary to try to characterize the pigmentation seen in basal cell carcinoma. In a "blink" you see colors, and that is all you need to know that the lesion with other criteria to make the diagnosis is a pigmented form of basal cell carcinoma.

- In many cases, structures such as blue ovoid nests or leaf-like structures are not identified.
- Do not be discouraged when you are presented with images at meetings, in books, or in the literature with descriptions of leaf-like structures that have no resemblance to any leaf you have ever seen. The term is a loose attempt to describe the structures, and some might consider it to be a misnomer.
- Just be aware that you might see black, brown, gray-blue, white, and pink colors in the form of dots, globules, blotches, or diffuse homogeneous areas.

PEARLS

- Dermoscopy is very helpful to diagnose tiny and/or feature-poor basal cell carcinoma.
- Be on the lookout for innocuous, translucent papules, and be sure to examine them with dermoscopy.

CASE 6

HISTORY
One of the patients multiple acquired and congenital melanocytic nevi has a definite change.

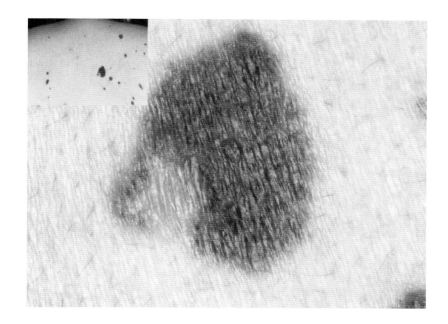

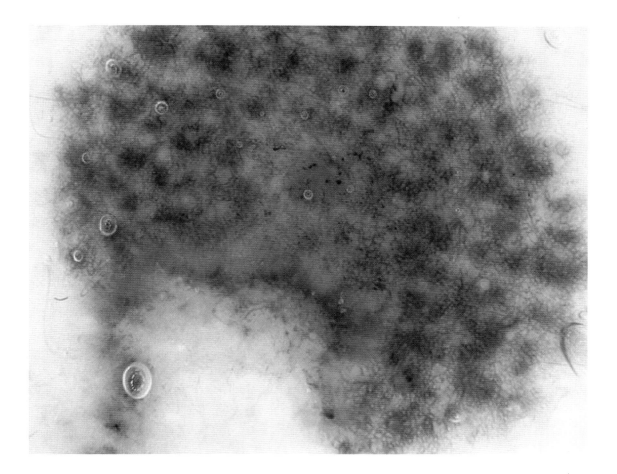

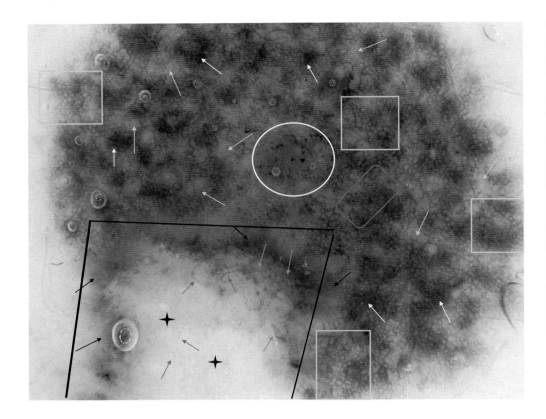

DIAGNOSIS:
Collision Tumor
Congenital Nevus/Pigmented Basal Cell Carcinoma

DERMOSCOPIC CRITERIA

Congenital nevus
- Regular pigment network (yellow boxes)
- Target network (red rectangle)
- Islands of normal skin (yellow arrows)
- Island of homogeneous brown color (white arrows)
- Deep blue blotch with irregular dots/globules (white circle)

Pigmented basal cell carcinoma
- Serpentine vessels (red arrows)
- Bluish-white color and blue dots (blue arrows)
- Brown stippling (light green arrow)
- Bony-white color (black stars)
- Gray homogeneous color (black arrows)

DISCUSSION

- Islands of normal skin, regular pigment network, and foci of brown homogeneous color symmetrically fill the lesion and make the diagnosis of a congenital melanocytic nevus.
- There is also a focus of target network that supports the diagnosis of a congenital melanocytic nevus.
- The central homogeneous blue blotch represents melanin deeper in the dermis (created by the Tyndall effect). This is commonly found in congenital melanocytic nevus.
  - Irregular dots and globules in the blue area are nonspecific and have no negative or positive diagnostic significance.
- The concept of dermoscopic differential diagnosis comes into play with this unusual lesion.
  - Could it be a melanoma arising in a congenital melanocytic nevus with bony-white color suggesting regression, polymorphous vessels, irregular bluish dots, and multiple colors?

- A collision tumor, in which 2 or more histopathologic entities, whether they lie next to each other or one within the other, is also in the differential diagnosis.
- The criteria to diagnose this pigmented basal cell carcinoma include serpentine vessels, bluish-dots, and gray homogeneous color.
- The bony-white color is nonspecific in that it may be seen in both melanoma and basal cell carcinoma.

PEARLS

- Always let your pathologist know that he or she might be dealing with a collision tumor, so that appropriate sections are made that can make the diagnosis.
- Sending digital dermoscopic images to your pathologist would be cutting-edge to give him or her a better understanding of what is going on.
- Pathologists are usually very appreciative to get digital dermoscopic images.

CASE 7

HISTORY
The patient was concerned about this dark spot in his scalp.

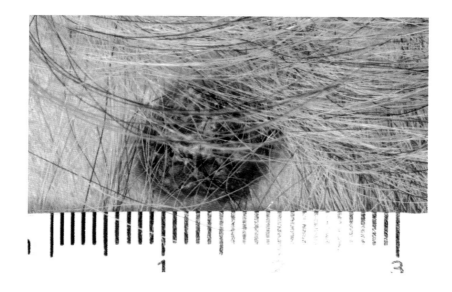

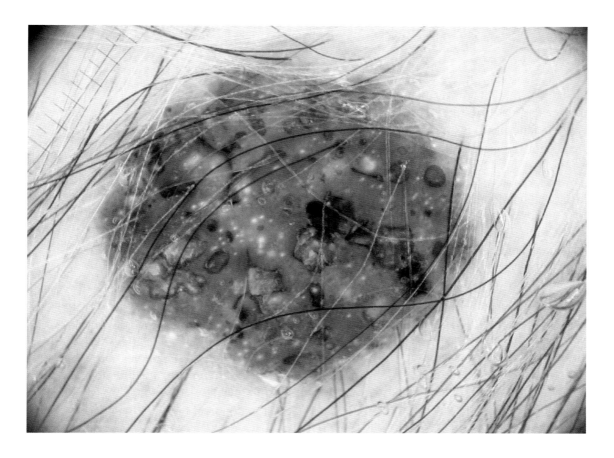

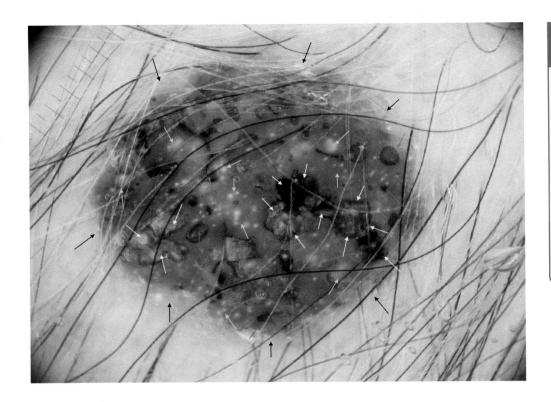

DIAGNOSIS:
Pigmented Seborrheic Keratosis

DISCUSSION

- The clinical differential diagnosis includes a pigmented seborrheic keratosis, pigmented basal cell carcinoma, and melanoma.
  - Fortunately for the patient, there are no criteria to suggest the diagnosis of pigmented basal cell carcinoma or melanoma.
- Milia-like cysts, pigmented and nonpigmented pseudofollicular openings, large keratin-filled crypts, and sharp border demarcation all combine to easily diagnose a seborrheic keratosis.
- Heavy pigmentation is a common, and often worrisome, feature seen in seborrheic keratosis.
- Milia-like cysts (epidermal horn cysts) are white or yellow, variously sized, roundish structures. They may appear opaque, or they may shine, like "stars in the sky." Both types are seen in this lesion, with a majority being stars in the sky.
- The lesion is also filled with pigmented and nonpigmented pseudofollicular openings (invaginations of the epidermis filled with keratin). Oxidized keratin gives them the dark color.
- Milia-like cysts and pseudofollicular openings may also be found in benign and malignant melanocytic lesions.
- There are 2 larger, irregular keratin-filled openings that are referred to as *crypts*.
- At times it is difficult to differentiate pigmented pseudofollicular openings from irregular dark dots and globules of a melanocytic lesion. It might also be difficult to differentiate irregular dark crypts from irregular blotches or ulceration.
- Fissures and ridges, fat fingers, and hairpin vessels, criteria used to diagnose seborrheic keratosis, are not found in this lesion.

PEARLS

- Be aware of seborrheic keratosis-like melanomas. Although rare, it is scary to know they do occur.
- Look for melanoma-specific criteria (eg, irregular pigment network, irregular streaks, bluish-white veil, irregular dots and globules, and bluish-black color) to help differentiate a pigmented seborrheic keratosis from melanoma.
- "If in doubt, cut it out!"

CASE 8

HISTORY
This lesion has been present for years without any changes.

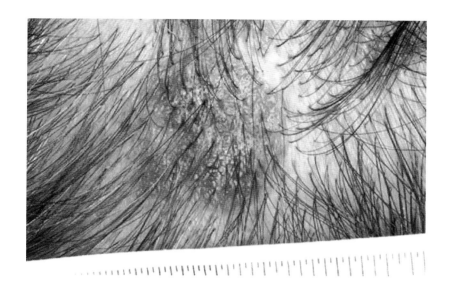

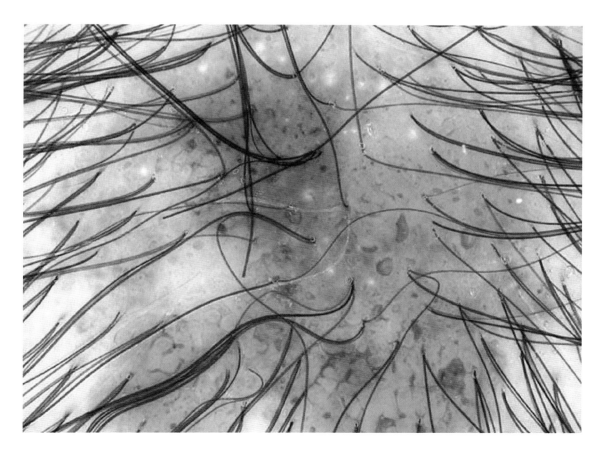

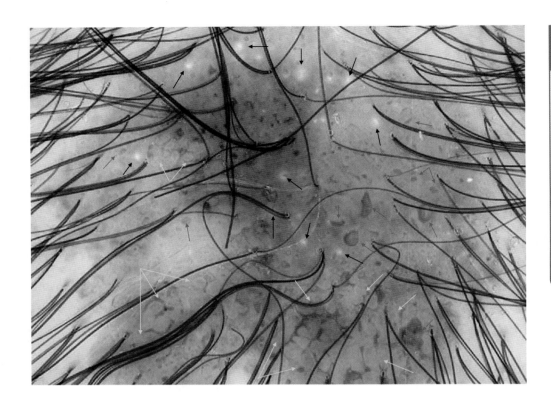

DIAGNOSIS:
Seborrheic Keratosis

DISCUSSION

- The history of no change for years plus the greasy brown clinical appearance of this pigmented well-demarcated plaque favor a benign diagnosis.
- Milia-like cysts, pigmented and nonpigmented pseudofollicular openings, fissures and ridges creating a brain-like pattern, diagnose a classic seborrheic keratosis.
- There are multiple milia-like cysts that are bright and shiny like stars in the sky.
- The pseudofollicular openings should not be confused with irregular brown dots and globules of a melanocytic lesion or follicular openings seen on the face.
- Thin, dark fissures and thick, light ridges, many with fat finger shapes in the lower section create the very commonly encountered classic cerebriform or brain-like pattern.

- The bluish color could be a red flag for concern for the novice dermoscopist; it has a differential diagnosis that includes inflammation and possibly a collision tumor (eg, melanoma and a seborrheic keratosis).
- Bluish-black color should always be a red flag for concern.
- Being filled with pigmented pseudofollicular openings is a positive sign that there is no high-risk pathology, unless you confuse the openings with the irregular dots and globules of a melanocytic lesion.

PEARLS

- Nonpolarized contact dermoscopy might make it easier to see milia-like cysts in seborrheic keratosis.
- You should pay special attention to black "seborrheic keratoses" and examine them with dermoscopy so as not to miss a seborrheic keratosis-like melanoma.

CASE 9

HISTORY
This was a solitary lesion on the right lower leg of a 69-year-old man.

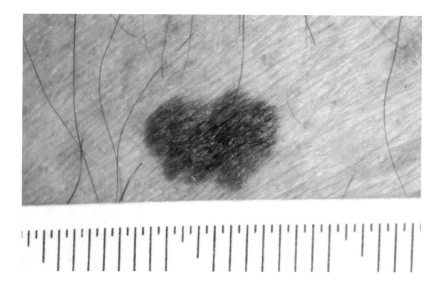

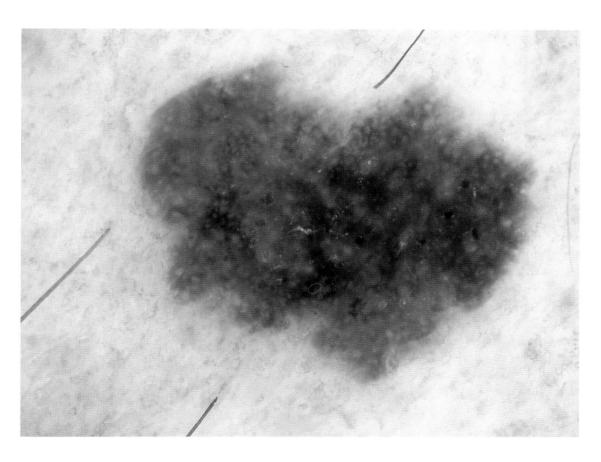

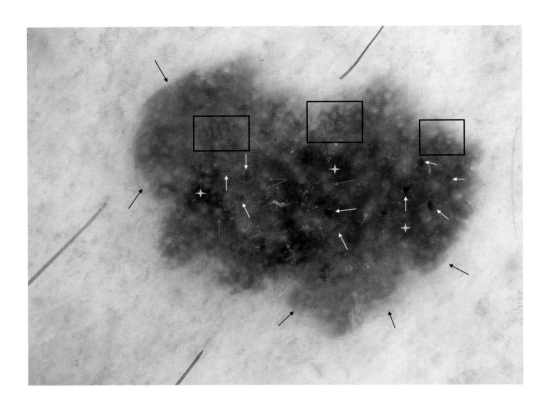

DERMOSCOPIC CRITERIA

- Asymmetry of color and structure
- Multicomponent global pattern
- Irregular pseudonet-work (boxes)
- Irregular black blotches (stars)
- Milia-like cysts (red arrows)
- Pigmented pseudofollic-ular openings (white arrows)
- Sharp border demarca-tion (black arrows)

DIAGNOSIS:
Pigmented Seborrheic Keratosis

DISCUSSION

- For the busy clinician, at first blush this lesion looks bad clinically and by dermoscopy.
  - There are irregular pigment network, asymmetry of color and structure, the multicomponent global pattern, irregular dark dots and globules, and irregular black blotches.
- On closer inspection things are looking better because there are multiple milia-like cysts, and the irregular dark dots and globules are really pigmented pseudofollicular openings.
  - Milia-like cysts and pseudofollicular openings can be found in seborrheic keratosis and melanocytic lesions.
- There appear to be foci of irregular pigment network. Seborrheic keratosis can have network-like structures created by hyperkeratosis and acanthosis and referred to as *pseudonetwork*.
- Sharp border demarcation further favors the diagnosis of a seborrheic keratosis.

- Bluish-black color should always be a red flag for concern in a "seborrheic keratosis," because it is one of the main dermoscopic features found in seborrheic keratosis-like melanomas.
- This lesion brings us into a gray zone that is neither clearly benign nor malignant. Rather, it has several high-risk features and deserves a histopathologic diagnosis.
- This could be considered a melanoma-like seborrheic keratosis. They are out there!

PEARLS

- Even for experienced dermoscopists, things will not always be clear.
- It is important to take your time and focus your attention to correctly identify what is going on in a given lesion.
- Be knowledgeable so that you can create a dermoscopic differential diagnosis when appropriate.

CASE 10

HISTORY
A 72-year-old woman was concerned about this spot on her face.

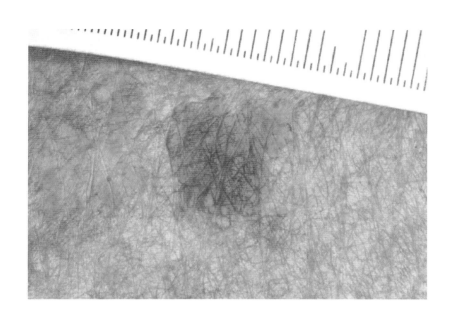

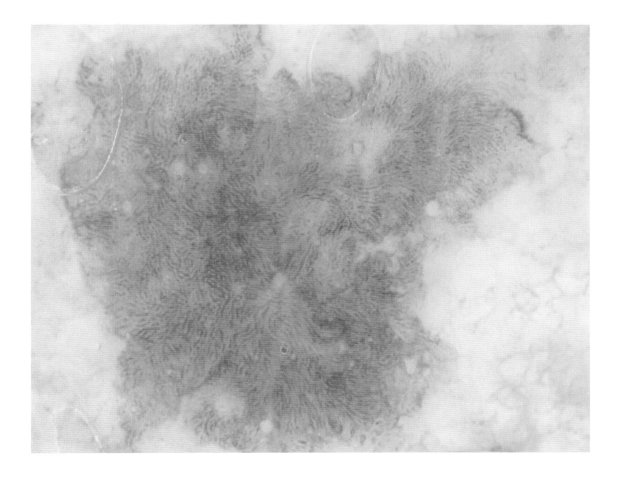

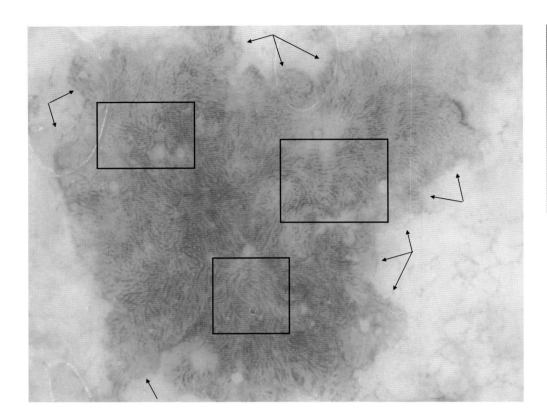

DERMOSCOPIC CRITERIA

- Fingerprint global pattern
- Parallel brown line segments (boxes)
- Moth-eaten borders (black arrows)
- Absence of reticulated pigment network

DIAGNOSIS:
Solar Lentigo

DISCUSSION

- This is a picture-perfect solar lentigo with sharp, concave moth-eaten borders and a very well-developed fingerprint pattern.
- The fingerprint pattern fills the lesion and is created by thin tan parallel line segments creating a swirl-and-whirl pattern similar to that of a fingerprint.
  - An appropriate metaphoric description of this criterion.
- Solar lentigo with this set of criteria can be found on any sun-exposed area.
- Things will not always be this clear, because in most cases the fingerprint pattern is not so well-developed.
- Beware; larger lesions, typically on the face, may have a mixture of criteria associated with solar lentigo, pigmented actinic keratosis, or lentigo maligna.
- Lentiginous melanoma not located on the face but on other sun-exposed areas might also have foci of the fingerprint pattern.

- It is important to differentiate the fingerprint pattern of a solar lentigo from the line segments of the pigment network of a melanocytic lesion that has reticulated/honeycomb-like line segments.
- There will be cases of solar lentigo that might have both features, a confounding dermoscopic finding.

PEARLS

- Facial pigmented lesions are some of the hardest to diagnose.
- Learn the criteria associated with benign and malignant facial pathology.
- It is essential to completely examine large facial lesions that might have a mixture of benign and malignant criteria.

CASE 11

HISTORY

This is one of many tan spots on the face of a 45-year-old woman.

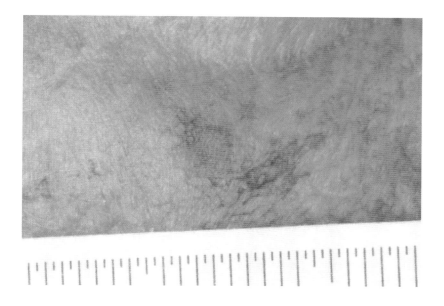

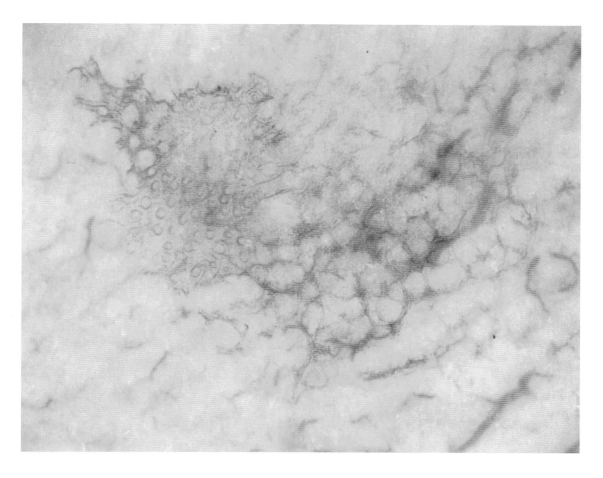

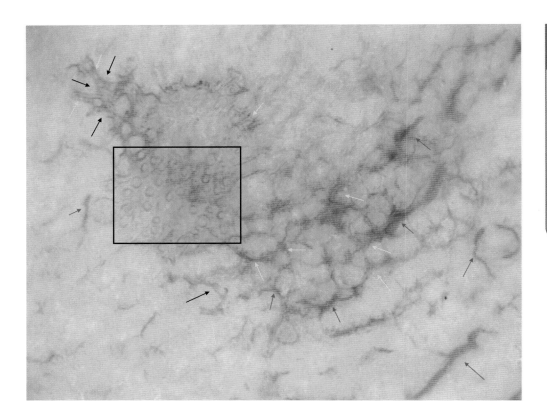

DERMOSCOPIC CRITERIA

- Fingerprint pattern
- Parallel brown line segments (yellow arrows)
- Moth-eaten borders (black arrows)
- Asymmetrical follicular pigmentation (box)
- Normal background skin vessels (red arrows)

DIAGNOSIS:
Solar Lentigo

DISCUSSION

- Clinically, but not dermoscopically, this is a banal tan macule.
- There are foci of poorly developed fingerprint pattern (as compared with the previous case) with fine, tan parallel line segments and moth-eaten, sharp concave borders. This suggests the diagnosis of a solar lentigo.
- There are areas with what looks like asymmetrical follicular pigmentation. However, when magnified, it becomes clearer that they are created by parallel line segments of the fingerprint pattern.
- The normal facial blood vessels seen here should not be confused with milky-red color seen in high-risk lesions.
- There is a large area of well-developed follicular openings that unfortunately reflect asymmetrical follicular pigmentation.
  - Asymmetrical follicular pigmentation is a primary criterion used to diagnose lentigo maligna. However, it is not diagnostic and may also be seen in a solar lentigo.

- Asymmetrical follicular pigmentation associated with lentigo maligna typically has more irregular and darker color partially surrounding follicular openings.
- The asymmetrical follicular pigmentation, created by uniform light tan color, in conjunction with the fingerprint pattern seen in this case, together favor the diagnosis of a solar lentigo.
- Any presentation of asymmetrical follicular pigmentation should be a red flag for concern, and for that reason this lesion should be biopsied.
- If you plan an incisional biopsy, it should be in the area of asymmetrical follicular pigmentation.

PEARLS

- Asymmetrical pigmentation seen, biopsy done!
- It might be a good idea to review the cases of lentigo maligna and lentigo maligna melanoma from Chapter 3 to refresh your memory on the criteria used to make these diagnoses.

CASE 12

HISTORY

This patient has diffuse actinic keratosis on his face. One area has a slightly raised scaly papule.

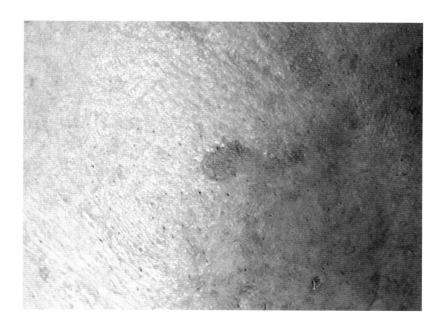

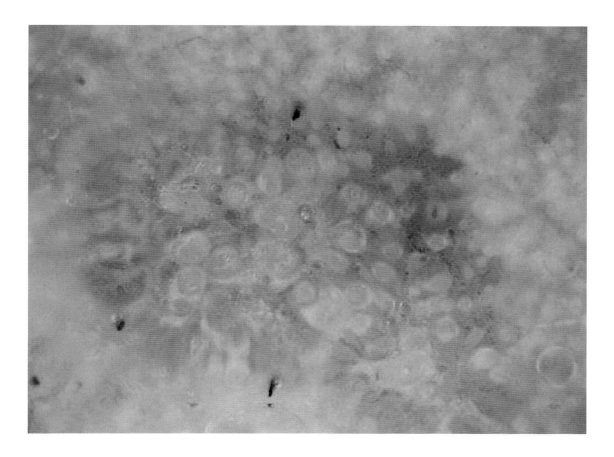

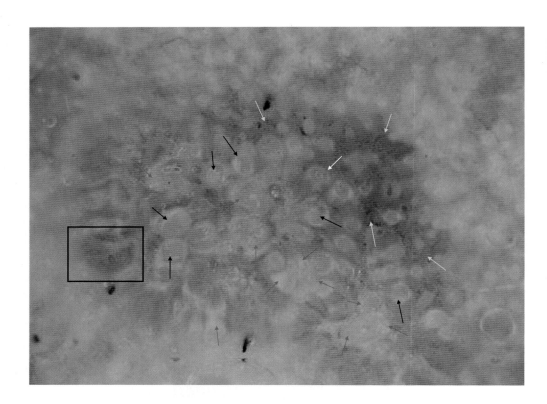

DIAGNOSIS:
Squamous Cell Carcinoma

DISCUSSION

- Clinically, the differential diagnosis of the scaly papule in an area of diffuse actinic keratoses includes a hypertrophic actinic keratosis versus early invasive squamous cell carcinoma.
- This lesion has dramatic white circles and featureless irregular homogeneous white areas associated with invasive squamous cell carcinoma.
- The hallmark of squamous cell carcinoma is keratinization, so white structureless areas are prevalent.
- The strawberry pattern associated with nonpigmented actinic keratosis is in the dermoscopic differential diagnosis. However, it would not be as dramatic as what is seen here.
- The strawberry pattern of a nonpigmented actinic keratosis consists of an irregular erythematous/pink pseudonetwork (created by arterioles) and follicular openings characterized by homogeneous, uniform, yellowish-white globules.

- Homogeneous brown pigmentation with irregular brown dots/globules can be seen in invasive squamous cell carcinoma.
- There is a focus of irregular hairpin vessels, which is an important clue that this is not an actinic keratosis.
  - Hairpin, comma, serpentine, pinpoint, or glomerular vessels may be found in invasive squamous cell carcinoma and are never seen in actinic keratosis.
- One circle within a circle was identified and is of no diagnostic significance.

PEARLS

- Clinically, it may be difficult to differentiate a hypertrophic actinic keratosis from early invasive squamous cell carcinoma.
- Learn the dermoscopic criteria to make the differentiation.
- When there are prominent white circles combined with larger irregular white areas, think invasive squamous cell carcinoma.

CASE 13

HISTORY
A 79-year-old man has this sore, nonhealing area on his face.

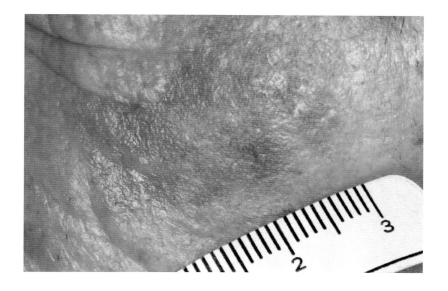

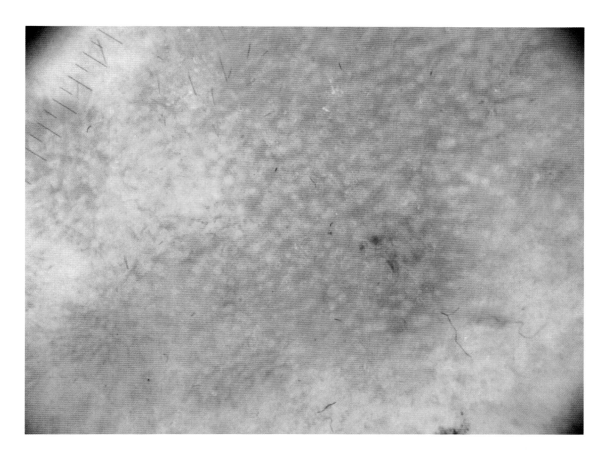

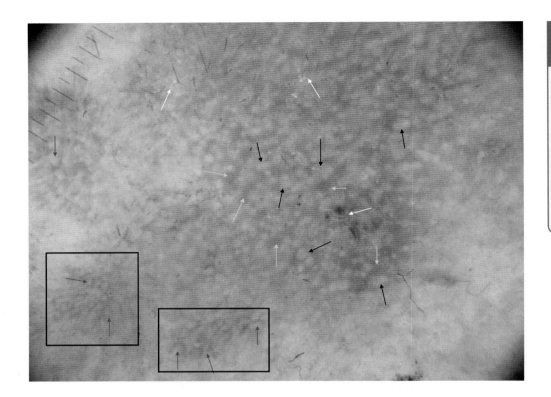

DERMOSCOPIC CRITERIA

■ Strawberry pattern
■ White circles
  (black arrows)
■ Erythematous pseudo-
  network (yellow arrows)
■ Asymmetrical follicular
  pigmentation
  (boxes, blue arrows)
■ Scale (white arrows)

DIAGNOSIS:
Actinic Keratosis

DISCUSSION

- Here you have it: the classic strawberry pattern of an actinic keratosis filling the majority of the lesion.
  - It is a good metaphor, and a pattern that you will see all the time if you look.
  - This pattern is only seen on the face.
- The strawberry pattern of a nonpigmented actinic keratosis consists of an irregular erythematous/pink pseudonetwork (created by arterioles) and follicular openings characterized by homogeneous, uniform yellowish-white globules.
  - Typically the pseudonetwork is spotty, whereas the follicular openings are uniform in shape and color.
- The lesion is large and sensitive; clinical findings suggestive of a squamous cell carcinoma.
- There are white circles that are uniform and small as compared with the dramatic and prominent white circles associated with invasive squamous cell carcinoma as presented in the previous case.

- There are 2 subtle foci of asymmetrical follicular pigmentation
  - Asymmetrical follicular pigmentation is considered a primary criterion to diagnose lentigo maligna. However, it is also a feature of actinic keratosis of the face.
- At times, it is impossible to differentiate a pigmented actinic keratosis from lentigo maligna if both contain prominent asymmetrical follicular pigmentation.

PEARLS

- You will be in for a surprise when you biopsy an actinic keratosis with the strawberry pattern and it turns out to be an amelanotic lentigo maligna.
  - Although amelanotic lentigo maligna is in the differential diagnosis, it occurs only rarely compared with pink actinic keratosis.
- "If it's pink, stop and think!"

CASE 14

HISTORY
This pink, scaly area was found on the forearm of a 50-year-old golfer.

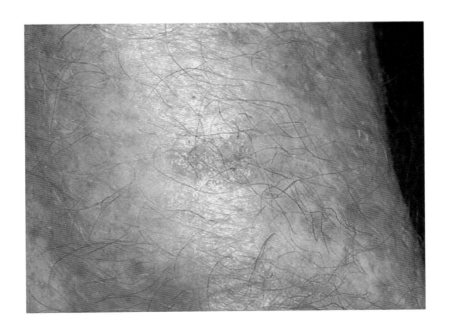

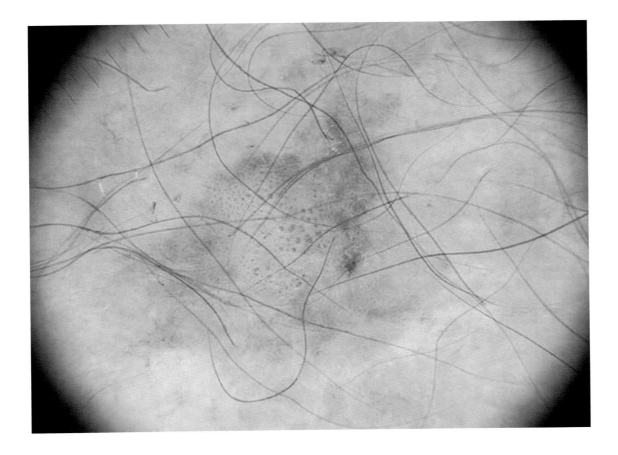

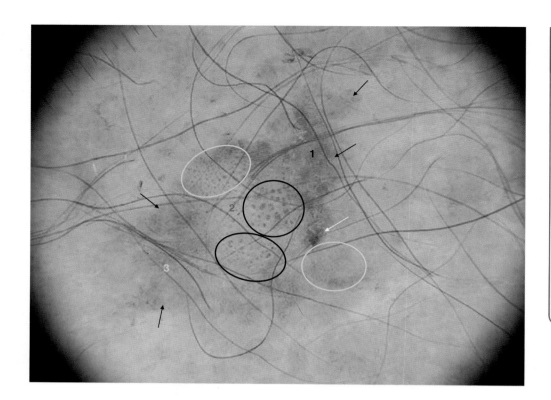

DIAGNOSIS:
Pigmented Bowen Disease

DISCUSSION

- In this case we find no criteria to diagnose a melanocytic lesion.
- There is, however, asymmetry of color and structure and the multicomponent global pattern. Both features are nonspecific.
- Pink lesions that lack melanoma-specific criteria usually have telangiectatic vessels that help make the diagnosis.
- Foci of pinpoint/dotted and glomerular/coiled vessels are seen. This puts Bowen disease at the top of the differential diagnostic list.
- There is also smudged tan color with foci of tiny brown dots representing the pigmentation associated with this pigmented Bowen disease.
- In most cases, Bowen disease presents as a pink scaly patch on sun-exposed skin in older patients with a history of excess sun exposure.

- Typically, it has a diffuse or spotty presentation of pinpoint and/or glomerular vessels, without pigment.
- With experience, the diagnosis of Bowen disease is made in a "blink," to be confirmed by biopsy.

PEARLS

- Vessels seen with dermoscopy are nonspecific yet have the possibility of suggesting a specific diagnosis.
  - Arborizing: Basal cell carcinoma
  - Pinpoint/glomerular: Bowen disease
  - Linear, curvilinear, circular pinpoint/glomerular vessels: Clear cell acanthoma
  - Polymorphous: Melanoma
  - Hairpin: Seborrheic keratosis
  - Comma: Nevus

CASE 15

HISTORY

This was a solitary asymptomatic lesion found on the forehead of a 92-year-old man. There is a no history of psoriasis.

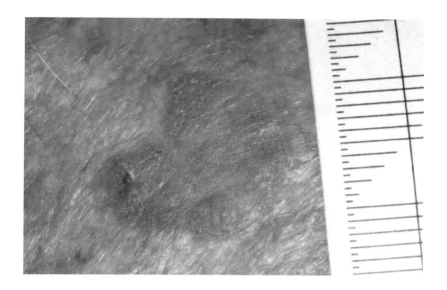

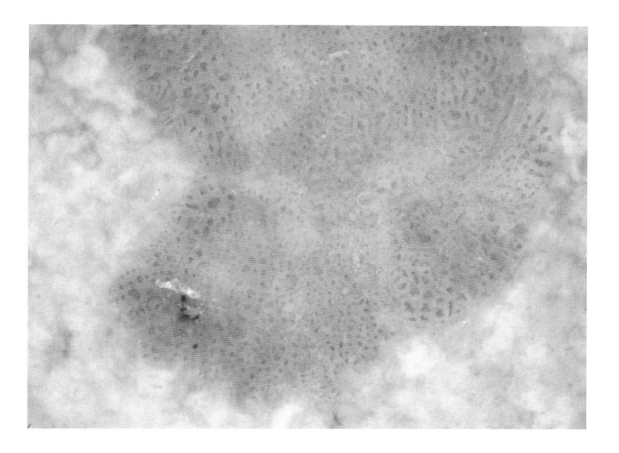

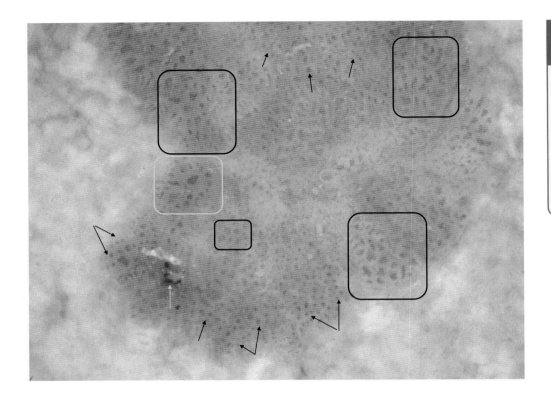

DERMOSCOPIC CRITERIA

- Glomerular vessels (black rectangles)
- Pinpoint/dotted vessels (black arrows)
- Pinpoint and glomerular vessels (yellow rectangle)
- Scab (yellow arrow)

DIAGNOSIS:
Bowen Disease

DISCUSSION

- This is a stereotypical example of Bowen disease.
- At first blush it appears to be full of coiled/round glomerular vessels.
- On closer inspection, there are also pinpoint/dotted vessels.
- Glomerular and pinpoint vessels are seen side by side.
  - In reality, pinpoint and glomerular shapes are a variation of the same vessel.
- There can be asymmetrical foci or a diffuse distribution of vessels in Bowen disease as opposed to a plaque of psoriasis, which typically has a diffuse distribution filling the lesion with only pinpoint/dotted vessels.
- Scattered throughout the lesion, some of the larger glomerular vessels have a linear appearance.

PEARLS

- Polarized dermoscopy using gel or mineral oil and minimal pressure gives you the best view of all telangiectatic vessels.
- The clinical impression of psoriasis can be confirmed in a "blink" by dermoscopy with the identification of pinpoint vessels filling multiple red scaly plaques—"inflammoscopy."

CASE 16

HISTORY
A 62-year-old man was concerned about this nonhealing lesion in his groin.

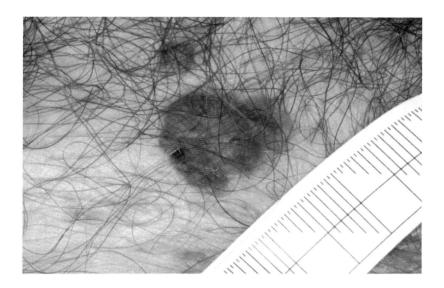

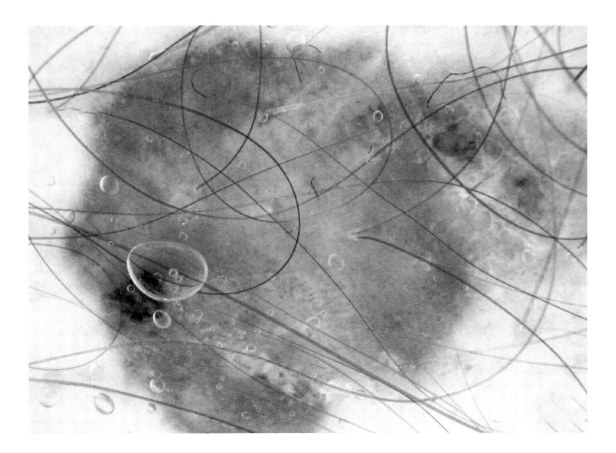

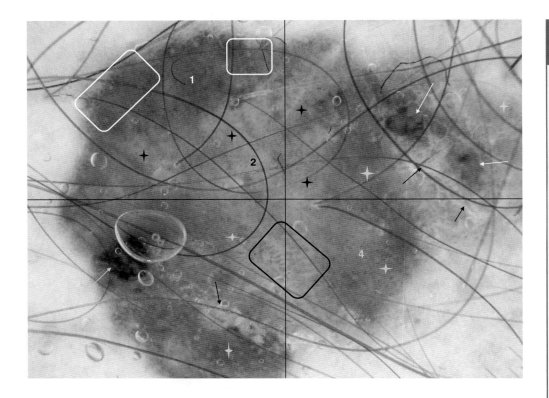

DIAGNOSIS:
Pigmented Bowen Disease

DERMOSCOPIC CRITERIA

- Asymmetry of color and structure (+)
- Multicomponent global pattern (1, 2, 3, 4, 5)
- Regression with "peppering" (black stars)
- Milky-red color and pinpoint vessels (yellow stars)
- Irregular black blotch (yellow arrow)
- White network (black rectangle)
- Brown dots (white rectangles)
- Scabs (white arrows)
- Hyperkeratosis (black arrows)
- Six colors (black, light/dark brown, white, gray, pink)

DISCUSSION

- Clinically, but not dermoscopically, this looks like a seborrheic keratosis. However, there are no dermoscopic criteria to suggest this could be a seborrheic keratosis.
- The entire lesion has an unusual grainy appearance that is not typical for melanocytic lesions—a red flag for concern.
  - There is asymmetry of color and structure and the multicomponent global pattern—nonspecific.
  - There are subtle foci of brown dots and globules that could define this as a melanocytic lesion.
    - Brown dots and globules can be seen in nonmelanocytic lesions (eg, basal cell carcinoma, Bowen disease).
  - The lesion is filled with what looks like regression with bony-white color and fine grayish dots and blotches.
  - The lesion also has milky-red color with subtle pinpoint vessels.

- There are 1 irregular black blotch, a focus of poorly defined white network, foci of scabs, and hyperkeratosis.
- This lesion has all of the criteria needed to diagnose an invasive melanoma, yet the criteria are presenting differently from how they would look in a typical invasive melanoma—in other words, the grainy look.
  - A biopsy diagnosed pigmented Bowen disease.
- Because the first consideration was invasive melanoma, the case was discussed and reviewed by our dermatopathologist. Pigmented Bowen disease was confirmed.

PEARLS

- It is worth the time and effort to take digital dermoscopic images of potentially high-risk lesions.
- Studying digital dermoscopic images allows you to see things more clearly and offers a better opportunity to analyze criteria in lesions that seem difficult to diagnose.

CASE 17

HISTORY
This is from the abdomen of a 19-year-old patient and has been getting scabby over a 3-month period.

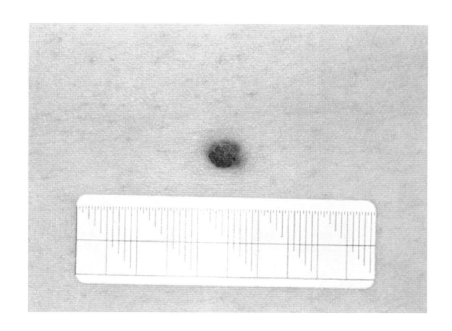

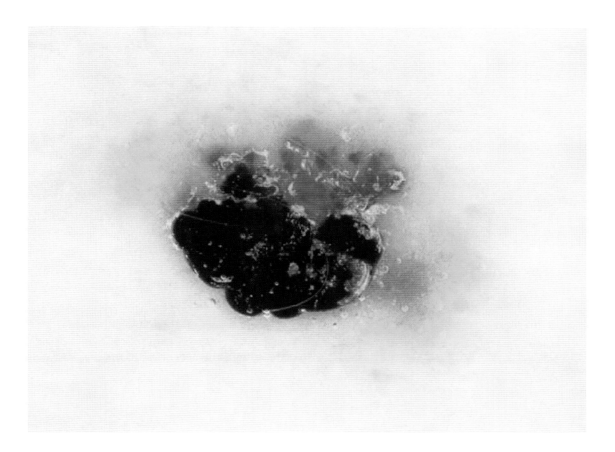

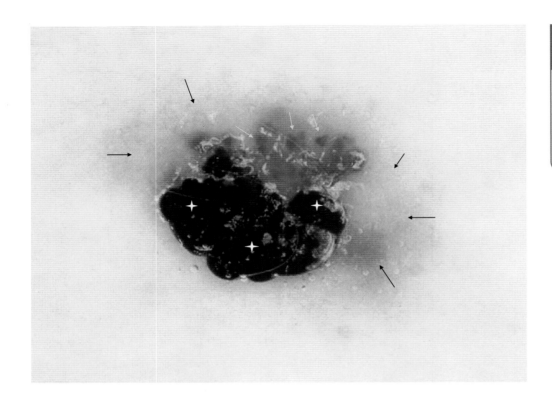

DIAGNOSIS:
Thrombosed Hemangioma

DISCUSSION

- This worrisome gray-zone lesion that could be an invasive melanoma turned out to be a thrombosed hemangioma.
- A hemorrhagic crust, remnants of lacunae, and peripheral erythema characterize the lesion.
- The lacunae represent what is left of the hemangioma.
- Milky-red color with milky-red globules of a melanoma are in the differential diagnosis of the hemangioma component.
- At times, it might be difficult to differentiate the sharply demarcated lacunae of a hemangioma from the out-of-focus milky-red globules seen in melanoma.
- The peripheral erythema represents inflammation and is a nonspecific finding.
- Potential melanoma dermoscopic analysis: the lesion is melanocytic by default. There is asymmetry of color and structure, the multicomponent global pattern, a large irregular black blotch, milky-red color, and milky-red globules.
- Melanoma can have ulceration and crust formation.
- A pyogenic granuloma, which is in the clinical differential diagnosis, would not have such a large hemorrhagic crust.

PEARLS

- A thrombosed angiokeratoma might also look like this, especially because there are areas of yellow color that represent hyperkeratosis.
- A positive stool guaiac test might help differentiate hemorrhagic crust (guaiac positive) from a nonulcerated black blotch in a melanoma (guaiac negative).
- The color seen in thrombosed vascular lesions is often as jet black as ever can be seen when using dermoscopy, with the exception of the black lamella.

CASE 18

HISTORY
A 43-year-old woman had this nonchanging, asymptomatic lesion on her right lower leg for 9 months.

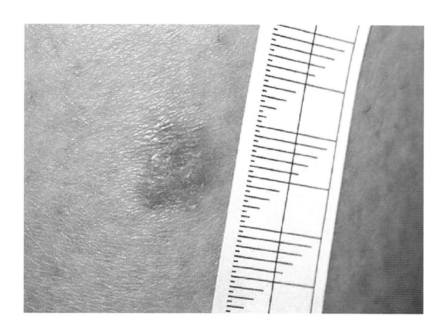

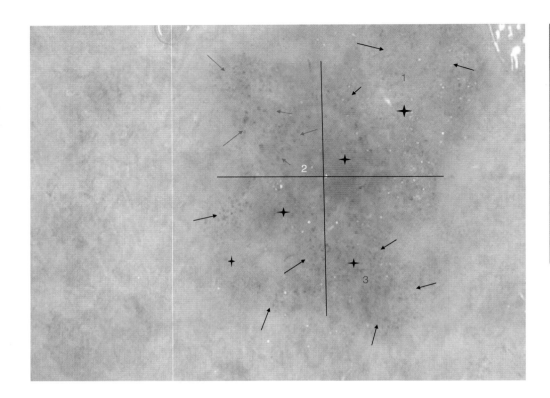

DERMOSCOPIC CRITERIA

- Asymmetry of color an structure (+)
- Multicomponent global pattern (1, 2, 3)
- Pinpoint/dotted vessels (red arrows)
- Homogeneous gray color and peppering (stars)
- Peppering (black arrows)

DIAGNOSIS:

Lichen Planus–Like Keratosis

DISCUSSION

- Regressive melanoma should be your first thought here.
  - Regression filling a lesion is always a very serious dermoscopic finding.
- The good news is the same regressive picture could also be associated with a chronic lichen planus–like keratosis.
- There is asymmetry of color and structure, the multicomponent global pattern, and regression made up of grayish-white color with the gray dots of peppering.
- Some of the foci of dots and globules have the suggestion of red color. They could represent dotted and glomerular vessels.
- There is also a suggestion of diffuse brownish and pink color seen clinically and with dermoscopy.
- Lichen planus–like keratosis can be acute, subacute, or chronic.
- **Acute lichen planus–like keratosis,** the most common presentation, is typically a pink lesion with greasy yellow scale that has milky-red/pink color with polymorphous vessels. This may be indistinguishable from amelanotic melanoma.

- **Subacute lichen planus–like keratosis** is characterized by dusky-red or violaceous color seen clinically along with irregularly pigmented shades of brown, gray, and/or white color and a variable amount of regression with prominent peppering.
- **Chronic lichen planus–like keratosis** typically is filled with peppering.
- A subset of lichen planus–like keratosis is thought to represent immunologically mediated regression of a preexisting benign lesion such as solar lentigo or seborrheic keratosis. Consequently, there might be residual foci of criteria associated with the previous lesion such as a fingerprint pattern in the case of a solar lentigo along with peppering.

PEARLS

- Put lichen planus–like keratosis in your differential diagnosis of regressive lesions with peppering, and you will not be too surprised when a lesion that you are concerned is a bad melanoma turns out not to be.
- The presence of greasy yellowish scales in a pink lesion is an important clue to diagnose acute lichen planus–like keratosis.

CASE 19

HISTORY
This firm papule was found on the right shin of a 48-year-old woman.

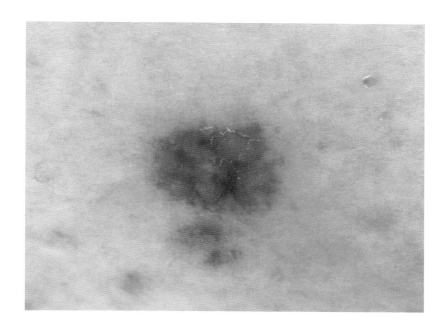

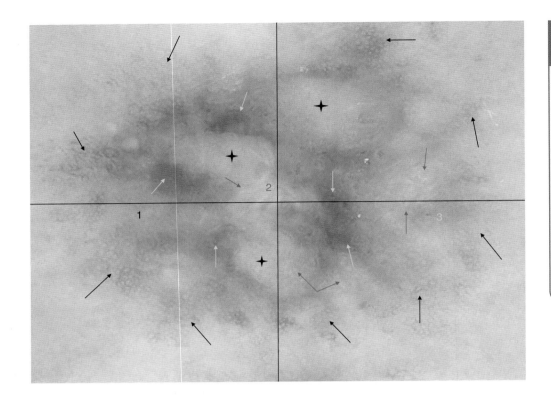

DIAGNOSIS:
Dermatofibroma

DISCUSSION

- The pigment network might be seen in a melanocytic lesion or in a dermatofibroma.
- Dermatofibroma is one of the nonmelanocytic lesions that can have pigment network.
- The irregular bony-white color could represent regression of a melanoma, or it could represent fibroplasia of dermatofibroma.
- The history of a longstanding, nonchanging lesion that is firm to palpation favors the diagnosis of a dermatofibroma.
- A classic dermatofibroma is made up of regular peripheral pigment network and a centrally located bony-white patch. Telangiectatic vessels may also be present.
- There are variations of the central white patch that could look like a white network or like crystalline structures.
  - There are foci of crystalline structures in the central white patch in this lesion.
  - When irregular, the white color of a dermatofibroma is indistinguishable from regression seen in melanomas.
- One must be aware that there are innumerable variations of morphology and color that can be found in a dermatofibroma. However, all dermatofibromas are by definition pathologically benign, regardless of whether the color appears regular or irregular.
- The diffuse erythema seen clinically blanches away with pressure and is a nonspecific finding.
- The irregular purplish-white blotches could represent deep pigmentation of a melanocytic lesion or vascularization that could be seen in a melanocytic lesion or a dermatofibroma.
- It is not the milky-red color typically seen in melanomas.

PEARLS

- Irregular-appearing dermatofibromas warrant a histopathologic diagnosis.
- Beware of dermatofibroma-like melanomas.
- A "dermatofibroma" with white network could actually be a melanoma.
- Learn how to differentiate crystalline structures from white network.
- White network is reticular, whereas crystalline structures are never reticular.
- Be sure to analyze all of the criteria in a lesion before making a diagnosis.

CASE 20

HISTORY
This was found on the back of an 88-year-old man.

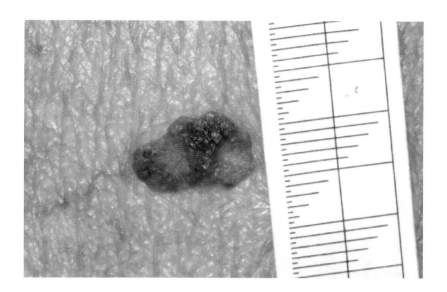

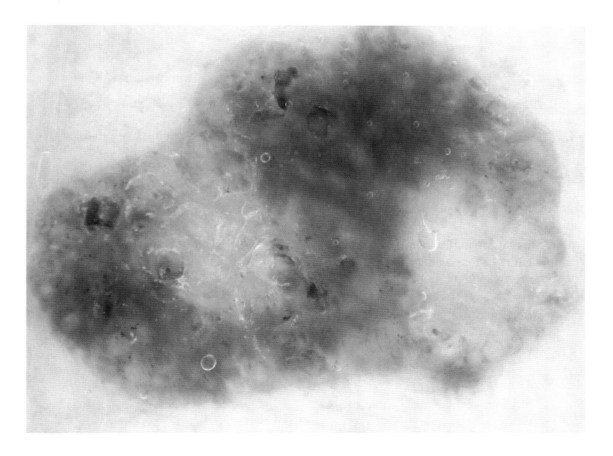

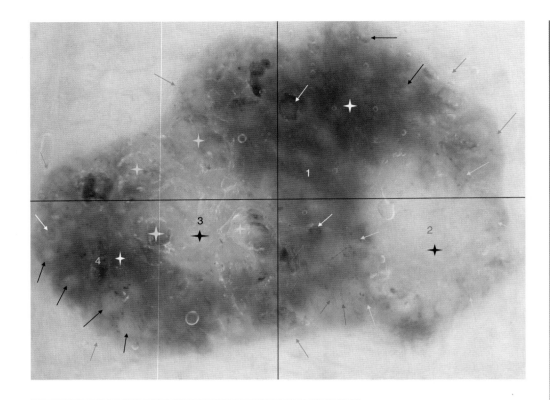

DIAGNOSIS:
Seborrheic Keratosis

DISCUSSION

- Do not let the 2 large areas with irregular pinkish-white color throw you off. Although white color is a red flag for concern, it is not always associated with high-risk pathology.
- There is asymmetry of color and structure and the multicomponent global pattern with 4 zones. These two features are also not always associated with high-risk pathology.
- Sharp border demarcation, multiple milia-like cysts, a few nonpigmented pseudofollicular openings, and greasy scale support the diagnosis of a seborrheic keratosis.
- Hairpin vessels, which may or may not be present, are associated with seborrheic keratosis. This lesion has a focus of serpentine vessels but no hairpin vessels.
- The pinkish-white area could represent fibroplasia (scarring) or giant milia-like cysts.
- In a small subset of seborrheic keratosis, milia-like cysts may be very large.

- There are foci of gray color with peppering that represent inflammation and are a common nonspecific finding in SK.
- Dark brown hyperpigmentation is also commonly found in seborrheic keratosis (pigmented seborrheic keratosis).
- Beware! Bluish-black color could be a clue that you are dealing with a seborrheic keratosis–like melanoma.
- There are no features to suggest this lesion is a collision tumor.

PEARLS

- Keep in the back of your mind that seborrheic keratosis is one of the most common pathologies associated with benign and malignant collision tumors.
- Hopefully, with a high index of suspicion you will not miss a seborrheic keratosis–like melanoma or a high-risk collision tumor (eg, seborrheic keratosis and squamous cell carcinoma, seborrheic keratosis and melanoma).

CASE 21

HISTORY

The patient's gynecologist was concerned about the irregular pigmentation on his patient's nipple.

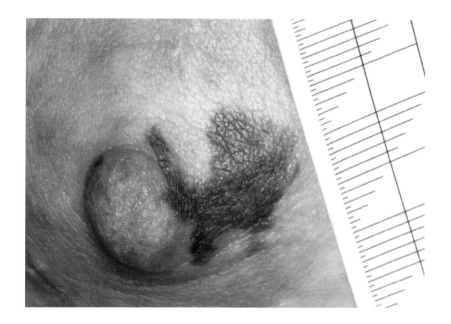

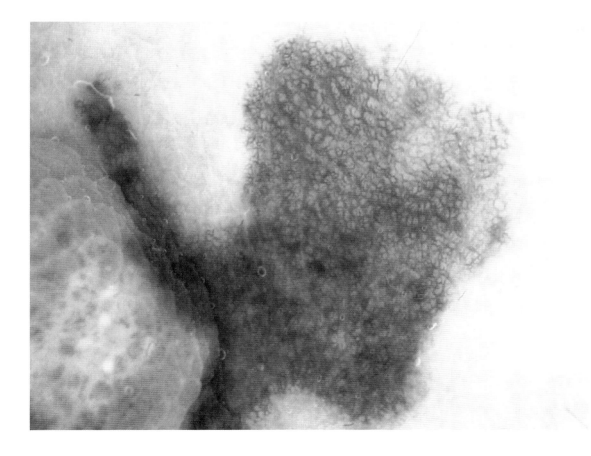

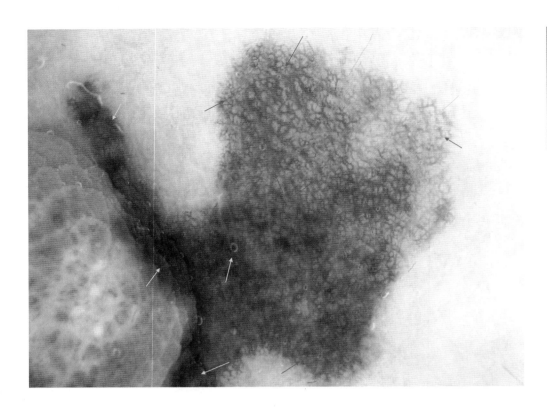

DIAGNOSIS:
Melanosis

DISCUSSION

- The differential diagnosis of eccentric pigmentation on the nipple and/or areola includes benign melanosis, pigmented Paget disease, and melanoma.
- Hyperpigmentation and regular pigment network diagnose benign melanosis of the nipple.
- This is another example of a nonmelanocytic lesion that has pigment network.
- Regular versus irregular dermoscopic criteria will point in the right direction.
- In this case there are no irregular dermoscopic criteria.
- Features of benign melanosis of the nipple/areola: a young woman in the 20- to 30-year-old age group, solitary lesion with eccentric, homogeneous brown color, regular pigment network or the cobblestone pattern, and stable over time.
  - One might see a cobblestone pattern due to the natural cobblestone pattern of the nipple.

- Histopathologically, there is hyperpigmentation of the basal layer without atypia with a normal to slightly increased number of melanocytes.
- The presence of melanoma-specific criteria brings into play the differential diagnosis of melanoma or pigmented Paget disease.
- Melanosis of the nipple/areola is part of the family of melanosis of the vulva, penis, lip, and oral cavity.

PEARLS

- Pigmentation on the nipple and/or areola should be examined with dermoscopy before any surgical procedure.
- If there are any melanoma-specific criteria, a histopathologic diagnosis should be made posthaste.

CASE 22

HISTORY
A 44-year-old woman has a tender nonhealing area on her right nipple.

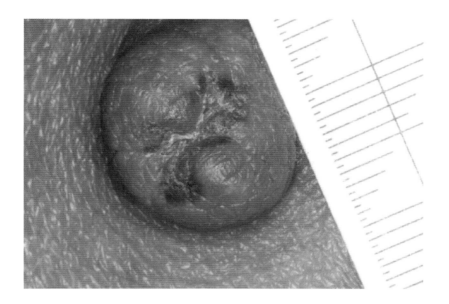

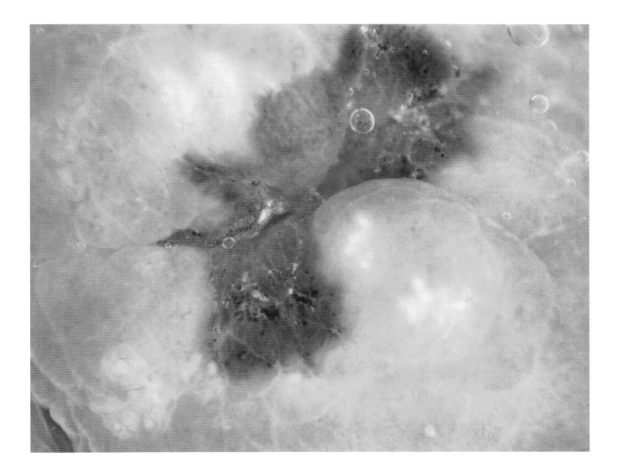

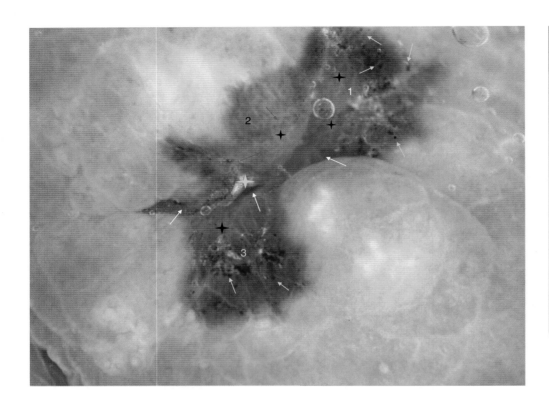

DERMOSCOPIC CRITERIA

- Asymmetry of color and structure
- Multicomponent global pattern (1, 2, 3)
- Scattered irregular brown dots and globules (yellow arrows)
- Milky-red color (black stars)
- Milky-red globules (red arrows)
- Fissure (white arrows)
- Scab (yellow star)
- Five colors (light/dark brown, pink, white, gray)

DIAGNOSIS:
Pigmented Paget Disease

DISCUSSION

- At first blush, compared with the previous case, this is looking bad.
- There is definite asymmetry of color and structure with the multicomponent global pattern—high-risk features.
- The exact number of zones is up for debate. Whether there are 3 or 4 zones, it does not make a difference.
- There are irregular milky-red areas with a suggestion of foci of milky-red globules. High-risk!
- Irregular brown dots and globules are scattered throughout the lesion. These could define a melanocytic lesion.
- An irregular, centrally located fissure and the presence of 5 colors round off the criteria in this pigmented Paget disease.

- "Blink"; there is nothing low-risk in this lesion, and a biopsy is indicated posthaste.
- It is not possible to differentiate this pigmented Paget disease from melanoma on clinical/dermoscopic grounds.

PEARLS

- Melanoma and pigmented Paget disease of the nipple/areola are both rare tumors.
- Contact dermoscopy using gel or oil will bring out the criteria in a scaly/dry lesion like this.
- A biopsy of any part of this lesion should make the diagnosis.

CASE 23

HISTORY
The physician of a 62-year-old woman noticed this nail discoloration and referred her for evaluation to rule out melanoma.

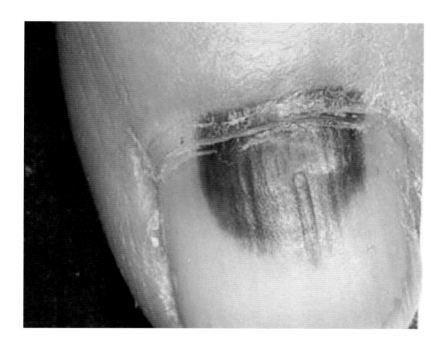

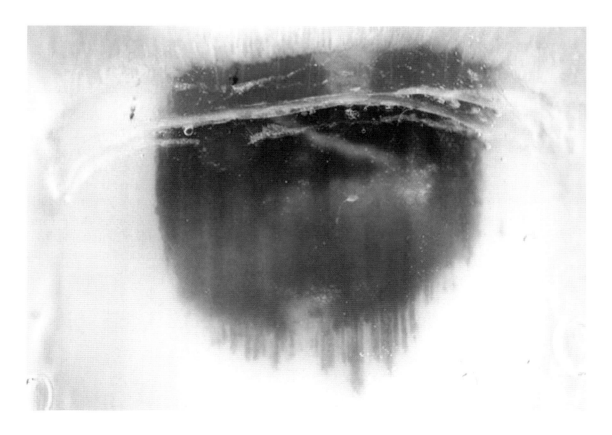

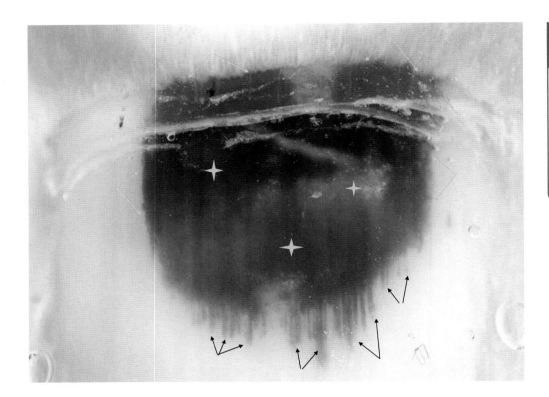

DERMOSCOPIC CRITERIA

- Homogeneous bluish-white color (stars)
- Well-demarcated proximal and lateral borders (yellow arrows)
- Purple filamentous distal border (black arrows)

DIAGNOSIS:
Subungual Hematoma

DISCUSSION

- This is a classic example of a subungual hematoma with bluish-white homogeneous color, well-demarcated lateral and proximal borders, and a purplish filamentous distal border.
  - The filamentous lines are solid and bear no resemblance to irregular hairpin vessels that can be seen in a malignant blue nevus.
  - Purple is not the only color seen as a result of subungual hemorrhage. Shades of black, blue, brown, green, and yellow often develop, depending on the stage of heme oxidation.
  - Irregular bony-white color secondary to trauma can also been seen, and it should not be confused with the bony-white color of regression.
  - Although not seen here, another very characteristic feature of subungual hematoma are blood spots, and blood pebbles, which look like irregular purple and/or red (not brown) dots and globules.

- A history of trauma is typical and strongly supports the diagnosis.
- Beware! It is essential to examine the entire nail to rule out melanoma-specific criteria, because blood itself may also be found in nail apparatus melanoma.

PEARLS

- Even though the solid purplish filamentous distal border and blood spots are not seen in every case, they are very typical and often are the major clues to diagnose subungual hematoma. Seek them out!
- Be cutting-edge and take digital clinical and dermoscopic images of subungual hematomas to document their expected migration and ultimate disappearance as the nail grows out distally.

CASE 24

HISTORY
A 34-year-old woman has had this dark brown pigmentation on her vulva for many years.

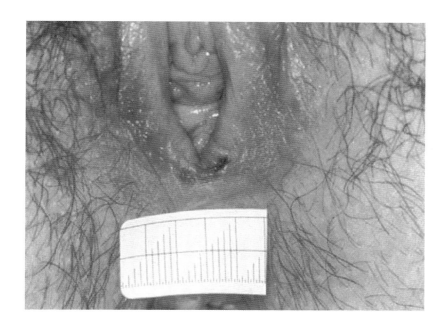

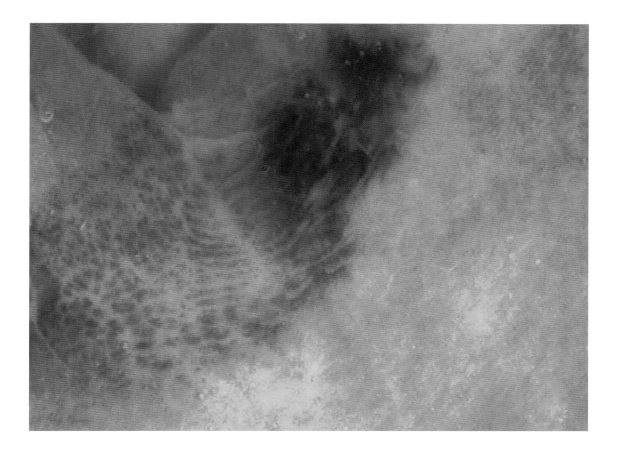

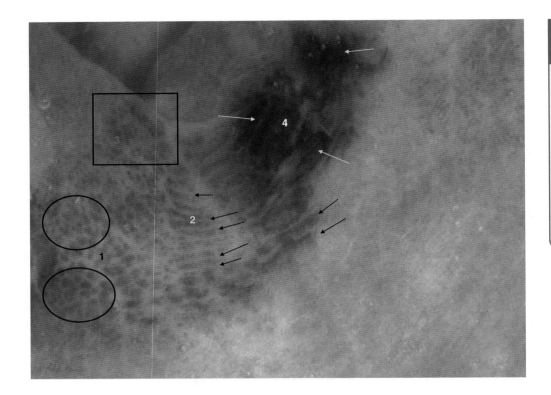

DIAGNOSIS:
Genital Lentigo

DISCUSSION

- The history is low-risk, whereas clinically and dermoscopically this genital lentigo has worrisome features.
- There is a multicomponent global pattern with 4 different areas that put melanoma in the differential diagnosis.
  - Globular pattern made up of regular brown dots and globules (zone 1).
  - Parallel pattern made up of regular thick parallel brown line segments (zone 2).
  - Homogeneous gray color (zone 3).
  - Irregular dark brown blotch (zone 4).
- Other than the prominent irregular dark brown blotch, which is the most worrisome feature, this lesion has a combination of benign patterns that can be seen in a genital lentigo.
- The focus of homogeneous gray color represents peppering than can result from inflammation or trauma.
- Black, blue, pink, and white colors in any form are the high-risk colors associated with melanoma in the genital area.

- The differential diagnosis includes a lentigo, inflamed lentigo, melanocytic nevus, and collision tumor (ie, lentigo and nevus, lentigo and melanoma).
- A histopathologic diagnosis is indicated.

PEARLS

- It is critical to address the fact that skin cancers can and do arise in the genital area.
- If is necessary to make a histopathologic diagnosis, one should select the most atypical dermoscopic area for an incisional biopsy or biopsies to avoid more aggressive surgical techniques.
  - To rule out a collision tumor, more than one incisional biopsy should be performed.
  - Alert your pathologist to be on the lookout for a possible collision tumor when one is in the differential diagnosis.

CASE 25

HISTORY
A 55-year-old woman was concerned about the discoloration in her genital area.

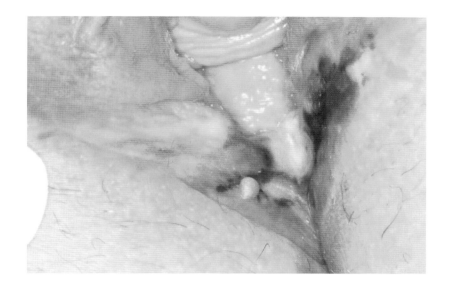

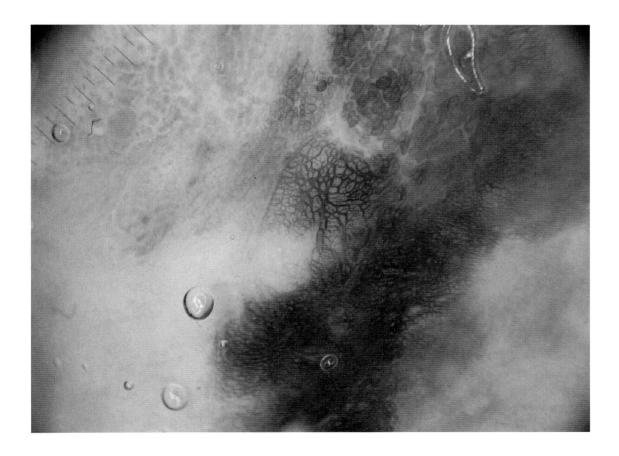

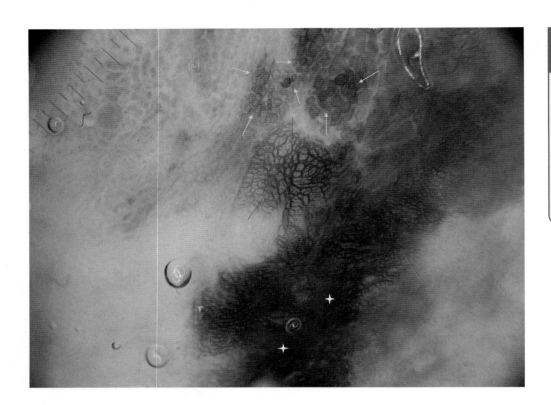

DIAGNOSIS:
Genital Lentigo

DISCUSSION

- The criteria are very well developed.
  - There are foci of ring-like structures.
    - Although not well studied criterion, ring-like structures have been associated with mucosal lentigines and Bowenoid papulosis. They can also be found in dermatofibromas and seborrheic keratosis.
  - The pigment network, although prominent, is nevertheless uniform and regular, and thus is considered low-risk.
  - The area of greater concern is the irregular black blotch with subtle blue color. This black blotch is an indication for a biopsy.

- Black, blue, pink, and white in any form are high-risk colors associated with melanoma in the genital area.
- The biopsy was consistent with mucosal lentigo without atypical features.

PEARLS

- Avoid contaminating your dermatoscope with mucosal lesions by using a noncontact technique.
  - Polyethylene food wrap film barrier (eg, Saran wrap) could be used as an interface between the genital mucosa and your dermatoscope to avoid contamination.

CHAPTER 5

Dermoscopy in General Dermatology

Aimilios Lallas, MD, MSc, PhD

General Instructions

- For each case, there is a short history along with a clinical and an unmarked dermoscopic image.
- Study the unmarked dermoscopic image and try to identify the global and local dermoscopic features.
- Make your diagnosis.
- Next, turn the page and the dermoscopic image will be presented again, this time marked with all the salient dermoscopic findings.
- On the same page you will also find the diagnosis along with a detailed discussion and a few pearls for your review.

CASE 1

HISTORY
These lesions were symmetrically located on the shins of a 70-year-old woman.

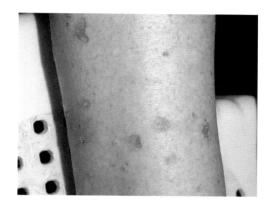

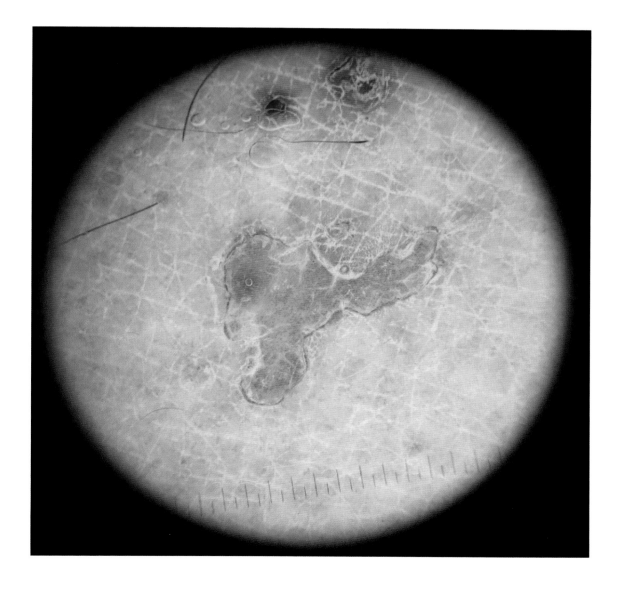

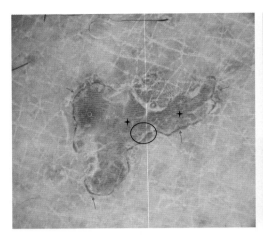
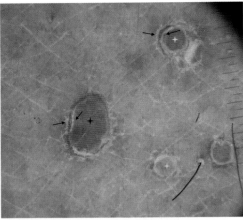

DERMOSCOPIC CRITERIA

- Peripheral white to brownish scaly rim ("white track") (red arrows)
- Double white track at some sites of the peripheral rim (black arrows)
- Multiple dotted/pinpoint (black stars) and a few short linear vessels (black circle)
- Homogeneous white-yellowish center in 2 lesions (yellow stars)

DIAGNOSIS:
Disseminated Superficial Actinic Porokeratosis

DISCUSSION

- The diagnosis is disseminated superficial actinic porokeratosis.
- The dermoscopic hallmark of disseminated superficial actinic porokeratosis is white track structures at the periphery.
  - These structures have also been described as "volcanic craters."
  - They may be singular or double.
  - They reflect the pathognomonic cornoid lamellae of disseminated superficial actinic porokeratosis seen on histopathology.
- Red dots, globules, and lines in the center correspond to the vessels of the superficial plexus that become visible as a result of the central atrophy typical of disseminated superficial actinic porokeratosis.

- White-yellowish homogeneous areas that correspond to acanthosis are rarely seen.
- Depending on the clinical subtype of porokeratosis, different dermoscopic features may be seen.
  - For example, porokeratosis of Mibelli is characterized by dark brown continuous lines circumscribing a central hypopigmented scar-like area. Brown globules/dots and red dots in the central area may also be found.

PEARL

- The peripheral white track structure in dermoscopy is a strong diagnostic criterion of any type of porokeratosis, because it is never seen in other dermatologic entities.

CASE 2

HISTORY
A 79-year-old man complained of swelling, redness, and itching on his face for the past year.

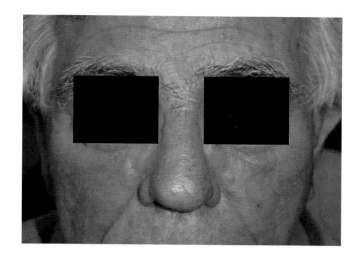

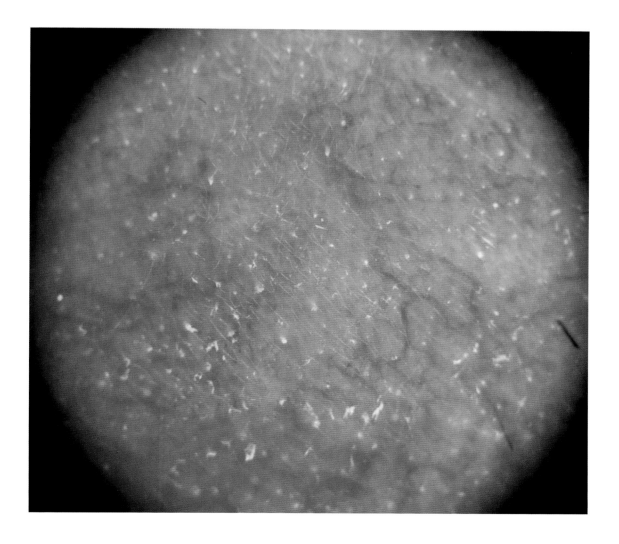

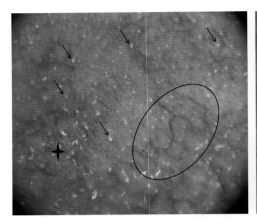 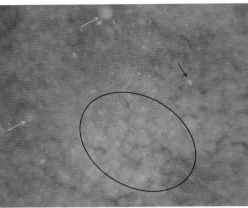

DIAGNOSIS:

Rosacea

DISCUSSION

- The diagnosis is type 1 (erythematotelangiectatic) rosacea.
  - Linear vessels arranged in a polygonal network (vascular polygons) are the dermoscopic hallmark.
  - Since the vascular polygons are not present in other skin diseases, they represent a very specific criterion for the diagnosis of rosacea.
  - Demodex tails, which correspond to the presence of *D. folliculorum*, are not always present.
  - White-yellowish globules correspond to the pustules and are a characteristic additional dermoscopic feature of type 2 (papulopustular) rosacea.
  - In type 2 rosacea, we usually observe the combination of vascular polygons and pustules.

- In type 4 (granulomatous/phymatous) rosacea, we also may see the following:
  - Orange-yellowish structureless areas, which histologically correspond to the presence of granulomas in the dermis and overlying fine arborizing vessels.
- White scales are an additional, albeit nonspecific, dermoscopic finding that may be present in all the clinical subtypes of rosacea.

PEARLS

- The linear vessels are not always arranged in a perfect polygonal network as seen in the present case. Rather, vessels may also present in a so-called zigzag vascular pattern of incomplete polygons.
- Microscopic identification of several Demodex mites (using a 15 blade and mineral oil) may help to guide your initial treatment by decreasing their prevalence and thereby potentially mitigate disease severity.

CASE 3

HISTORY

A 49-year-old woman was referred by her primary care physician to diagnose and treat this lesion that has been present for 6 months.

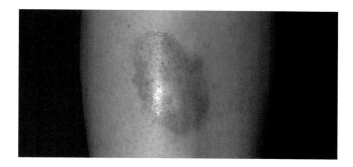

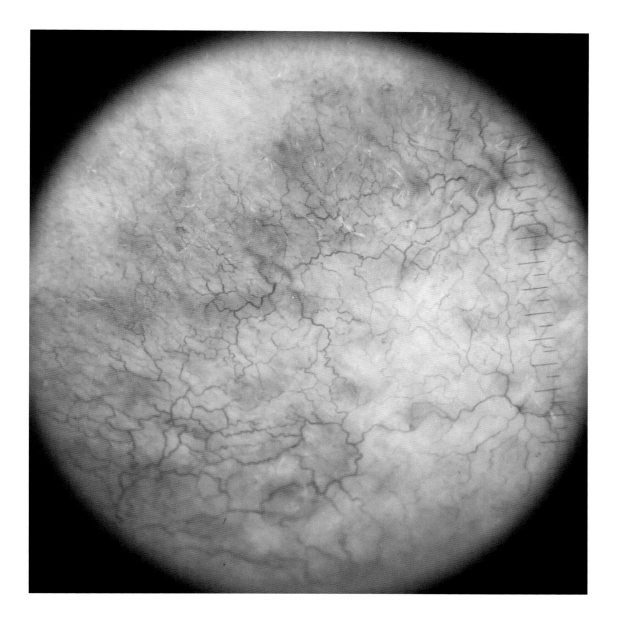

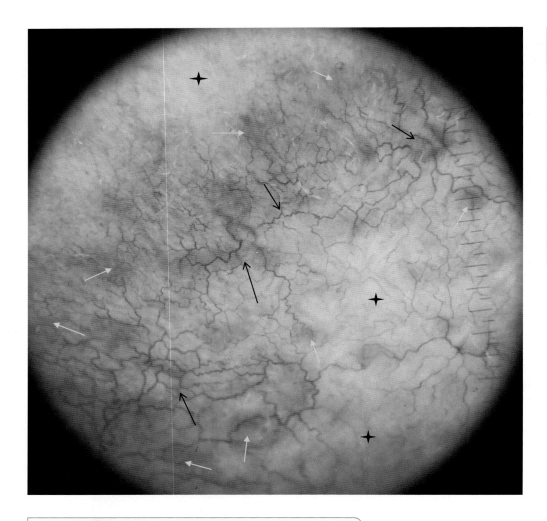

DIAGNOSIS:
Necrobiosis Lipoidica

DISCUSSION

- Necrobiosis lipoidica is a granulomatous dermatosis, which exhibits a characteristic dermoscopic pattern, characterized by a prominent vascular network and orange-yellowish structureless areas in the background.
  - The orange-yellowish structureless areas seen by dermoscopy correspond histologically to granulomas within the dermis.
  - The vascular network, consisting of linear arborizing vessels, represents a valuable feature for the differential diagnosis of necrobiosis lipoidica from other granulomatous dermatoses which characteristically lack them.
- White structureless areas, mainly located in the central part of the lesion, correspond to dermal fibrosis.

- Erosions, ulcerations, and crusts represent additional dermoscopic features, most commonly seen in the perforating subtype of necrobiosis lipoidica.

PEARLS

- Structureless orange-yellowish color seen with dermoscopy—think granulomatous disease.
- The arborizing vessels of necrobiosis lipoidica must be differentiated from the arborizing vessels seen in basal cell carcinoma.
  - Vessels of basal cell carcinoma typically reveal ramification of thinner branches, ending in very thin capillaries.
  - Vessels of necrobiosis lipoidica do not show significant variation in diameter.

CASE 4

HISTORY

These lesions were found on the knee of a 45-year-old woman.

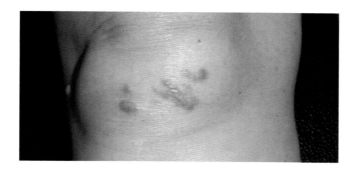

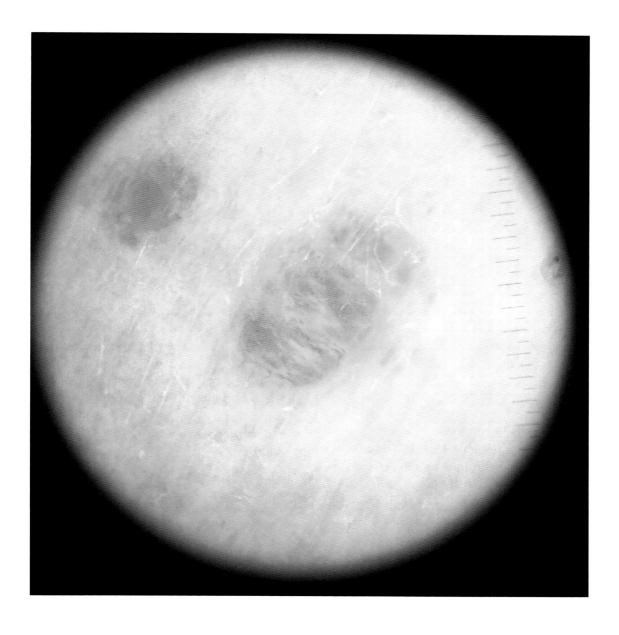

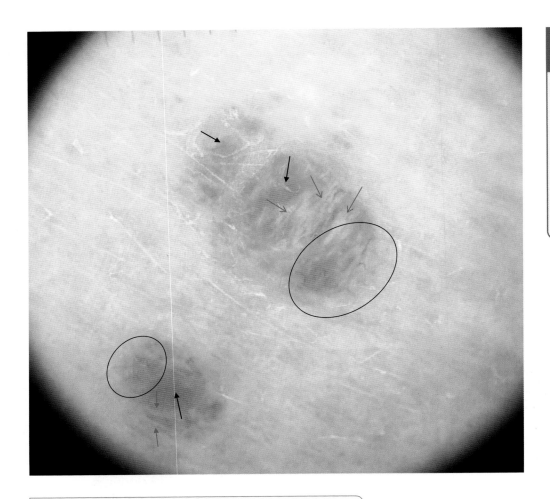

DERMOSCOPIC CRITERIA

- Orange-yellowish structureless areas (black arrows)
- Subtle, fine, linear, and partially branching vessels (black circles)
- White lines/bony-white color/crystalline structures (red arrows)

DIAGNOSIS:
Sarcoidosis

DISCUSSION

- Sarcoidosis is a granulomatous dermatosis that is dermoscopically characterized by the presence of structureless orange-yellowish patchy areas with subtle, fine linear, and branching vessels.
  - The translucent orange-yellowish patchy areas seen with dermoscopy histologically represent granulomas in the dermis.
  - White lines (crystalline structures) and pinkish and/or whitish structureless areas are an additional common dermoscopic feature seen in sarcoidosis, which represent focal dermal fibrosis.

PEARLS

- Structureless orange-yellowish color seen with dermoscopy—think granulomatous disease.
- The dermoscopic pattern of sarcoidosis is not pathognomonic, because it may be seen in various granulomatous dermatoses including cutaneous tuberculosis and granulomatous rosacea.
- A final diagnosis is based on consideration of all clinical, dermoscopic, histologic, and laboratory findings.

CASE 5

HISTORY

This asymptomatic lesion was found on a 28-year-old man while performing a total-body skin examination.

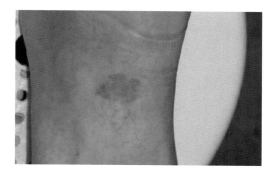

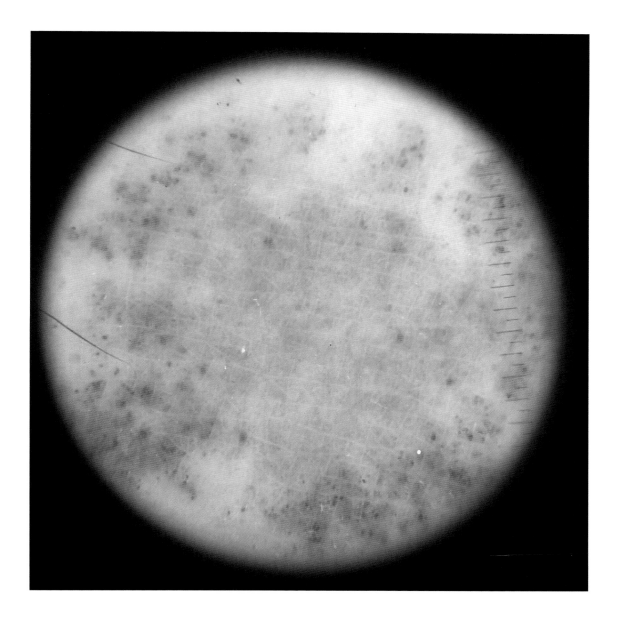

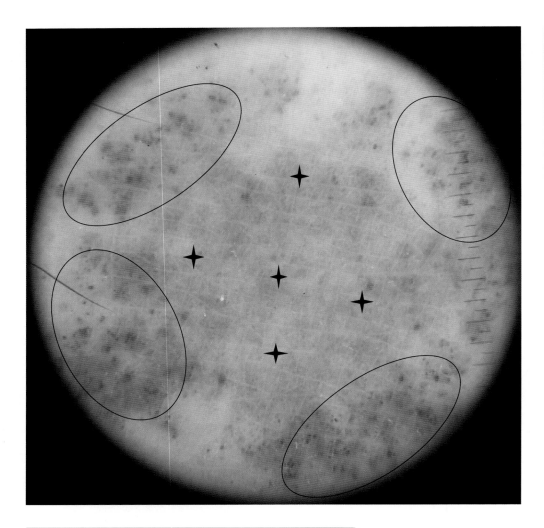

DERMOSCOPIC CRITERIA

- Orange-brown structureless background (black stars)
- Round-to-oval purple dots/globules (black circles) more evident at the periphery of the lesion

DIAGNOSIS:
Pigmented Purpuric Dermatosis (Lichen Aureus)

DISCUSSION

- The group of pigmented purpuric dermatoses includes 5 main entities:
  - Progressive pigmented purpuric dermatosis (Schamberg disease).
  - Purpura annularis telangiectodes (Majocchi disease).
  - Lichen aureus.
  - Pigmented purpuric lichenoid dermatosis (Gougerot-Blum).
  - Eczematid-like purpura of Doucas and Kapetanakis.
  - The dermoscopic pattern of all pigmented purpuric dermatosis entities consists of an orange-brown structureless background (similar to granulomatous diseases) and multiple reddish dots and globules.
  - The orange-brown background reflects hemosiderin deposition.

- The reddish purpuric dots and globules reflect extravasation of erythrocytes.

PEARLS

- Of note, rare presentations of mycosis fungoides have been reported to share similar clinical and dermoscopic features to that of pigmented purpuric dermatosis. However, such overlap between the 2 disorders is regarded as exceedingly rare.
- Nevertheless, healthy caution should be maintained when confronted with uncommon presentations of pigmented purpuric dermatosis and appropriate diagnosis and management should be undertaken accordingly, including a histopathologic diagnosis if clinical suspicion warrants.

CASE 6

HISTORY
A healthy 25-year-old man developed these itchy lesions over a 2-week period.

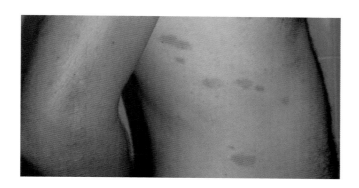

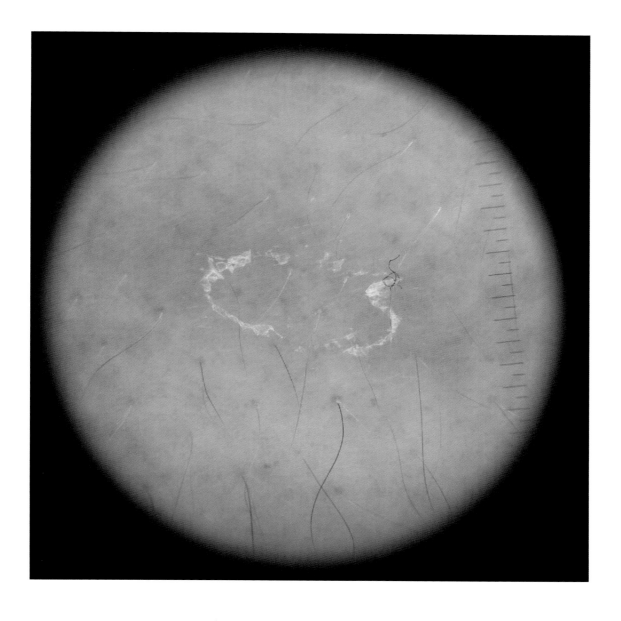

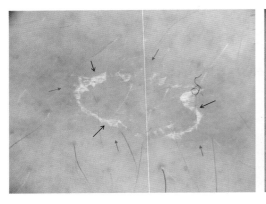
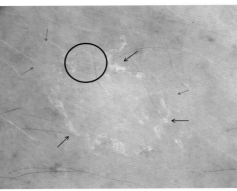

DERMOSCOPIC CRITERIA

- White scale at the periphery, the so-called collarette sign (black arrows)
- Yellowish background (red arrows)
- Dotted vessels (circle)

DIAGNOSIS:
Pityriasis Rosea

DISCUSSION

- Pityriasis rosea is dermoscopically characterized by the combination of white scales localized at the periphery of the lesion (collarette sign) and a yellowish, structureless background.
- A few subtle red dots/dotted vessels may be seen.
- The sparse dotted vessel pattern significantly differs from the dotted vessels seen in psoriasis, which fill the lesion.

PEARL

- Although the presence of peripheral scales is a strong clue for pityriasis rosea, the overall dermoscopic pattern is not strictly pathognomonic, and it should be considered in context along with the clinical history, morphology, and distribution of the lesions.
- Similar white scales can be seen in lesions of secondary syphilis. Biett's collarette, Biett's sign.

CASE 7

HISTORY

A 68-year-old man has had an itchy rash on his legs for many years. There is no personal or family history of psoriasis.

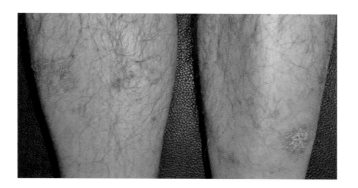

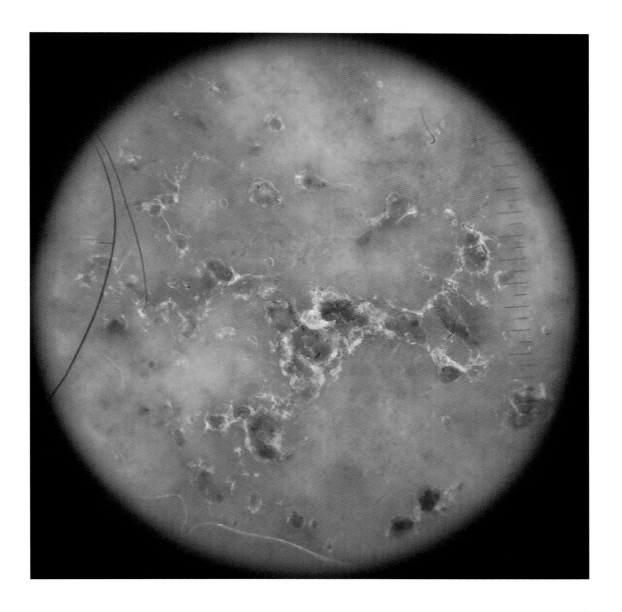

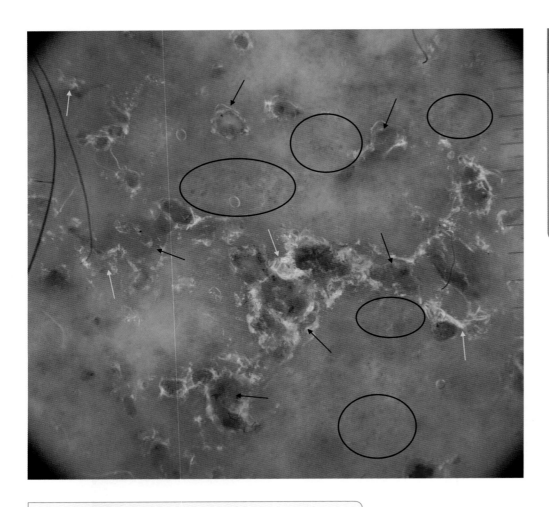

DIAGNOSIS:
Dermatitis

DISCUSSION

■ The most common dermoscopic features of dermatitis in general, whether it be contact dermatitis, nummular eczema, generalized dermatitis, or seborrheic dermatitis, include dotted/pinpoint vessels in a patchy distribution and yellow sero-crusts and scaling.
  ■ The underlying spongiosis is responsible for the dermoscopic pattern of dermatitis. Yellow crusts/ scales correspond to dried exudated serum admixed with keratin masses.
  ■ Focal whitish scales are sometimes visible, especially in subacute and chronic subtypes, but always in combination with yellow structures.
■ Depending on the stage and the clinical subtype of the disease, dermatitis may display some differences.
  ■ For example, acute exudative lesions are characterized by a predominance of yellow scale/crusts, whereas chronic and lichenified lesions predominantly display dotted/pinpoint vessels in a patchy distribution with yellow and sometimes whitish scales.

PEARLS

■ The dotted/pinpoint vessels of dermatitis are identical to those seen in psoriasis, but unlike in psoriasis in which they fill the lesion, their distribution in dermatitis is more focal, creating an irregular, patchy pattern.
■ Additionally, in psoriasis there is a predominance of white, as opposed to yellowish, scales.
■ The presence of yellow sero-crusts represents a strong clue for the diagnosis of dermatitis.

CASE 8

HISTORY
These were seen on the arms and trunk of a 49-year-old man.

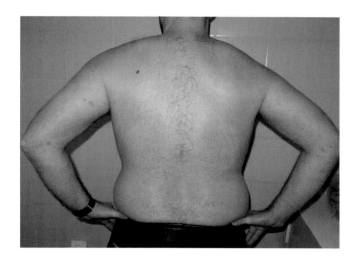

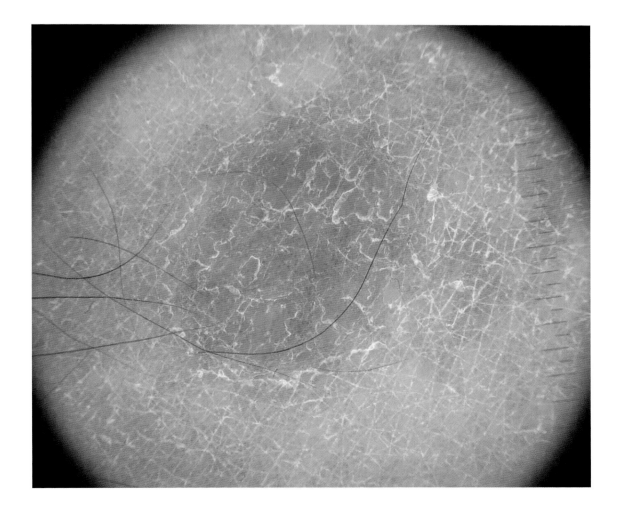

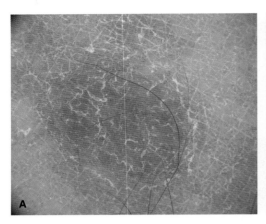

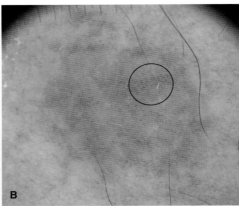

DERMOSCOPIC CRITERIA

- Diffuse white scales (A)
- Regularly distributed dotted/pinpoint vessels (black circle) that become more evident after the application of an alcohol-based solution that makes the scales translucent (B)
- Light erythematous background

DIAGNOSIS:
Psoriasis

DISCUSSION

- Dermoscopy of psoriasis displays diffuse white scales and regularly distributed red dots on a light or dull red background.
- The red dots histologically correspond to the vertically oriented, dilated, and looped vessels of the dermal papillae.
- The regular distribution of the vessels is explained by the regular acanthosis and papillomatosis of the epidermis, resulting in an even elongation of the rete ridges.

PEARLS

- In chronic plaque psoriasis, the presence of marked parakeratotic scales might impede the visualization of the underlying structures, including the dotted vessels.
- Removal of scales with the application of an alcohol-based solution may be necessary to reveal the underlying characteristic vascular pattern.
- Removal of scales may also result in the development of the so-called dermoscopic Auspitz sign, which is the appearance of hemorrhagic dots in dermoscopy.

CASE 9

HISTORY

A healthy 23-year-old woman presented with these lesions on her trunk and extremities.

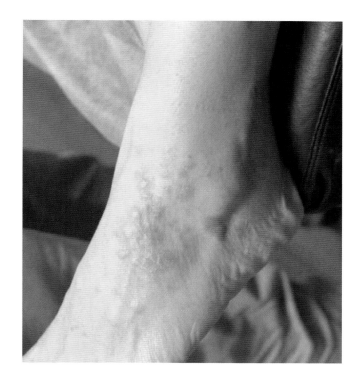

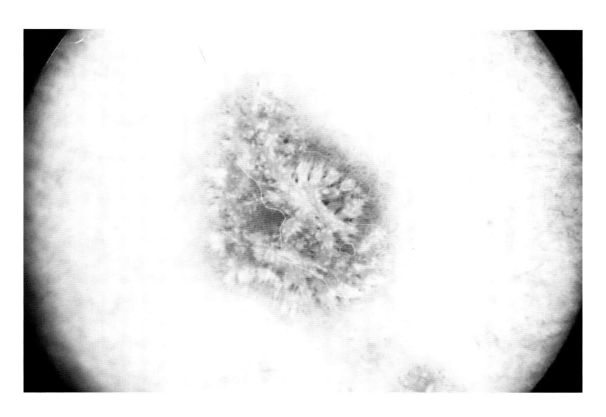

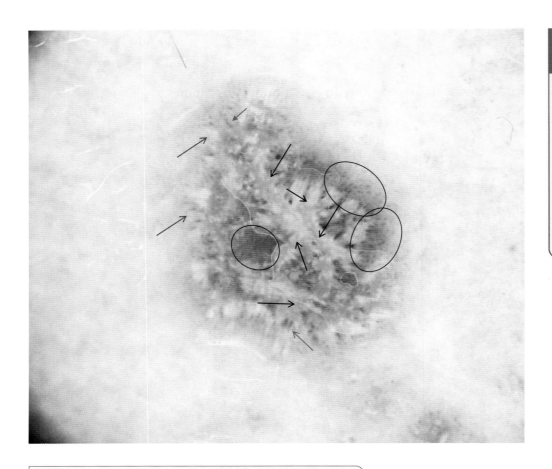

DIAGNOSIS:
Lichen Planus

DISCUSSION

- Wickham striae (white crossing lines) are the dermoscopic hallmark of lichen planus, irrespective of disease subtype.
- Wickham striae consist of crossing white strands. Histopathologically, this feature corresponds to hypergranulosis.
- Vessels of mixed morphology (short linear and dotted) may be present and more prevalent at the periphery of the lesion.

- Brown granules/dots may also be found in late stages of the disease, histopathologically corresponding to the presence of melanophages ("peppering") in the upper dermis.

PEARL

- Wickham striae are a highly specific dermoscopic clue for the diagnosis of lichen planus.

CASE 10

HISTORY
Topical antibiotics did not clear the "rosacea" on the nose of a 58-year-old woman.

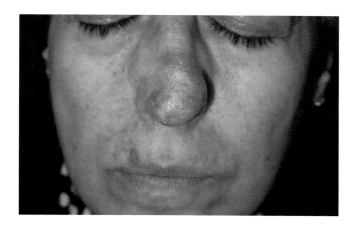

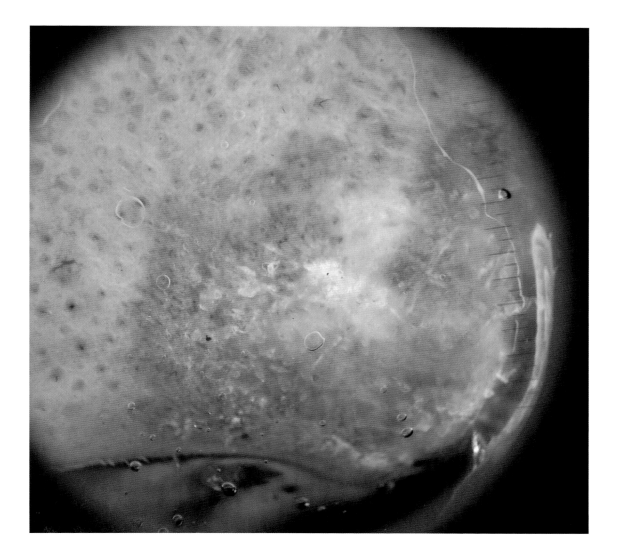

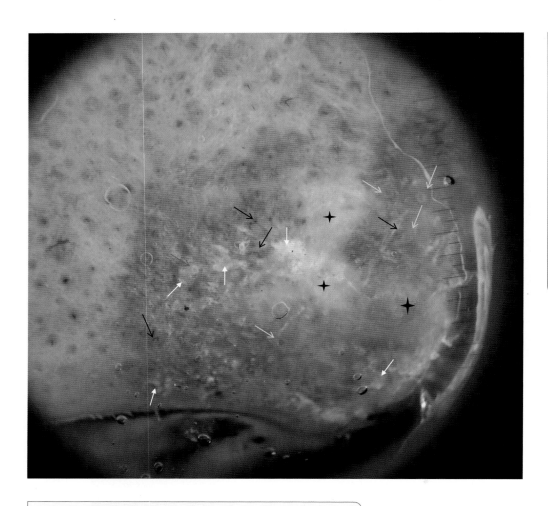

DERMOSCOPIC CRITERIA

- Short linear vessels (black arrows)
- Follicular keratotic plugs (yellow arrows)
- White scales (white arrows)
- Perifollicular whitish halos (red arrows)
- Whitish structureless areas/scarring (stars)
- Erythematous background

DIAGNOSIS:
Discoid Lupus Erythematosus

DISCUSSION

- Dermoscopy of discoid lupus erythematosus displays different features depending on the stage of the disease.
  - Erythema, perifollicular whitish halos, follicular keratotic plugs, short linear vessels, and white scales dermoscopically characterize early stages.
  - Whitish structureless areas/scarring, hyperpigmentation, and blurred telangiectasias (linear branching vessels) are mostly seen later in the course of the disease.
  - In intermediate stages (as in the currently presented case), we may observe a mixture of the aforementioned features.

- Of note, the zigzag and/or polygonal vessels typical of rosacea are not seen in this case.

PEARLS

- The dermoscopic pattern of discoid lupus erythematosus is highly specific and is useful for the discrimination of discoid lupus erythematosus from other dermatoses, especially for lesions involving the face.
- Do not forget that dermoscopy is very useful for rashes, not only skin tumors.

CASE 11

HISTORY
A 17-year-old female patient developed itchy unilateral pink papules in her left axilla.

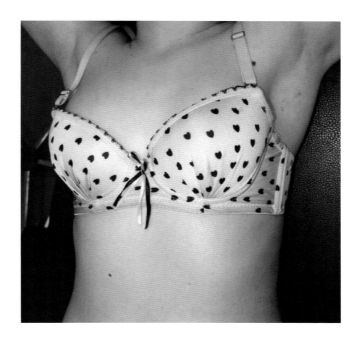

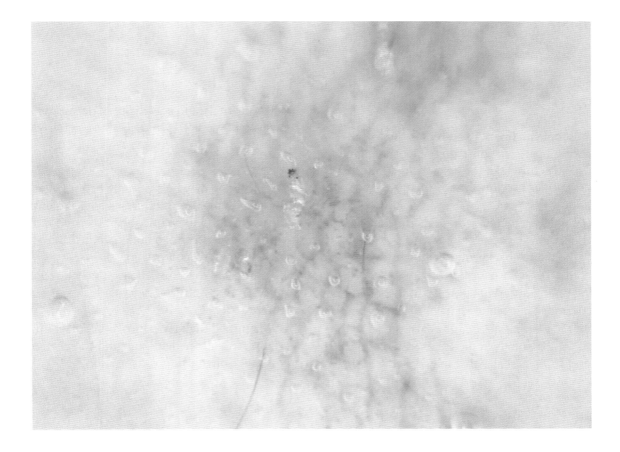

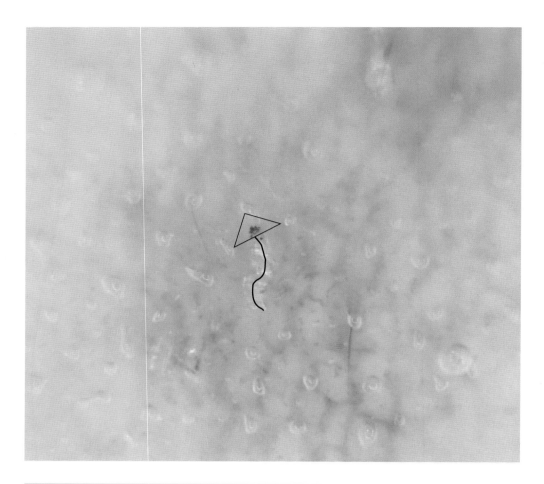

DIAGNOSIS:
Scabies

DISCUSSION

- The dermoscopic hallmark of scabies is the so called jet with contrail pattern, consisting of a triangular dark brown structure (aka the delta sign) combined with whitish scales in a linear or S- or zigzag-shaped arrangement.
  - The triangular structure represents the parasite.
  - The white scales represent the burrow.
  - The erythematous background is not always present. It represents a local inflammatory reaction.
- Depending on the different clinical variants of scabies, different dermoscopic features may be seen.
  - In Norwegian scabies, recognition of the jet with contrail sign is not always easy, given the typically thick and copious scales that may obscure seeing the sign.

- The sensitivity and specificity of dermoscopy to diagnose scabies are 91% and 86%, respectively.

PEARLS

- Dermoscopy may be especially helpful when diagnosing scabies in young children such as infants and toddlers who tend to be uncooperative and move around while you are trying to obtain your scabies prep to make the microscopic diagnosis.
- Bear in mind that the delta sign may be challenging to detect at first until you have gained experience finding it in practice.
  - Magnified digital dermoscopic images may help to detect a true delta sign and thereby reduce the chance of a false-positive finding.

Trichoscopy/Hair

Antonella Tosti, MD

General Instructions

- For each case, there is a short history along with a clinical and an unmarked dermoscopic image.
- Study the unmarked dermoscopic image and try to identify the global and local dermoscopic features.
- Make your diagnosis.
- Next, turn the page and the dermoscopic image will be presented again, this time marked with all the salient dermoscopic findings.
- On the same page you will also find the diagnosis along with a detailed discussion and a few pearls for your review.

CASE 1

HISTORY

This is a 72-year-old woman who complains of progressive patches of alopecia associated with pain for 6 months. Treatment with topical steroids produced no improvement.

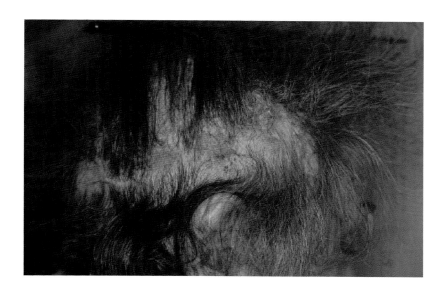

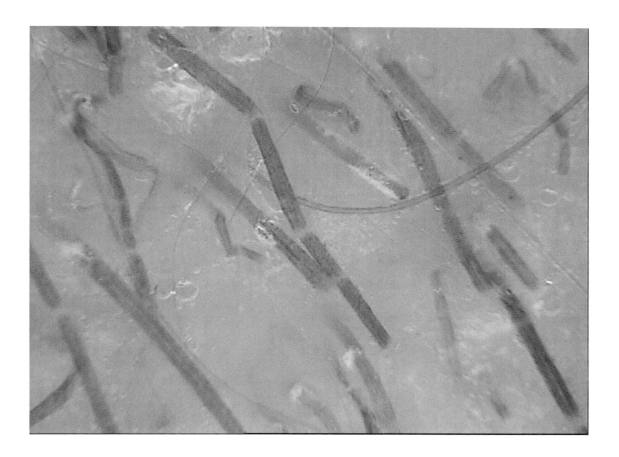

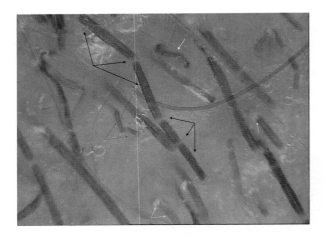

DERMOSCOPIC CRITERIA

- Comma hair (white arrow)
- "Morse" hair (black arrows)
- Zigzag hair (red arrows)
- Broken hair with cast (yellow arrows)

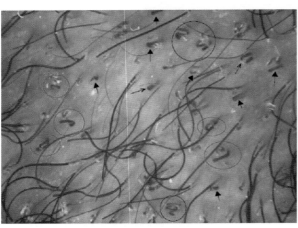

DERMOSCOPIC CRITERIA

- Comma hairs (red circles)
- Corkscrew hairs (black circles)
- Broken hairs with different lengths (black arrows)

DIAGNOSIS:
Tinea Capitis

DISCUSSION

- Dermoscopic examination/trichoscopy allows for fast, noninvasive diagnosis of tinea capitis.
  - Clinical differential diagnosis includes dissecting cellulitis and discoid lupus.
  - Alopecia areata is excluded by the intense inflammatory changes.
- Dermoscopy shows different types of broken hairs that are characteristic of tinea capitis.
- Dermoscopic criteria for diagnosis include:
  - Comma-shaped hair: broken, very short hair that bends like a comma.
  - Corkscrew hair (in patients with curly hair): broken and coiled hair resembling a corkscrew.
  - Black dots (in patients with black hair): follicular openings are black created by broken hair shafts at or below follicular openings.
  - Morse hair/Morse code–like hair (aka bar-code hairs): irregularly broken and curved or angulated hairs. Light color is seen where the hairs bend.
  - Zigzag hair: broken, short Z-shaped hairs.
  - Broken hair with peripilar casts.
    - Peripilar casts: white concentric scales surrounding the hair shafts.

PEARLS

- Use dermoscopy to select specific hairs suitable for microscopic examination or culture.
- All of the distorted hairs reflect the presence of dermatophyte infection.
- Lymphadenopathy (submandibular, occipital, or postauricular) in the setting of alopecia and/or scaling suggests tinea capitis.
- You can start treatment based on dermoscopic findings.
- Dermoscopic examination is also useful when screening possible contacts.

CASE 2

HISTORY

A 14-year-old girl had a history of tinea capitis successfully treated with systemic antifungals. Three months later she developed diffuse hair shedding and mild thinning.

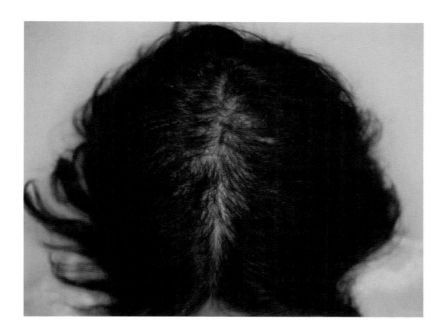

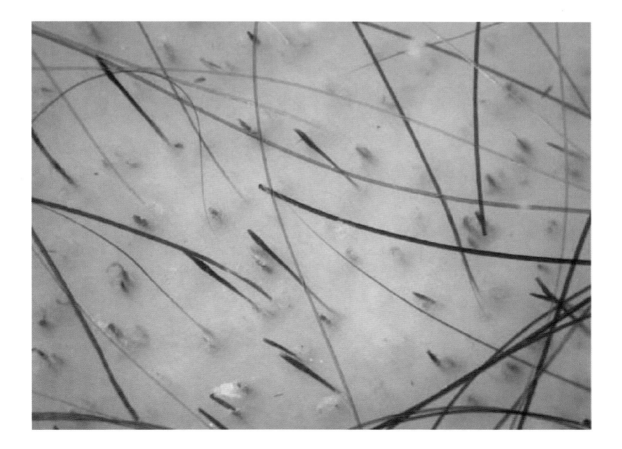

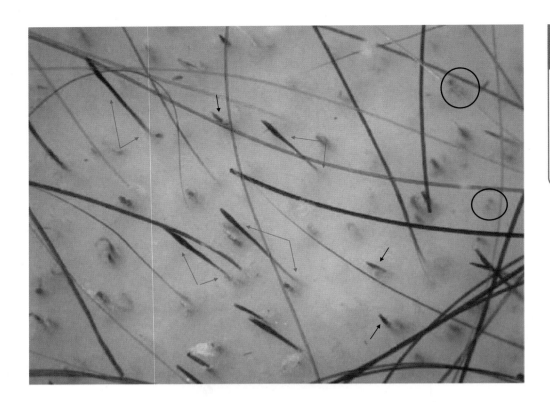

DIAGNOSIS:
Diffuse Alopecia Areata

DISCUSSION

- Trichoscopy/dermoscopy demonstrates broken hairs with different lengths.
- Broken hairs with different lengths may be seen in alopecia areata, chemotherapy-induced alopecia, tinea capitis, and trichotillomania.
- There are also exclamation mark hairs characterized by the following:
  - Dark thick and possibly frayed tips.
  - Proximal portions are pale and tapered.
- Exclamation mark hairs are almost exclusively seen in alopecia areata.
  - The only other condition where they are seen is in chemotherapy-induced alopecia.
- There are black dots/macules corresponding to hair shafts broken off at the skin surface.
- Black dots are also commonly found in tinea capitis. This suggests the tinea might still be active.
- Yellow dots corresponding to infundibula filled with sebum and keratinous debris and circle hairs (short, regularly coiled, fine vellus hair forming circles) can also be seen in alopecia areata.

PEARLS

- Dermoscopic examination should be used for obvious and not-so-obvious cases of hair loss.
- Dermoscopic examination can often give you a clue or clues to make the correct diagnosis with difficult or atypical presentations.
- It is essential to learn the definitions and dermoscopic appearances of the important trichoscopic criteria.

CASE 3

HISTORY
This is an 83-year-old woman who reports progressive alopecia associated with scalp erythema and severe itching.

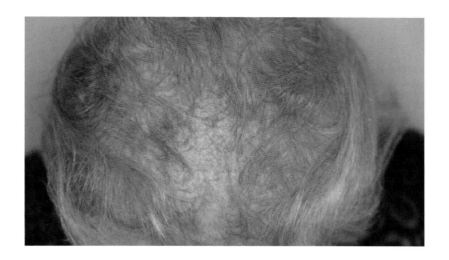

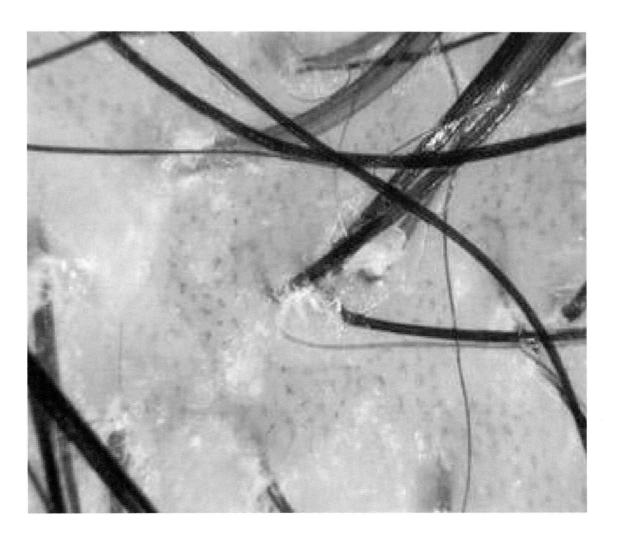

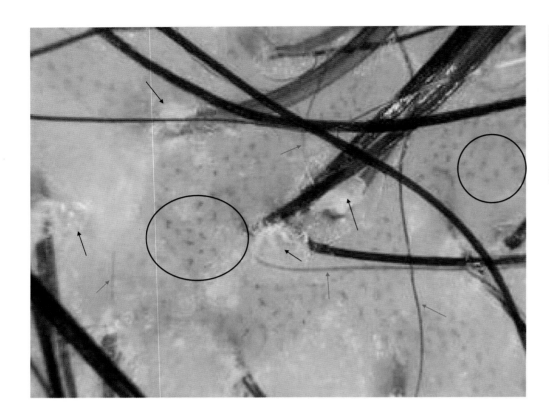

DIAGNOSIS:
Psoriasis and Androgenic Alopecia

DISCUSSION

- Hair loss and severe scalp pruritus are common features of scalp psoriasis. Interestingly, dermoscopy in this case shows both the hair shaft variability found in androgenic alopecia and the dotted/glomerular vessels typical of psoriasis.
- Dermoscopic criteria for diagnosis of psoriasis include the following:
  - White scales localized to both the perifollicular and interfollicular compartments.
  - Dotted/glomerular vessels at 10× magnification.
  - Twisted capillary loops, which reflect coiled capillaries of different shapes but regular thickness at 40× magnification.
- Principle dermoscopic criteria for androgenic alopecia include the following:
  - More than 20% hair shaft variability. This means that more than 20% of the hairs have a reduced thickness.

PEARLS

- How to differentiate seborrheic dermatitis from psoriasis by dermoscopy?
  - Vascular patterns help make the diagnosis.
  - Dermoscopy of scalp psoriasis shows pinpoint or glomerular vessels similar to skin plaques.
  - Seborrheic dermatitis lacks pinpoint or glomerular vessels but has arborizing and polymorphous vessels.

CASE 4

HISTORY
A 17-year-old adolescent girl presents with a 6-month history of diffuse hair shedding.

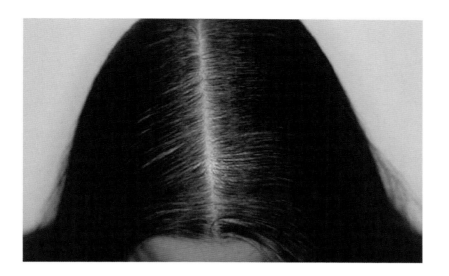

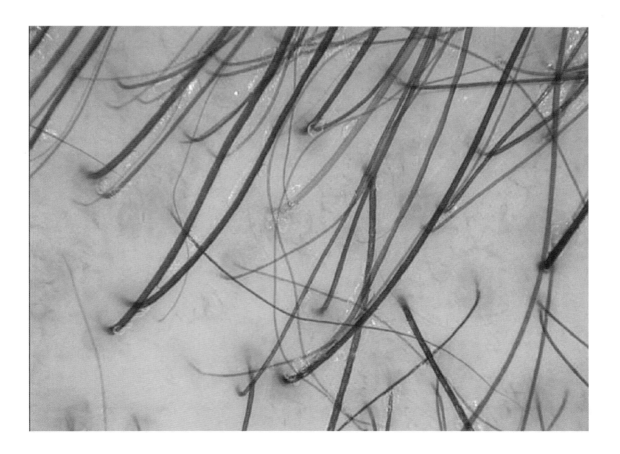

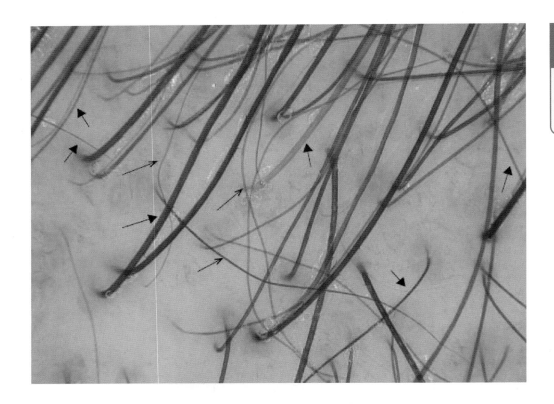

DIAGNOSIS:
Androgenic Alopecia

DISCUSSION

■ Trichoscopy/dermoscopy demonstrates more than 20% diversity in the diameter of the hair shafts.

■ Diversity/variability indicates the presence of hair shafts with different thickness.

■ The presence of more than 20% variability is diagnostic of androgenic alopecia (aka pattern hair loss, male-pattern hair loss, female-pattern hair loss.

■ Androgenic alopecia is the most common cause of hair loss.

■ Widening of the central parting of the scalp is a clue to suggest the diagnosis of androgenic alopecia.

■ Thinned hair shafts indicate hair follicle miniaturization.

■ It occurs in both men and women and can start at an early age, as seen in this case.

■ Do hair counts. Determining percentages are rough estimates.

■ For example, normal and total hairs (30 and 40, respectively).

■ Ten hairs are thinner than normal.

■ Calculate the percentage of the abnormal hairs.

■ In this case it is 25%.

■ Yellow dots (advanced cases) indicate severe miniaturization, which reflects hair follicle ostia lacking any hairs (empty hair follicles). The yellow color represents active sebaceous lobules.

■ Peripilar sign: brown coloration at skin level surrounding hair shafts thought to represent perifollicular inflammation is seen in early cases of androgenic alopecia.

PEARLS

■ Dermoscopy allows for the early diagnosis of androgenic alopecia.

■ Biopsy may be needed to exclude other causes of hair loss that may be found in conjunction with androgenic alopecia.

CASE 5

HISTORY

This is an 11-year-old girl with a 6-year history of progressive alopecia associated with scalp itching.

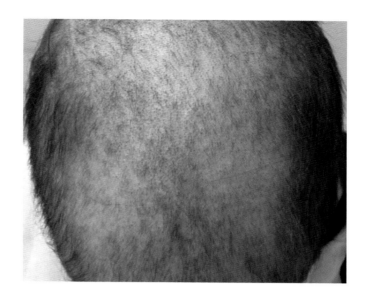

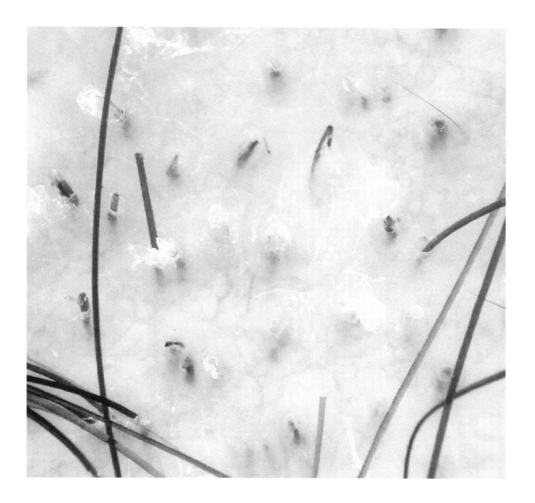

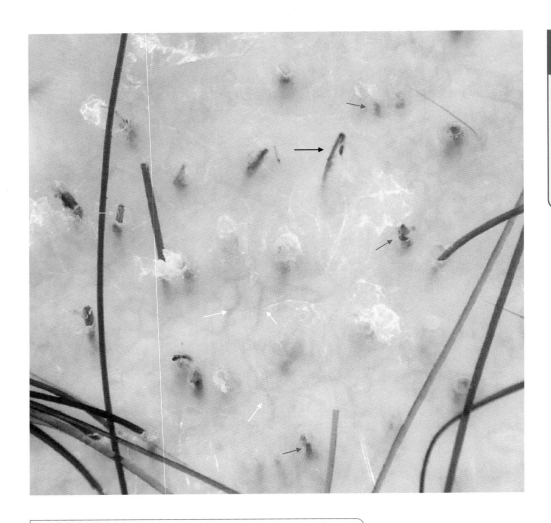

DIAGNOSIS:
Trichotillomania

DISCUSSION

- Clinical differential diagnosis includes alopecia areata and hair shaft disorders with increased fragility.
- Dermoscopic criteria for diagnosis include the following:
  - Question mark hair: broken hair with a coiled tip resembling a question mark.
  - Broken hairs of different lengths with tip of same thickness as rest of the shaft.
  - Flame hairs: very short (less than 1-mm) pigmented hair with a thin wavy distal tip resembling the flame on a match point (pathologically correspond to pigmented casts).
- Although broken hairs and flame hairs can be seen in alopecia areata, the presence of the question mark hair indicates a diagnosis of trichotillomania.

PEARLS

- Trichotillomania and alopecia areata share numerous dermoscopic features.
- Look for exclamation mark hairs (seen in alopecia areata but not in trichotillomania) and question mark hairs (seen in trichotillomania but not in alopecia areata).
- Patient affect and historical clues are essential to clinch this important diagnosis.

CASE 6

HISTORY
This is a 45-year-old man reporting a single patch of alopecia associated with scalp itching and pain.

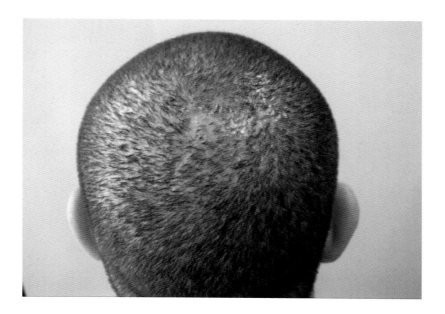

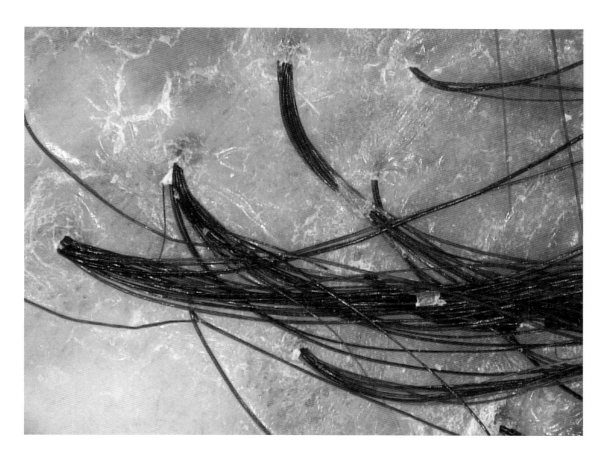

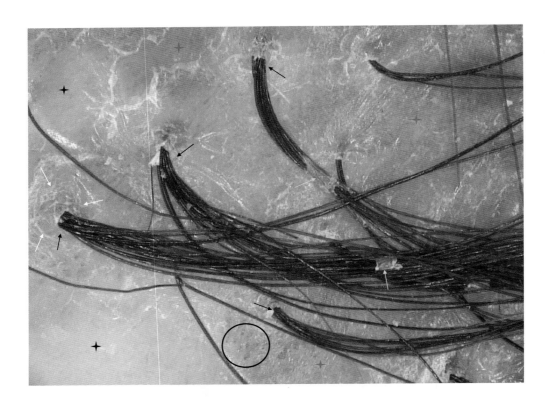

DIAGNOSIS:

Folliculitis Decalvans

DISCUSSION

- The diagnosis is folliculitis decalvans, aka tufted folliculitis.
- It is an inflammatory alopecia (erythema/scales/pustules around hair follicles).
- Dermoscopic criteria include the following:
  - Loss of follicular openings: sign of scarring alopecia (bony-white color).
  - Tufts of 7 to up to 100 hairs emerging together (toothbrush sign) and surrounded by a peripilar cast.
    - Peripilar casts are white-to-yellow scales, at times clumped, which are irregular in size/shape and are concentrically arranged around emerging hair shafts.
  - Hair casts: small cylindrical white structures that encircle the hair shaft.
    - Dotted/ glomerular vessels may be seen.

PEARLS

- Presence of tufts containing more than 7 hairs is diagnostic.
- It is essential to perform bacterial and fungal cultures in a patient with this clinical picture.
- Scalp biopsies to rule out tinea may also be helpful.

CASE 7

HISTORY

A 61-year-old woman has a 2-year history of hair loss and scalp itching.

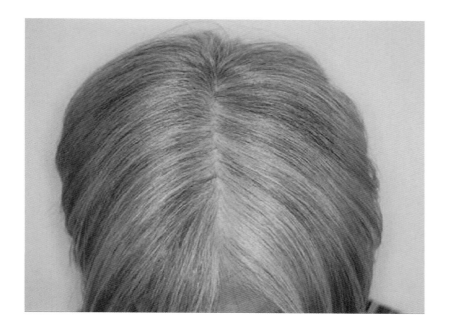

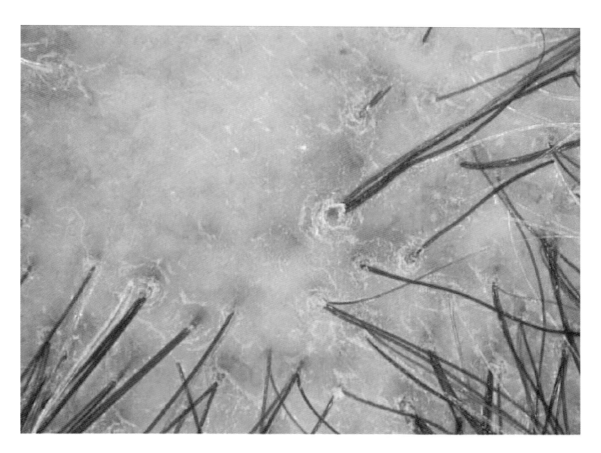

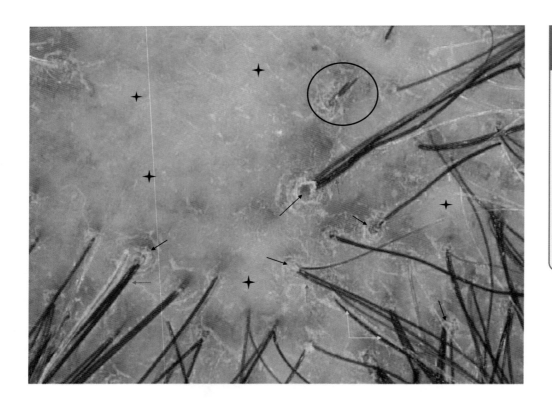

DIAGNOSIS:
Lichen Planopilaris

DISCUSSION

- Lichen planopilaris is one of the most common causes of scarring alopecia.
- It may be associated with lichen planus.
- Multifocal/diffuse smooth white patches of hair loss without visible hair follicles.
  - White patches correspond to areas of scarring.
- Symptoms are variable: itch, pain, tenderness, discomfort, burning.
- Biopsy demonstrates lymphocytic folliculitis.
- Trichoscopy/dermoscopy shows loss of follicular openings and bony-white color indicating scarring alopecia.
- The emerging hair shafts show peripilar casts (white-to-yellow scales, at times clumped, which are irregular in size/shape and are concentrically arranged around emerging hair shafts).
- Peripilar casts surrounding a group of 2 to 4 hairs emerging together are very suggestive of lichen planopilaris.
- Peripilar casts surrounding broken hair shafts are also suggestive of lichen planopilaris.
- Blue-gray dots ("peppering") can be seen around follicular ostia and represent melanophages, which are a result of the lymphocytic folliculitis.

PEARLS

- Definitive diagnosis requires a biopsy because other scarring alopecias may present similar findings.
- The best biopsy site is an area showing tufted hairs with peripilar casts.
  - Use dermoscopy to select your optimal site for biopsy.

CASE 8

HISTORY
A 36-year-old man reported multiple inflammatory patches of alopecia associated with pain.

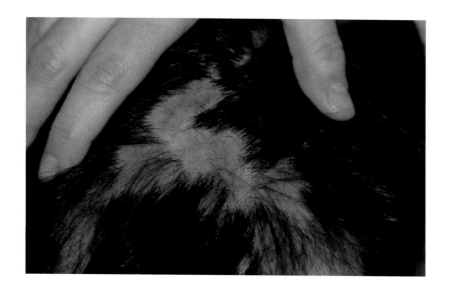

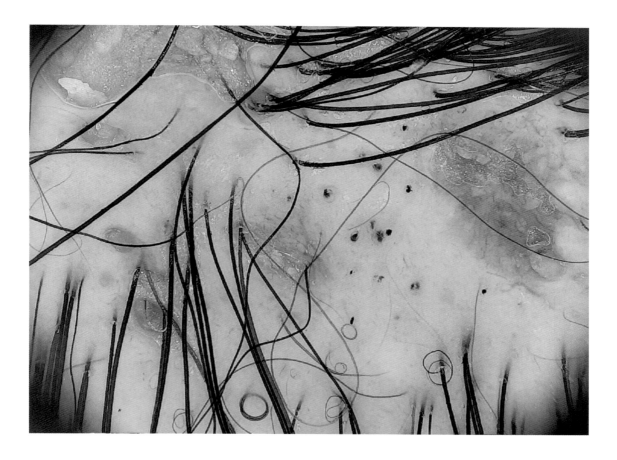

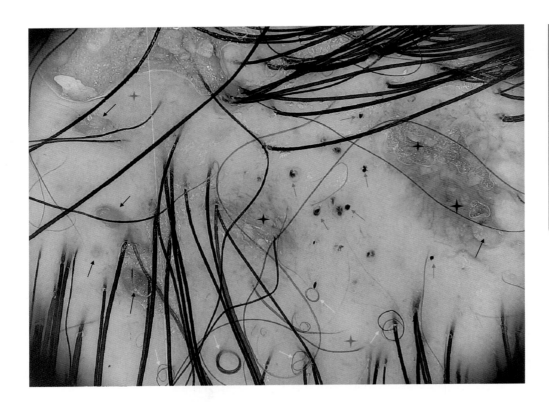

DERMOSCOPIC CRITERIA

- Black dots (red arrows)
- Circle hairs (yellow arrows)
- Keratotic plugs (black arrows)
- Yellowish exudate (red stars)
- Scalp erythema (black stars)

DIAGNOSIS:
Dissecting Cellulitis

DISCUSSION

- Clinical differential diagnosis of dissecting cellulitis includes tinea capitis and discoid lupus. Alopecia areata is excluded by the intense inflammatory changes.
- Dermoscopy shows features of nonscarring alopecia.
- Dermoscopic criteria for diagnosis include the following:
  - Black dots (in patients with black hair): follicular openings are black created by broken hair shafts at/below follicular opening.
  - Circle hairs.
  - Keratotic plugs: large, irregular yellow plugs that cover enlarged follicular openings.

- The presence of large yellow keratotic plugs is diagnostic.
  - Yellow dots may also be seen in alopecia areata. However in alopecia areata, they tend to be smaller and more monomorphous in shape.
- Scalp erythema: patchy erythema of the scalp.
- Yellowish exudate: scalp is covered by a yellow irregular layer that may be difficult to see.

PEARLS

- In this clinical context, the presence of large keratotic plugs helps to distinguish dissecting cellulitis from tinea capitis or alopecia areata.
- Hair regrowth is achievable with proper treatment in early disease.

CASE 9

HISTORY
This is a 56-year-old woman who reports hair loss and loss of eyebrows (madarosis).

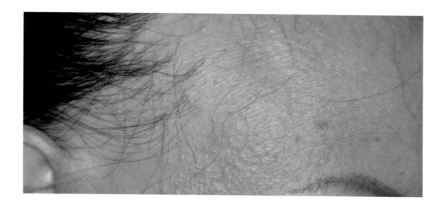

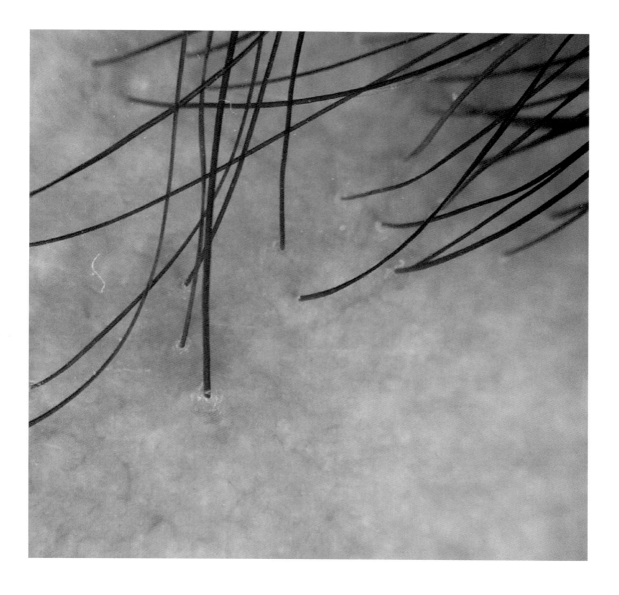

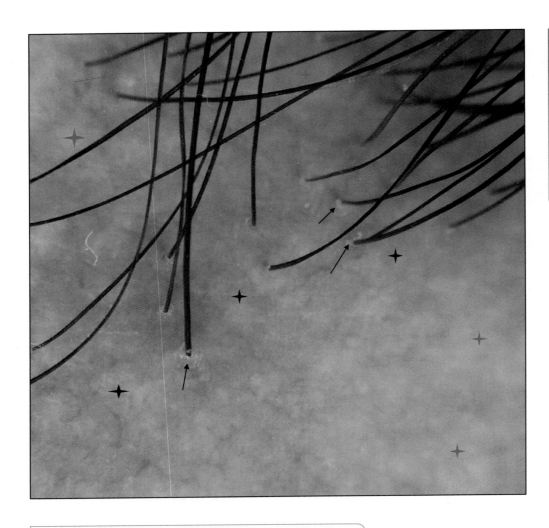

DERMOSCOPIC CRITERIA

- Peripilar casts (black arrows)
- Peripilar erythema (red arrows)
- Absence of vellus hairs (black stars)
- Scarring (red stars)

DIAGNOSIS:
Frontal Fibrosing Alopecia

DISCUSSION

- Frontal fibrosing alopecia is typically diagnosed in postmenopausal women older than 50.
- It presents as a symmetrical band of hair loss at the front/sides of the scalp.
- Clinical differential diagnosis includes androgenic and traction alopecia.
- Dermoscopic criteria for diagnosis include the following:
  - Absence of vellus hairs at the new hairline—the hairline only contains terminal hairs.
  - Peripilar casts: white concentric scales surrounding terminal hair shafts.
  - Peripilar erythema: erythema around hair shafts.
  - Bony-white patches of scarring.
- Skin biopsy makes the diagnosis: scarring and lichenoid infiltrate around affected hairs.
  - This is characteristic of frontal fibrosing alopecia, because the disease targets vellus and intermediate thickened hairs.

PEARLS

- Loss of vellus hairs distinguishes frontal fibrosing alopecia from androgenic and traction alopecia, in which vellus hairs are preserved.
- The presence of thin peripilar casts around terminal hairs at the new hairline confirms the diagnosis.
- Always look for presence/absence of vellus hairs at the hairline in patients complaining of hair loss.

CASE 10

HISTORY
This is a 51-year-old woman reporting a single patch of alopecia.

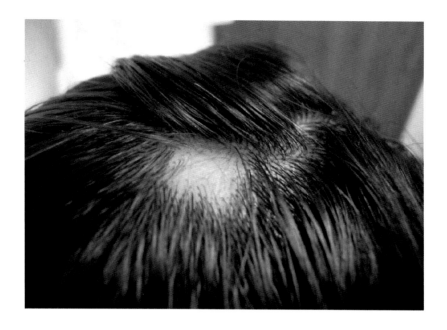

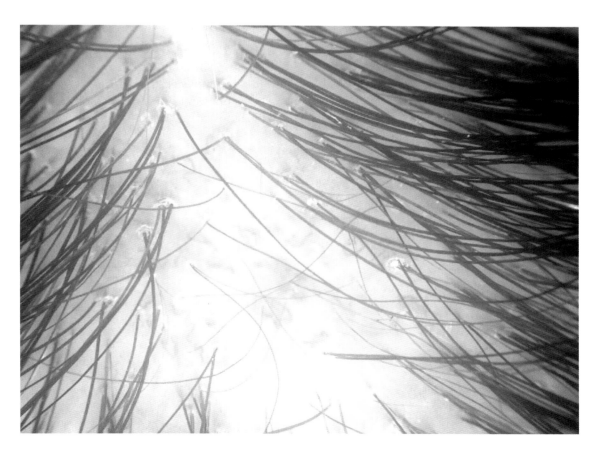

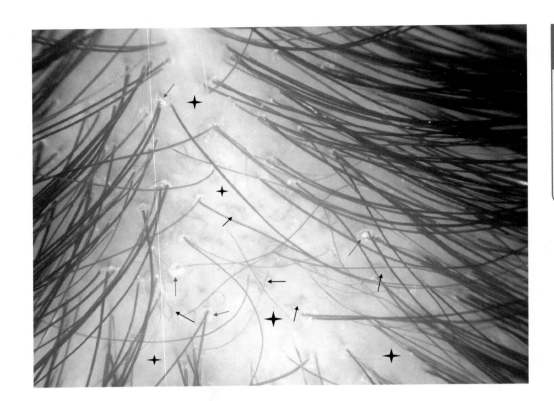

DERMOSCOPIC CRITERIA

- Loss of follicular openings/scarring (stars)
- Peripilar casts (red arrows)
- Enlarged tortuous vessels (black arrows)

DIAGNOSIS:
Discoid Lupus and Erythematosus

DISCUSSION

- Clinical differential diagnosis includes alopecia areata.
- Dermoscopic differential diagnosis includes lichen planopilaris.
- Dermoscopic criteria for diagnosis include the following:
  - Loss of follicular openings: sign of scarring alopecia.
  - Peripilar casts: white concentric scales surrounding the hair shafts.
  - Enlarged tortuous vessels seen at higher magnification.
  - Gray dots representing melanophages (peppering) in the papillary dermis can be seen and are referred to as a speckled pattern.
- Keratotic plugs/keratin material occluding the dilated infundibular openings can also be seen in discoid lupus erythematosus.
- One does not need to see all of these features to diagnose discoid lupus erythematosus.

PEARLS

- Enlarged tortuous vessels are characteristically seen in connective tissue disorders.
- Presence of tortuous vessels helps to distinguish discoid lupus erythematosus from lichen planopilaris.

CASE 11

HISTORY
A 33-year-old African American woman has a 2-year history of progressive hairline thinning, particularly in the temporal regions. There is a patchy alopecia surrounded by a rim of preserved hairs.

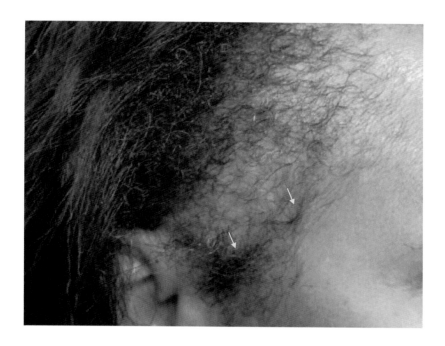

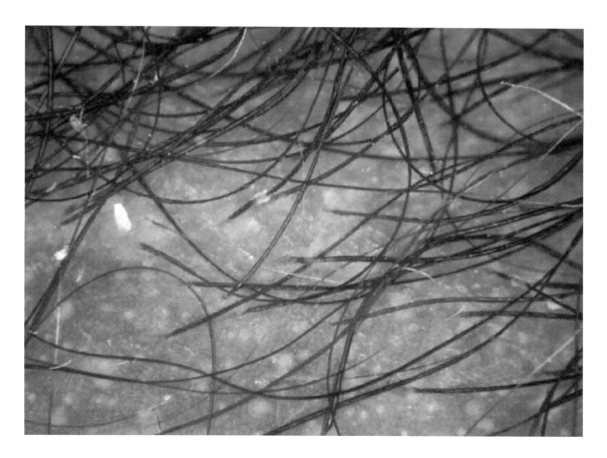

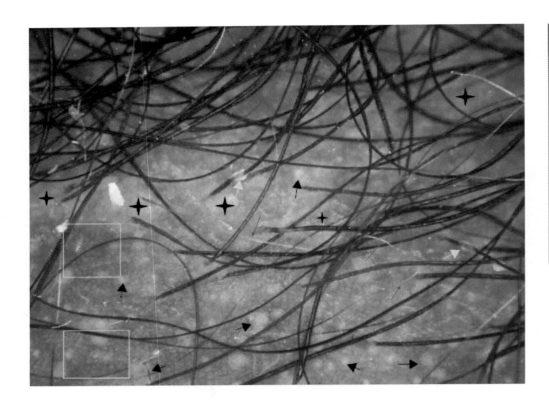

DIAGNOSIS:
Traction Alopecia

DISCUSSION

- Traction alopecia is a clinical diagnosis that can be confirmed with trichoscopy/dermoscopy.
- Hair loss is reversible if caught early.
- The presence of hair along the margins of alopecia is a diagnostic clue: the so-called fringe sign.
- In this case, there are hair casts around terminal hairs.
    - Small cylindrical white structures that encircle the proximal hair shaft.
    - Hair casts are not exclusively found in traction alopecia. They may also be seen in tinea capitis, psoriasis, and folliculitis decalvans.
- Trichoscopy/dermoscopy also demonstrates white dots.
    - White dots are a normal feature in darker-skinned persons.
    - They represent follicular/sweat gland openings.
- There is also a suggestion of scarring with larger areas of bony-white color.
- Vellus hairs are typically preserved even in long-standing cases.
- Vellus hairs are very fine and short and cannot be pulled.
- A few broken hairs are commonly seen.
- The honeycomb/pigment network pattern is seen in darker-skinned persons.

PEARLS

- Warn your patients you consider at risk of developing traction alopecia about the deleterious effects of tight braids, cornrows, weaves, and/or chemical processing.
- In many cases, traction alopecia is a diagnosis of exclusion.

CHAPTER 6 Trichoscopy/Hair   **297**

CASE 12

HISTORY

This is a 22-year-old woman who reported a patch of alopecia associated with itching. It was treated with intralesional steroids with no improvement.

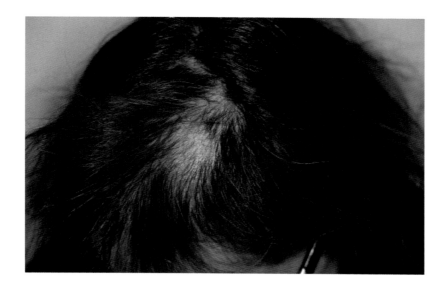

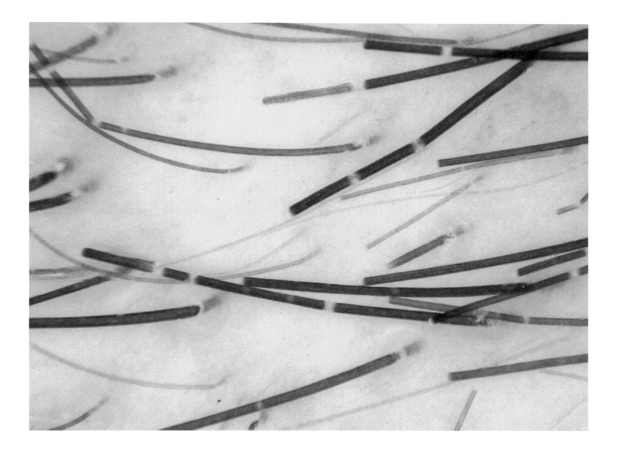

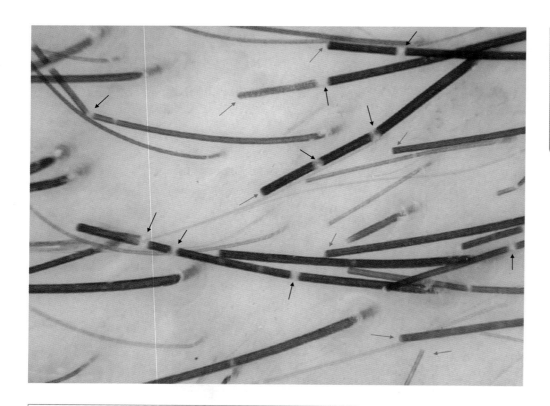

DERMOSCOPIC CRITERIA

- Trichorrhexis nodosa (black arrows)
- Hair shaft breakage (red arrows)

DIAGNOSIS:
Friction Alopecia

DISCUSSION

- This is a case of frictional alopecia causing trichorrhexis nodosa, which results in defects in the hair shaft characterized by thickening or weak points (nodes) that cause the hair to break off easily.
  - This phenomenon contributes to the appearance of hair loss, diminished hair growth, and/or damaged-looking hair.
- Clinical differential diagnosis includes alopecia areata and trichotillomania.

- Dermoscopic criteria for diagnosis include the following:
  - There are multiple, irregularly distributed, small white foci along the length of hair shafts.
  - There is also the presence of hair shaft breakage at irregular intervals.

PEARLS

- Chronic friction due to scratching tends to cause a proximal trichorrhexis nodosa.
- Hair weathering tends to cause trichorrhexis nodosa that affects the distal hair shaft.

CASE 13

HISTORY

A 2-year-old girl has diffuse hair thinning. Her mother says that her hair has always been this way.

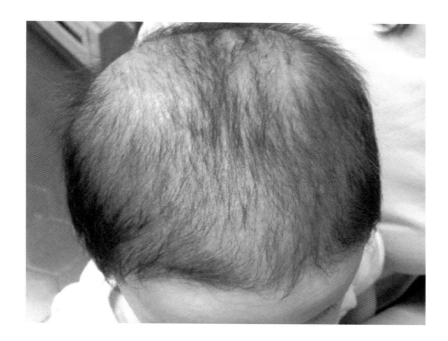

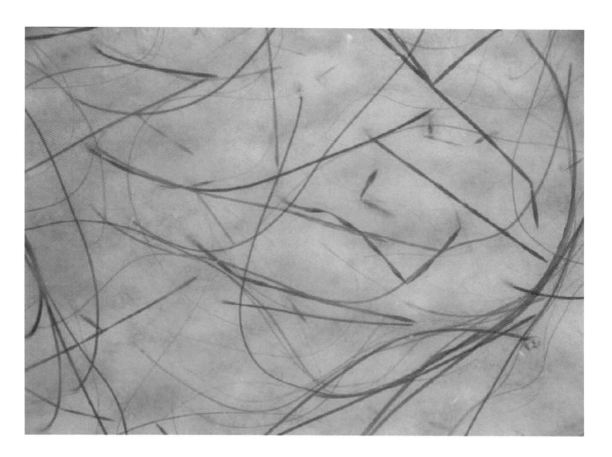

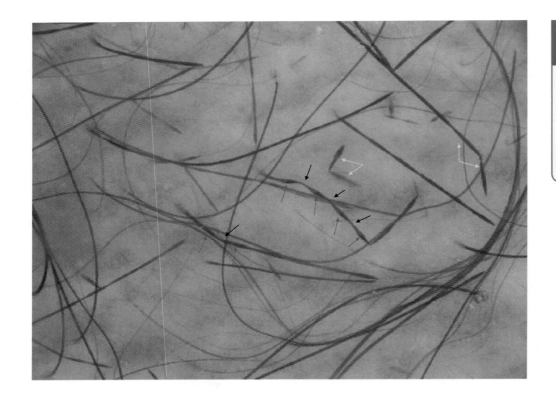

DERMOSCOPIC CRITERIA

- Regular interval beading (red arrows)
- Thin internodes (black arrows)
- Bending hairs (yellow arrows)

DIAGNOSIS:
Monilethrix

DISCUSSION

- The presence of hair beading is diagnostic of monilethrix.
- Monilethrix results in alopecia characterized by short, fragile, and broken beaded hairs.
- Scalp hair, eyebrows and eyelashes all may be affected.
- Dermoscopic criteria for diagnosis include the following:
  - The affected hair shafts show elliptical nodes and intermittent constrictions at regular intervals.
  - Breakage occurs at the internode level.
  - The thin internode is where the pathology lies.
  - Affected hairs can bend in different directions.
- Dermoscopy allows one to evaluate the severity of monilethrix.
- In this patient, only few hair shafts show the abnormality, and breakage is minimal.

- In severe cases, most hair shafts including vellus hairs are affected, and broken hairs are extensive.
- Pseudo-monilethrix is seen in alopecia areata and chemotherapy-induced alopecia.
  - In the latter condition, beading is found at irregular, rather than regular, intervals.

PEARLS

- Trichoscopy allows for the fast diagnosis of many congenital and acquired genetic hair shaft disorders.
- Avoidance of trauma is the most effective method to manage monilethrix.
- Avoid weathering and cosmetic damage (eg, sunlight exposure, dyeing, bleaching, perming, curling).

Glossary

ABCD rule of dermatoscopy: A semiquantitative algorithm that evaluates symmetry or asymmetry (A), sharp border demarcation (B), multiple colors (C), and structural components in a lesion (D). The criteria in each group are given a point and then multiplied by cofactors to determine the total dermatoscopy score (TDS). A score × 1.3 + B score × 0.1 + C score × 0.5 + D score × 0.5 = TDS. TDS greater than 5.45 is highly suggestive of a melanoma.

Acrosyringia: Monomorphous round white structures found only in the ridges on the palms and soles. They represent the intraepidermal eccrine ducts and are said to look like a string of pearls.

Anisotrichosis: The presence of hairs with variable thickness as seen in androgenic alopecia.

Annular-granular structures: Brown or gray fine dots that surround follicular openings. These are seen only on the face, nose, and ears (site-specific) and represent melanophages and/or atypical melanocytes.

Arborizing vessels: Thick and/or thin in-focus red tree-like branching telangiectatic blood vessels.

asymmetry within a lesion: Using the mirror image technique, a lesion is bisected by 2 lines that are placed 90 degrees to each other. There is asymmetry of color and/or structure if the color and/or structure on the left side are different from the right side and lower half is different from the upper half.

Basal cell carcinoma, criteria: Absence of pigment network, arborizing blood vessels, pigmentation, ulceration, spoke-wheel structures.

Black dots, hair: Black dots are inside the follicular openings and represent broken hair shafts.

Biett's Collarette: "Biett's sign". White scale at the periphery of lesions found in secondary syphilis. Similar to the scale found in pityriasis rosea.

Black dots, skin: Round structures smaller than globules that represent melanin and/or atypical melanocytes that are in the epidermis.

Black lamella: A superficial, thin black shiny area seen in flat benign nevi that represents pigmented parakeratosis. Tape stripping can remove the black lamella, and hidden local criteria such as pigment network may or may not then become visible.

Blanch test: Diffuse erythema seen in a lesion blanches away with direct pressure using dermoscopic instrumentation. What remains are the nonerythematous features of a lesion.

Blood pebbles: One component of a subungual hematoma characterized by irregular purple dots and/or globules that represent blood.

Blotch, irregular: Irregular in shape, asymmetrically located, structureless (ie, absence of network, dots, or globules); shades of black, brown, or gray color; bigger than dots and globules.

Blotch, regular: Uniform, symmetrically located, structureless (ie, absence of network, dots, or globules); shades of black, brown, or gray color; bigger than dots and globules.

Blue ovoid nests: One of the shapes of pigmentation seen in basal cell carcinoma.

Blue-white veil: Irregular, structureless area of confluent blue color that does not fill the entire lesion with an overlying whitish ground-glass appearance.

Central white patch: Centrally located, homogeneous, bony-white, scar-like area seen in some but not all dermatofibromas.

Circle hairs: Thin, short vellus hairs that form a circle.

Circle within a circle: Seen on the face, nose, or ears (site-specific) and is composed of a central hair shaft (inner circle) and gray pigmentation (atypical melanocytes and/or "peppering") that surrounds the hair shaft (outer circle).

Clear cell acanthoma: A benign tumor characterized by glomerular or pinpoint vessels that can be linear or serpiginous or form round necklace-like shapes.

Cobblestone global pattern: Larger angulated brown globules filling the lesion; said to resemble street cobblestones.

Coiled hairs: Telogen/catagen broken hairs that can coil back.

Collarette sign: White scales localized at the periphery of the lesions of pityriasis rosea. Similar scales can be seen in lesions of secondary syphilis, referred to as Biett's collarette, Biett's sign.

Collision tumor: Typically 2, rarely 3 different pathologies identifiable adjacent to each other or one within another (eg, seborrheic keratosis and basal cell carcinoma, hemangioma and nevus, melanoma and seborrheic keratosis, nevus and basal cell carcinoma).

Colors: Depend on the location of melanin in the skin. Upper epidermis: black; dermoepidermal junction: light-to-dark brown; papillary dermis: gray; reticular dermis: steel blue, white scarring; red/pink: neovascularization, inflammation; purple: hemorrhage; and yellow: hyperkeratosis.

Combined nevus: The association of a blue nevus and another melanocytic nevus characterized by variations of blue and brown color.

Comedo-like openings: Variously-sized, pigmented or nonpigmented, sharply-demarcated roundish or irregular structures that represent keratin-filled invaginations of the epidermis. Also called pseudofollicular openings. A primary criterion used to diagnose seborrheic keratosis that can also be found in papillomatous nevi and melanoma.

Comma hairs: Short C-shaped broken hair shafts with ectothrix parasitization.

Comma-like blood vessels: Resembling the shape of a comma.

Corkscrew blood vessels: Irregular thick coiled vessels.

Corkscrew hair: Short spiral-shaped broken hair shafts.

Cotton balls: White scar-like areas seen around the nail apparatus in scleroderma.

Coudability hair: Exclamation mark hairs seen at the periphery of an area of alopecia in alopecia areata.

Crista profunda intermedia: The epidermal rete ridges underlying the ridges of the skin markings on acral skin where atypical melanocytes proliferate in acral melanomas (parallel ridge pattern).

Crista profunda limitans: Epidermal rete ridges underlying the surface furrows on acral skin markings. Benign melanocytes favor this site to proliferate and form several benign patterns (ie, parallel furrow pattern).

Crown vessels: Arborizing-type vessels seen in sebaceous gland hyperplasia that are said not to enter the center of the lesion. This term is a misnomer.

Crypts: Irregular in size and shape, large keratin-filled invaginations of the epidermis. A variation of smaller pseudofollicular openings.

Crystalline structures: Shiny, bright white, linear streaks, or other shapes that are only seen with polarized dermoscopy.

Default criteria, melanocytic lesion: A lesion should be considered melanocytic by default when there is an absence of criteria for a melanocytic lesion, seborrheic keratosis, basal cell carcinoma, vascular lesion, or dermatofibroma.

Delta structure: A tiny gray triangular speck that represents the anterior section of the scabies mite with the head and legs.

Demodex tails: Short, white, spine-like projections seen on the face in patients with rosacea.

Dermatofibroma, criteria: Central white patch and peripheral pigment network.

Dermatoglyphics: Parallel ridges and furrows on the fingers, palms, toes, and soles that form whorls, loops, and arches, also known as *fingerprints*.

Dimple sign: Pinching a dermatofibroma produces a central dell/depression/dimple.

Dots and globules: Black, brown, gray, or red roundish structures distinguished only by their relative sizes. Dots (0.1 mm) are smaller than globules (greater than 0.1 mm).

Dots and globules, irregular: Roundish structures with different sizes, shapes, and shades of color usually asymmetrically located within the lesion.

Dots and globules, regular: Roundish structures where the size, shape, and color are more or less the same with an even distribution within the lesion.

Dotted/pinpoint blood vessels: Telangiectatic blood vessels resembling tiny dots that can be diffuse, grouped, or isolated.

Eleven-point checklist: A melanocytic algorithm used to diagnose melanoma that contains 2 negative features (symmetry of pattern, presences of a single color) and 9 positive features (blue-white veil, multiple brown dots, pseudopods, radial streaming, scar-like depigmentation, peripheral black dots/globules, multiple colors, blue-gray dots, broadened network). To diagnose melanoma, both negative features should not be present and 1 or more of the 9 positive features are identified.

Empty follicles: Skin-colored small depressions seen on the scalp without hairs.

Erythronychia: Longitudinal single or multiple pinkish bands seen in a single or multiple nail plates.

Exclamation mark hairs: Dark thick and possibly frayed tips with proximal portions that are pale and tapered.

Exophytic projections: Ridges forming elevations in papillomatous lesions.

Featureless lesion: A lesion in which there are no identifiable dermoscopic criteria.

Feature-poor lesion: A lesion in which the local criteria are not well-developed and are difficult to identify.

Fibrillar acral pattern: A benign pattern with uniform brown parallel lines that run in an oblique (///////) direction.

Fibrous septae: Linear and/or patchy white or bluish-white color commonly seen in hemangiomas.

Fingerprint pattern: Thin brown parallel line segments that resemble fingerprints, forming swirls, whorls, and arches; or can appear broken up and look like fungal hyphae.

Fish-scale pattern: A benign pattern seen on mucosal surfaces (eg, genitalia) characterized by areas of inverted V and/or U-shaped structures.

Flame hairs: Wavy cone-shaped hair residues seen in trichotillomania and which represent pigmented hair casts.

Follicular keratotic plugging: Keratotic masses plugging follicular ostia.

Follicular pigmentation, asymmetrical: Black, brown, or gray color irregularly outlining follicular openings on the face, nose, or ears (site-specific). Seen in melanoma, solar lentigo, and pigmented actinic keratosis.

Follicular red dots: Erythematous concentric structures in and around follicular ostia representing dilated vessels and extravasated blood.

Fried-egg appearance: Seen in nevi, dysplastic nevi, and melanoma; characterized by a larger light brown macular component and a regular or irregular darker roundish area, which is said to have the appearance of a fried egg.

Fringe sign: Hairs located along the periphery of a patch of alopecia, seen in traction alopecia.

Furrows/fissures and ridges: Furrows/fissures (sulci) created by clefts in the epidermis and ridges (gyri), raised areas created by the fissures. Seen in seborrheic keratosis and some papillomatous melanocytic nevi.

Glabrous skin: Non–hair-bearing areas of the skin (eg, palms, soles, mucosa).

Global pattern: The overall dermoscopic pattern of a lesion.

Globular global pattern: Regular or irregular brown dots and/or globules filling most of the lesion.

Glomerular vessels: Diffuse or clustered fine coiled telangiectatic vessels (capillary loops).

Hair powder: Small dots representing hair shaft residue.

Hair tufting: Multiple hairs emerging from the same ostium.

Hairpin blood vessels: Thin and elongated telangiectatic vessels (capillary loops) resembling hairpins.

Homogeneous global pattern: Diffuse pigmentation filling most of the lesion in the absence of local criteria such as pigment network, dots, and globules.

Honeycomb network: A term used to describe a fine brown pigment network seen on the scalp in darker-skinned persons.

Hutchinson sign: Clinically visible dark brown or black pigmentation seen at the nail cuticle.

Hutchinson sign, micro: Dark brown or black pigmentation seen at the nail cuticle that is better seen with dermoscopy.

Hypopigmentation: Tan light color that may or may not contain local criteria (eg, pigment network, dots, and globules).

Ink spot lentigo: Black macule seen on sun-exposed areas with a thickened black pigment network as the only criterion.

Jelly sign: A rarely-seen feature of seborrheic keratosis in which there is a global appearance of apple jelly with contact dermoscopy.

Keratotic plugs: Large irregular yellow plugs that cover enlarged follicular openings in the scalp.

Lacunae: The most commonly-used term to describe the well-demarcated vascular spaces seen in hemangiomas/vascular lesions.

Lagoons: One of the uncommonly-used terms to describe the well-demarcated vascular spaces seen in hemangiomas/vascular lesions.

Lattice-like acral pattern: A benign acral pattern with brown parallel lines in the furrows and brown lines running perpendicular to the furrows forming a ladder-like picture.

Leaf-like pattern: Brown to grayish-blue discrete bulbous extensions forming a leaf-like pattern seen in basal cell carcinoma. A dermoscopic misnomer.

Melanocytic lesion, criteria: Pigment network, brown globules, homogenous blue global pattern, parallel acral patterns, by default.

Melanoma-specific criteria: High-risk criteria that can be seen in both benign and malignant lesions but are more sensitive and specific for melanoma.

Melanoma-specific criteria, face, nose, ears (site-specific): Asymmetrical follicular pigmentation, annular-granular structures, rhomboid structures, circle within a circle.

Melanoma-specific criteria, palms and soles (site specific): Parallel-ridge, nonspecific, diffuse variegate, and multicomponent patterns.

Melanoma-specific criteria, trunk and extremities (site-specific): Asymmetry of color and structure, multicomponent global pattern, nonspecific global pattern, irregular pigment network, irregular dots/globules, irregular streaks, irregular blotches, blue and/or white color, regression, 5 to 6 colors, polymorphous vessels, milky-red areas, pink color.

Melanonychia striata, irregular: Nail plate brown, black, and/or gray parallel longitudinal lines or bands with different shades of color and irregular spacing and thickness. There can also be loss of parallelism (broken up line segments).

Melanonychia striata, regular: Single or multiple longitudinal nail plate brown parallel lines or bands with uniform color, spacing, and thickness. There is no loss of parallelism (broken-up line segments).

Milky-red areas: Localized or diffuse pinkish-white color with or without reddish and/or bluish out-of-focus/fuzzy globular structures that can represent neovascularization.

Milia-like cysts: Single or multiple variously-sized white or yellow roundish structures that can appear opaque or bright like stars in the sky (epidermal horn cysts). A primary criterion used to diagnose seborrheic keratosis that can also be found in papillomatous nevi and melanoma.

Monilethrix: The affected hair shafts show elliptical nodes and intermittent constrictions at regular intervals. The constrictions represent the pathology. Individual hairs appear beaded like the beads of a necklace.

Mirror-image technique: This technique is used to determine symmetry or asymmetry of color and/or structure within a lesion by bisecting the lesion with two lines that are placed 90 degrees to each other. One has to determine whether the color/structure on the left side is similar/a mirror image of the right side and the lower half is similar/a mirror image of the upper half. Note that there is rarely perfect symmetry of color and/or structure in nature.

Morse hair/Morse code–like hair (a.k.a. bar-code hairs): Irregularly interrupted hairs with ectothrix parasitization. Paler narrow spots are seen where the hairs are bent.

Moth-eaten borders: Well-demarcated, concave borders that are felt to resemble a moth-eaten garment. A primary criterion used to diagnose a solar lentigo.

Mountain-valley pattern: Seen in seborrheic keratosis in which there are roundish ridges and furrows rather than the brain-like pattern.

Multicomponent global pattern: Three or more different-appearing areas within a lesion. Each zone can be composed of a single criterion or multiple criteria.

Negative network: White network–like structures (reverse of the typical brown pigment network), also called white network or reticular depigmentation. A criterion that can be seen in dermatofibromas, nevi, Spitz nevi, and melanoma.

Neighborhood sign: The presence of multiple similar lesions (neighbors) is an important clinical clue used to differentiate pigmented actinic keratosis from lentigo maligna on the face, nose, or ears. Pigmented actinic keratoses tend to have several similar lesions in the same area (a positive neighbor sign).

Nonspecific global pattern: None of the defined (reticular, globular, cobblestone, homogeneous, starburst, multicomponent) global patterns can be identified.

Orange-yellowish structureless areas: Orange-yellowish structureless areas that correspond histologically to granulomas within the dermis.

Parallel furrow pattern: One of the benign acral melanocytic patterns seen on the palms and soles, characterized by pigmentation in a linear fashion located in the skin furrows (crista profunda limitans). One can see combinations of single or double lines with or without brown dots and/or globules.

Parallel ridge pattern: Pigmentation seen in the ridges of the palms or soles (crista profunda intermedia). The major pattern used to diagnose acral melanomas.

Parallelism, loss of: Pigmented longitudinal nail plate bands in which there are broken-up line segments. A criterion seen in acral melanomas.

Parallelism, nail plate: Pigmented longitudinal nail plate bands forming parallel lines.

Pattern analysis: A melanocytic algorithm in which one has to identify the criteria in a lesion and put them into recognizable diagnostic patterns.

Pebbles on the ridges: Purplish/reddish dots and/or globules seen in the ridges of acral skin and represent blood, not melanocytes.

Peppering: Fine and/or coarse grayish granules/dots, which represent melanophages and/or free melanin in the papillary dermis.

Peripilar casts: Concentrically-arranged scales encircling emerging hair shafts.

Peripilar sign: Brown macules surrounding follicular openings caused by inflammation.

Peripilar white halo: Grayish-white macules surrounding follicular ostia created by fibrosis.

Pigment network/network: Honeycomb-like, reticular, web-like line segments (elongated and hyperpigmented rete ridges) with hypopigmented holes (dermal papillae).

Pigment network, irregular: Line segments that are thickened, branched, and broken up (enlarged, fused rete ridges) and asymmetrically located in the lesion.

Pigment network, regular: Honeycomb-like (web-like, reticular) line segments that have uniform color, thickness, and holes.

Polygonal network: Polygonal-shaped vessels seen on the face in rosacea. May or may not be well developed. When poorly developed the vessels have a zigzag appearance.

Polymorphous blood vessels: Three or more different shapes of telangiectatic blood vessels in a lesion (arborizing, dotted/pinpoint, glomerular, linear, hairpin, comma, corkscrew).

Pseudofollicular openings: Variously-sized, pigmented or nonpigmented, sharply demarcated roundish or irregular-shaped structures (keratin-filled invaginations of the epidermis). Also called comedo-like openings. A primary criterion used to diagnose seborrheic keratosis that can also be found in papillomatous nevi and melanoma.

Pseudonetwork/pseudopigment network: Network-like structures seen only on the face, nose, or ears (site-specific) created by follicular openings penetrating areas of brownish pigmentation. It is different from the true pigment network seen on the trunk and extremities created by elongated and hyperpigmented rete ridges.

Pseudopods/streaks: Linear projections of pigment at the periphery of the lesion with bulbous ends (may represent the radial growth phase of melanoma) that can be an extension of the pigment network, a dark blotch, or stand alone. They are also referred to as *streaks*.

Pyogenic granuloma: The dermoscopic features of pyogenic granuloma include homogeneous milky-red/pink color with the possibility of bleeding, ulceration, and peripheral collarette of scale. Vessels are not seen.

Question mark hairs: The proximal part of a hair shaft is coiled and looks like a question mark; seen in trichotillomania.

Radial streaming/streaks: Thin linear projections of pigment at the periphery of the lesion (may represent the radial growth phase of melanoma) that can be an extension of the pigment network, a dark blotch, or stand alone. They are also referred to as *streaks*.

Reflection artifact: Extraneous debris (eg, oil droplets, fabric strands) not related to the primary pathology seen with dermoscopy.

Regression: Milky/bony-white scar-like depigmentation (fibrosis) with or without gray pepper-like granules "peppering" (free melanin and/or melanophages in the dermis).

Reticular global pattern: Regular or irregular pigment network filling most of the lesion.

Rhomboid structures: Irregular black and/or brown pigmentation completely surrounding follicular openings (atypical melanocytes) on the face, nose, and ears (site-specific). True rhomboids are rarely formed. This term is a misnomer.

Ring-like pattern: Grouped circular brown structures seen in dermatofibromas (variation of the pigment network), seborrheic keratosis, genital lentigines, or bowenoid papulosis.

Saccules: One of the uncommonly-used terms to describe the well-demarcated vascular spaces of a vascular lesion.

Seborrheic keratosis, criteria: Milia-like cysts, pseudofollicular openings (comedo-like openings), fissures/furrows and ridges, "fat fingers," hairpin vessels, sharp border demarcation.

Seven-point checklist: A melanocytic algorithm that uses a point system with major and minor criteria. Major criteria receive 2 points (irregular pigment network, blue-white color, polymorphous vessels). Minor criteria receive 1 point (irregular streaks, irregular dots/globules, irregular blotches, regression). By simple addition of the points, a minimal score of 3 suggests the diagnosis of melanoma.

Speckled pattern: Gray dots representing melanophages ("peppering") in the papillary dermis can be seen in discoid lupus erythematosus on the scalp.

Spitzoid: A lesion is said to be spitzoid if it has one of the 6 patterns that can be found with Spitz nevi.

Spoke-wheel structures: Well-defined pigmented radial projections (islands of pigmented basal cell carcinoma) meeting at a darker central globule/central axle/hub. These are only seen in basal cell carcinoma.

Starburst (spitzoid) global pattern: Streaks and/or dots and globules at the periphery of the lesion. The central component of the lesion can be very dark, bluish, or contain a negative/white pigment network.

Stars in the sky: Mila-like cysts that appear bright and shiny like stars in the sky.

Streaks, false: Foci of linear projections of pigmentation not associated with a melanocytic lesion (eg, basal cell carcinoma, seborrheic keratosis).

Streaks, irregular: Foci of black and/or brown linear projections of pigment irregularly distributed at the periphery of a lesion. They do not symmetrically surround the lesion. They can be freestanding, associated with a pigment network, or a dark irregular blotch. The shape of the streaks does not determine if they are irregular, rather their spotty distribution at the periphery of the lesion.

Streaks, regular: Black and/or brown linear projections of pigment seen at all points along the periphery of the lesion. They can be freestanding or associated with a pigment network or dark blotch. The shape of the streaks does not determine if they are regular, rather their symmetrical distribution around the entire lesion.

String of pearls: Monomorphous, evenly-spaced, linear, round white dots created by acrosyringia (intraepidermal sweat ducts) in the ridges of acral skin said to look like a string of pearls.

Symmetry within a lesion: Using the mirror-image technique, a lesion is bisected by 2 lines that are placed 90 degrees to each other. There is symmetry of color and/or structure if the color and/or structure on the left side are more or less similar to the right side and lower half is similar to the upper half. The lines should be visualized in the direction that would create the most symmetry.

Tape stripping: Scotch tape is used to remove/strip away pigmented parakeratosis that creates the black lamella. If successful, black specks will be seen on the tape and the underlying structures (ie, pigment network) hidden by the black lamella may become visible.

Three-point checklist: A simplified screening algorithm used to diagnose high-risk melanocytic lesions (dysplastic nevi/melanoma) or basal cell carcinoma that mimics melanoma. One looks for asymmetry of color and/or structure, irregular pigment network, and blue and/or white color. If 2 out of 3 criteria are present, the lesion should be excised.

Toothbrush sign: Many hairs coming out of a single follicular opening. This is seen in folliculitis decalvans, aka tufted folliculitis.

Train tracks: Genital lentigines can have multiple parallel brown line segments. When there are only 2 parallel line segments, they are said to look like train tracks.

Triangle structure/delta structure: A tiny gray triangular speck that represents the anterior section of the scabies mite with the head and legs.

Trichorrhexis nodosa: There are multiple, irregularly-distributed small white foci along the length of hair shafts. There is also hair shaft breakage at irregular intervals. Brush like hair fractures and frayed nodes.

Trichoscopy: Dermoscopic examination of the scalp skin, hair, and blood vessels.

Tumoral melanosis: A nodular or plaque-like accumulation of melanin-laden macrophages in the dermis. There are no melanocytes. This has been associated with partial or complete melanoma regression.

Twisted red loops: Seen on the scalp, multiple red dots at low magnification (×10, ×20) and polymorphous beaded lines at higher magnification (×40) representing capillaries in the papillary dermis.

Tyndall effect: Light scattering by particles of melanin at different levels in the skin will determine the colors we see with dermoscopy: black in the epidermis, brown at the dermoepidermal junction, gray in the papillary dermis, and blue in the reticular dermis.

Ulceration: Single or multiple areas, where there is loss of epidermis with oozing blood or congealed blood and crusts.

V sign: Two hairs emerging from the same follicular opening. It is seen in trichotillomania.

Vascular lesion, criteria: Red lacunae (lagoons, saccules), well demarcated reddish-blue vascular spaces, and fibrous septae.

Vellus hairs (aka peach fuzz): Short, fine, light colored hairs that are barely visible.

White network/negative network/reticular depigmentation: White network-like structures.

White track: Single or double fine pigmented lines seen at the periphery of lesions of porokeratosis. Threadlike borders.

White patches: Well-demarcated white patches seen in scarring alopecia.

Wobble sign: Used to differentiate fixed lesions from pliable lesions. Instrumentation is placed over the lesion (usually a papule) and moved from side to side. A soft lesion will easily move from side to side (+ wobble sign), whereas a fixed lesion will not move (-wobble sign).

Yellow dots: Round or polycyclic yellow to yellow-pink dots representing infundibula plugged with sebum and keratin. May be devoid of hairs or contain miniaturized, cadaverized, or dystrophic hairs.

Zigzag hair: Z-shaped broken hair shafts with ectothrix parasitization.

Index

Page numbers followed by *f* indicate figures; those followed by *t* indicate tables.